Molecular Advances in Abiotic Stress Signaling in Plants: Focus on Atmospheric Stressors

Molecular Advances in Abiotic Stress Signaling in Plants: Focus on Atmospheric Stressors

Guest Editors

Mateusz Labudda
Philippe Jeandet

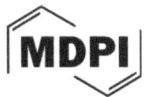

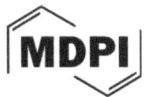Basel • Beijing • Wuhan • Barcelona • Belgrade • Novi Sad • Cluj • Manchester

Guest Editors

Mateusz Labudda
Department of Biochemistry
and Microbiology
Warsaw University of Life
Sciences-SGGW
Warsaw
Poland

Philippe Jeandet
Department of Biology
and Biochemistry
University of Reims
Reims
France

Editorial Office
MDPI AG
Grosspeteranlage 5
4052 Basel, Switzerland

This is a reprint of the Special Issue, published open access by the journal *International Journal of Molecular Sciences* (ISSN 1422-0067), freely accessible at: www.mdpi.com/journal/ijms/special_issues/K7RU8RIY4E.

For citation purposes, cite each article independently as indicated on the article page online and using the guide below:

Lastname, A.A.; Lastname, B.B. Article Title. *Journal Name* **Year**, *Volume Number*, Page Range.

ISBN 978-3-7258-3478-5 (Hbk)
ISBN 978-3-7258-3477-8 (PDF)
https://doi.org/10.3390/books978-3-7258-3477-8

Contents

About the Editors

Mateusz Labudda

Prof. Dr. Mateusz Labudda is currently working as an Associate Professor at the Department of Biochemistry and Microbiology, Institute of Biology, Warsaw University of Life Sciences—SGGW. He holds a Doctor of Philosophy (Biochemistry) (2017) and a Doctor of Science (Biochemistry and Ecophysiology) (2021) from the Warsaw University of Life Sciences—SGGW. He was a Research Assistant of biochemistry and plant physiology at the Plant Breeding and Acclimatization Institute. He has widely published in leading peer-reviewed international journals. His scientific interests involve the molecular, biochemical, physiological, and structural responses of plants to environmental stresses.

Philippe Jeandet

Prof. Dr. Philippe Jeandet was born on 18 April, 1960, in Beaune, France, in the heart of the Burgundy wine-growing area. He studied biological sciences and specialized in plant sciences as well as in organic chemistry in the Faculty of Sciences at the University of Bourgogne. He earned his PhD degree in plant physiology and biochemistry in 1991 and 1996, respectively, from the same university. He then started his research on natural products, namely resveratrol, a phytoalexin from the Vitaceae. His PhD thesis on resveratrol was the first of its kind to be defended in a French university. His work was supervised by Prof. Dr. Roger Bessis. He received an Associate Professor position at the University of Bourgogne in 1993. Philippe Jeandet spent several months as a Visiting Scientist at the Federal Agronomic Station of Changins, Switzerland, in 1994 and as a Visiting Professor at the University of Kentucky, USA, in 1997. He was then appointed in 1997 as a Full Professor of Food Chemistry and Chairman of the Laboratory of Oenology and Applied Chemistry at the University of Reims (1997–2013). During this period, his research activities focused on the role of macromolecules on the physico-chemistry of wine, the wine proteome, and wine microbiology while continuing some research activities on resveratrol and related stilbenes. He has been the Director (2003–2007) and Deputy Director (2008–2012) of the research unit "Vine and Wine of Champagne" and Adjunct to the Director of Research and Technology (2004–2010) in the Champagne-Ardennes area (French ministry of research).

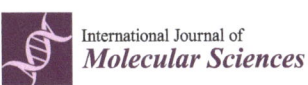

International Journal of
Molecular Sciences

Editorial

Molecular Advances in Abiotic Stress Signaling in Plants: Focus on Atmospheric Stressors

Mateusz Labudda [1],* and Philippe Jeandet [2]

[1] Department of Biochemistry and Microbiology, Institute of Biology, Warsaw University of Life Sciences—SGGW, Nowoursynowska 159, 02-776 Warsaw, Poland
[2] Research Unit "Induced Resistance and Plant Bioprotection", UPRES EA 4707, Department of Biology and Biochemistry, Faculty of Sciences, University of Reims, CEDEX 02, P.O. Box 1039, 51687 Reims, France; philippe.jeandet@univ-reims.fr
* Correspondence: mateusz_labudda@sggw.edu.pl; Tel.: +48-22-5932571

1. Introduction

Plants face many abiotic stresses that significantly impact their growth and survival, requiring intricate mechanisms in order to adapt and thrive. These responses occur at multiple levels of plant organization, beginning with changes in biochemical processes such as respiration, photosynthesis, and transpiration, which form the basis of stress adaptation. On a broader scale, these biochemical alterations lead to morphological and anatomical changes in plant organs, thereby enabling improved resilience to environmental challenges. Underlying these adaptations is a sophisticated molecular signaling network that acts as an early warning system, allowing the plants to perceive and respond to external abiotic stimuli effectively. This signaling machinery integrates various molecular pathways to initiate appropriate physiological and structural changes. Understanding the interplay between molecular signals and plant responses provides valuable insights into the complex nature of abiotic stress tolerance. Such knowledge is crucial for developing strategies to enhance crop resilience in the face of global environmental changes [1–4].

This Special Issue presents a collection of 12 original and review articles that explore the key thematic areas highlighted within this SI.

2. Experimental Articles

Crocus sativus L., a plant renowned for its cultivation of saffron—the most expensive spice in the world—was examined in order to evaluate the effects of pre-sowing treatments on plant performance and saffron quality [5]. The treatments included cold plasma (CP), vacuum, and electromagnetic field (EMF) applications, influencing sprouting kinetics, growth parameters, trichome density, and secondary metabolite content. CP treatment was found to negatively affect plant growth and metabolite content, while EMF treatment notably increased flower length and levels of various metabolites. Although vacuum treatment improved germination uniformity, it had minimal impact on stigma compounds compared to both CP and EMF. Among the treatments, EMF was the most effective at enhancing secondary metabolites, significantly raising the concentrations of crocin, picrocrocin, and safranal. While all treatments preserved corm viability, they induced stressor-specific alterations in plant traits. EMF treatment shows promise for improving saffron quality by enhancing the concentrations of bioactive compounds.

During photosynthesis, reactive oxygen species (ROS) such as hydrogen peroxide (H_2O_2) and singlet oxygen ($^1O_2$) are generated, with $^1O_2$ playing a crucial role in signaling through its reaction products, including lipid peroxides and reactive electrophile species

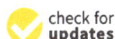
check for updates

Received: 26 January 2025
Revised: 15 February 2025
Accepted: 18 February 2025
Published: 22 February 2025

Citation: Labudda, M.; Jeandet, P. Molecular Advances in Abiotic Stress Signaling in Plants: Focus on Atmospheric Stressors. *Int. J. Mol. Sci.* 2025, 26, 1878. https://doi.org/10.3390/ijms26051878

(RES). Pancheri et al. [6] investigated the function of ROS in the high light (HL) acclimation of *Chlamydomonas reinhardtii*, focusing specifically on GreenCut2 genes that are unique to photosynthetic organisms. RNA sequencing analyses revealed that HL significantly influenced the expression of 131 GreenCut2 genes, with more than half of the HL-upregulated genes also responding to RES. Key upregulated genes included *RBCS1*, *PSBS1*, and *LHCSR1*, whereas downregulated genes comprised *CAO1*, *MDH2*, and *PGM4*. The impact of H_2O_2 and β-cyclocitral on gene expression was found to be limited, underscoring the specific role of $^1O_2$ in HL responses. Signaling by $^1O_2$ under HL conditions enhances photoprotection and carbon assimilation while downregulating primary metabolic pathways. These findings indicate that RES-mediated signaling is essential for photosynthetic acclimation to HL conditions.

Selenium nanoparticles (SeNPs) and melatonin (MT), both recognized as biostimulants, significantly influence the growth of plants. However, the combined effects of these treatments had not been previously reported. In an article by Kang et al. [7], two melon cultivars were treated with SeNPs, MT, and a combination of both, after which their physiological and biochemical responses were analyzed. While individual and combined treatments did not yield significant changes in plant height or stem diameter, both SeNPs and MT notably increased levels of soluble sugars (by 6–63%) and sucrose (by 11–88%), as well as enhanced the activity of sucrose phosphate synthase (by 171–237%) in leaves. Additionally, there were significant increases in key enzymes and mRNA levels associated with the phenylpropanoid metabolism pathway. Notably, the combined treatment was more effective than either individual treatment, resulting in higher activities of antioxidant enzymes, including superoxide dismutase (SOD), catalase (CAT), and peroxidase (POD). These findings suggest that SeNPs and MT can enhance melon seedling growth by improving carbohydrate metabolism, phenylpropanoid activity, and antioxidant capacity.

The mechanisms through which MT safeguards plants against cadmium (Cd) toxicity are still not fully understood, particularly at the molecular level. Lee et al. [8] successfully identified and cloned a novel serotonin N-acetyltransferase 3 (*SNAT3*) gene in rice (*Oryza sativa*); this gene is a pivotal enzyme involved in MT biosynthesis. *OsSNAT3* converts serotonin and 5-methoxytryptamine into N-acetylserotonin and MT, respectively. The suppression of *OsSNAT3* via RNA interference (RNAi) resulted in reduced MT levels and Cd tolerance in transgenic rice, alongside a decreased expression of endoplasmic reticulum chaperone genes (*BiP3*, *BiP4*, and *BiP5*). In contrast, the overexpression of *OsSNAT3* (referred to as SNAT3-OE) led to elevated MT levels and enhanced stress tolerance to Cd, as demonstrated by improved seedling growth, lower malondialdehyde (MDA) content, and increased chlorophyll levels. Additionally, SNAT3-OE lines displayed a higher expression of *BiP4* compared to wild-type plants. These findings indicate that engineering MT production through OsSNAT3 could boost crop resilience to Cd stress, thereby improving yields in contaminated agricultural fields.

Elevated atmospheric CO_2 levels play a significant role in global warming and can negatively impact plants' physiological and biochemical processes, even though CO_2 is crucial for photosynthesis. Li et al. [9] investigated the physiological and proteomic responses of the tetraploid *Robinia pseudoacacia* to high CO_2 concentrations (5%). The results showed that elevated CO_2 levels hindered growth and development, resulted in severe leaf damage, and diminished photosynthetic parameters (*Pn*, *Gs*, *Tr*, and *Ci*), respiration rates, and chlorophyll content. Additionally, chlorophyll fluorescence parameters (*Fm*, *Fv*/*Fm*, *qP*, and *ETR*) showed reductions, while the levels of ROS (H_2O_2 and $O2^{\cdot-}$) increased, accompanied by the decreased activity of antioxidant enzymes. The accumulation of ROS and nitric oxide (NO) in guard cells triggered stomatal closure. Proteomic analysis revealed 1652 differentially abundant proteins (DAPs) linked to redox activity, catalytic functions, and various metabolic pathways, including photosynthesis and the biosynthesis of secondary metabolites. These findings offer valuable insights into the adaptation mechanisms of tetraploid *R. pseudoacacia* under conditions of high CO_2 stress.

Transcription factors are essential for regulating plant responses to external stimuli, and the WRKY protein superfamily plays a pivotal role in mediating stress responses to conditions such as cold, heat, salt, drought, and pathogen attacks. The number and functions of WRKY transcription factors have evolved throughout the evolution of angiosperms, with different plant species retaining varying quantities of WRKY family members based on their evolutionary backgrounds. The WRKY family is categorized into three major groups in angiosperms, distinguished by their conserved domains and structural similarities. These transcription factors facilitate plant adaptation to environmental stresses by engaging in ROS and hormone signaling pathways and regulating enzyme activity, stomatal closure, and leaf shrinkage. Wu et al. [10] examined the evolution and functional roles of WRKY factors in angiosperms, particularly emphasizing Magnoliaceae plants. This article offers insights into the functional diversity of the WRKY family and its evolutionary importance. The findings provide theoretical and experimental guidance for understanding the molecular mechanisms underlying environmental stress tolerance in plants.

LESION-SIMULATING DISEASE1 (LSD1) is a vital regulator of cell death in *Arabidopsis thaliana* [11]. Mutations in *LSD1*, leading to the *lsd1* phenotype, result in runaway cell death (RCD) under various stress conditions. The manifestation of the *lsd1* mutant phenotype is influenced by ENHANCED DISEASE SUSCEPTIBILITY 1 (EDS1), PHYTOALEXIN-DEFICIENT 4 (PAD4), and salicylic acid (SA) and ROS signaling pathways. Notably, the conditional RCD phenotype of *lsd1* varies between controlled laboratory settings and field environments, indicating the involvement of different regulatory mechanisms. Transcriptome analysis has identified METACASPASE 8 (MC8) as a potential regulator of RCD associated with *lsd1*. In the *mc8/lsd1* double mutant, the RCD phenotype was mitigated under UV radiation, mirroring the outcomes observed in the double mutants *lsd1/eds1* and *lsd1/pad4*. This study highlights the positive role of MC8 in the EDS1- and PAD4-dependent regulation of cell death in the absence of LSD1 function. A working model has been proposed, positioning MC8 as an essential component of the LSD1-EDS1-PAD4 regulatory hub. These findings provide new insights into the molecular mechanisms governing plant stress-induced cell death [11].

OsBBTI5, a member of the Bowman–Birk inhibitor (BBI) family, is involved in the plant's stress responses and has been shown to bind specifically to the salt stress-related gene *OsAPX2*. Lin et al. [12] explored the role of the *OsBBTI5* gene in enhancing salt tolerance in rice by employing RNAi to inhibit its expression selectively. Transgenic *OsBBTI5*-RNAi plants demonstrated altered responses to brassinosteroid and gibberellin (GA) treatments, exhibiting reduced growth under high concentrations of GA3. When subjected to salt stress (40–60 mM NaCl), these plants showed increased activities of POD and SOD, along with a decreased MDA content, indicating enhanced stress tolerance. Transcriptomic analysis revealed the significant upregulation of photosynthesis-related genes in transgenic plants compared to wild-type plants under salt stress conditions. The findings suggest that *OsBBTI5* plays a role in the brassinosteroid signaling pathway and interacts with *OsAPX2* to improve stress tolerance. This study offers novel insights into the molecular mechanisms underlying salt tolerance in rice.

3. Review Articles

Green leaf volatiles (GLVs) have traditionally been linked to protecting plants from pests and pathogens. However, recent evidence suggests that GLVs also play a significant role in helping plants defend against abiotic stresses such as heat, cold, drought, light, and salinity. Although the molecular mechanisms behind this protective function remain largely unclear, it is evident that the production of GLVs is closely connected to the physical damage caused by these stresses. This damage acts as a primary trigger for GLV synthesis. Engelberth [13] summarized current knowledge regarding GLVs in relation to abiotic stress and proposed a model for their multifunctionality. GLVs appear to mediate plant responses to various stresses, underscoring their broader significance in promoting plant resilience. Further research is necessary to clarify the molecular pathways involved in the stress protection provided by GLVs.

Ultraviolet (UV) radiation presents a significant challenge by causing cellular damage, necessitating robust DNA repair mechanisms supported by histone acetyltransferases (HATs). HATs are vital in regulating chromatin structure and gene expression, facilitating chromatin relaxation and transcriptional activation, which are essential for development and stress responses. Boycheva et al. [14] examined the function of HATs in photomorphogenesis, chromatin remodeling, and gene regulation, emphasizing their significance in light responses and stress adaptation. They underscored the necessity for further research into individual HAT family members and their interactions with other epigenetic factors. Advanced genomic and genome-editing technologies offer promising avenues for enhancing crop resilience and productivity through the targeted modulation of HAT activities.

Drought stress poses a significant challenge to agricultural productivity due to its increasing frequency and intensity and the extensive losses it incurs. Sorghum (*Sorghum bicolor*), a C4 plant, exhibits a range of morphological, physiological, and biochemical adaptations that enable it to thrive in arid conditions [15]. These adaptations encompass improved water uptake, minimized water loss, osmotic potential adjustments, the scavenging of ROS, and the heightened activity of antioxidant enzymes. Moreover, specific genes in sorghum show downregulation in response to drought stress. Liu et al. [15] presented the mechanisms underlying sorghum's drought tolerance, focusing on its morphological traits, physiological processes, and the identification of functional genes. Implementing modern biotechnological and molecular strategies is essential for enhancing sorghum's resistance to drought.

Atmospheric stressors such as CO_2, NO_x, sulfur compounds, extreme temperatures, ozone, UV-B radiation, and acid rain significantly impact plants, particularly those of agricultural importance. Although NO and hydrogen sulfide (H_2S) were once viewed solely as toxic pollutants, they are now recognized as vital signaling molecules in plant stress responses [16]. These gasotransmitters enhance enzymatic and non-enzymatic antioxidant systems, strengthening the plant's defense mechanisms. They play crucial roles in alleviating the effects of various environmental stresses, including those posed by atmospheric conditions. Corpas [16] described the endogenous metabolism of NO and H_2S within plant cells and underscored their significance in stress signaling pathways. Additionally, the potential of applying NO and H_2S exogenously to enhance crop resilience has been discussed.

4. Conclusions

Research into plant responses to abiotic stress reveals a complex network of molecular, physiological, and biochemical mechanisms essential for adaptation and resilience. Studies have highlighted the promise of innovative treatments—such as EMF, SeNPs, and MT—in enhancing stress tolerance and boosting secondary metabolite production in crops like saffron, melon, and rice. Similarly, investigations into key genes, including *OsSNAT3* and *OsBBTI5*, have demonstrated their roles in stress mitigation by activating crucial biochemical pathways and stress signaling. Additional insights into transcription factors like WRKY and signaling molecules such as NO and H_2S have emphasized their importance in regulating adaptive responses. Mechanistic studies on ROS and histone acetyltransferases shed light on the plant's capacity for stress signaling and chromatin-level regulation under HL and UV stress conditions. Future research should aim to explore these molecular pathways in more depth, advance genome-editing technologies, and utilize these insights to develop sustainable agricultural solutions that enhance crop resilience in the face of a rapidly changing climate.

Author Contributions: Conceptualization, P.J. and M.L.; formal analysis, M.L.; writing—original draft preparation and editing, M.L. All authors have read and agreed to the published version of the manuscript.

Funding: This research received no external funding.

Institutional Review Board Statement: Not applicable.

Data Availability Statement: Not applicable.

Acknowledgments: I would like to convey my heartfelt gratitude to the authors of the referenced articles for their invaluable contributions to enhancing our understanding of plant responses to abiotic stresses. I also sincerely thank the reviewers for their meticulous evaluations, constructive feedback, and guidance, which have greatly enriched the quality of this SI. Furthermore, I wish to pay tribute to my dear friend, Philippe Jeandet, whose recent passing has profoundly saddened me. His unwavering support, generosity, openness, and friendship inspired me throughout my academic journey. His memory will forever reside in my heart, reminding me of the lasting impact of kindness and camaraderie in my personal and professional activities.

Conflicts of Interest: The authors declare no conflicts of interest.

References

1. Labudda, M.; Dziurka, K.; Fidler, J.; Gietler, M.; Rybarczyk-Płońska, A.; Nykiel, M.; Prabucka, B.; Morkunas, I.; Muszyńska, E. The Alleviation of Metal Stress Nuisance for Plants—A Review of Promising Solutions in the Face of Environmental Challenges. *Plants* **2022**, *11*, 2544. [CrossRef] [PubMed]
2. Matamoros, M.A.; Becana, M. Molecular Responses of Legumes to Abiotic Stress: Post-Translational Modifications of Proteins and Redox Signaling. *J. Exp. Bot.* **2021**, *72*, 5876–5892. [CrossRef] [PubMed]
3. Paes de Melo, B.; Carpinetti, P.d.A.; Fraga, O.T.; Rodrigues-Silva, P.L.; Fioresi, V.S.; de Camargos, L.F.; Ferreira, M.F.d.S. Abiotic Stresses in Plants and Their Markers: A Practice View of Plant Stress Responses and Programmed Cell Death Mechanisms. *Plants* **2022**, *11*, 1100. [CrossRef] [PubMed]
4. Zhang, Y.; Xu, J.; Li, R.; Ge, Y.; Li, Y.; Li, R. Plants' Response to Abiotic Stress: Mechanisms and Strategies. *Int. J. Mol. Sci.* **2023**, *24*, 10915. [CrossRef] [PubMed]
5. Mildažienė, V.; Žūkienė, R.; Fomins, L.D.; Naučienė, Z.; Minkutė, R.; Jarukas, L.; Drapak, I.; Georgiyants, V.; Novickij, V.; Koga, K.; et al. Effects of Corm Treatment with Cold Plasma and Electromagnetic Field on Growth and Production of Saffron Metabolites in Crocus Sativus. *Int. J. Mol. Sci.* **2024**, *25*, 10412. [CrossRef]
6. Pancheri, T.; Baur, T.; Roach, T. Singlet-Oxygen-Mediated Regulation of Photosynthesis-Specific Genes: A Role for Reactive Electrophiles in Signal Transduction. *Int. J. Mol. Sci.* **2024**, *25*, 8458. [CrossRef]
7. Kang, L.; Jia, Y.; Wu, Y.; Liu, H.; Zhao, D.; Ju, Y.; Pan, C.; Mao, J. Selenium Nanoparticle and Melatonin Treatments Improve Melon Seedling Growth by Regulating Carbohydrate and Polyamine. *Int. J. Mol. Sci.* **2024**, *25*, 7830. [CrossRef] [PubMed]
8. Lee, H.-Y.; Back, K. Melatonin-Regulated Chaperone Binding Protein Plays a Key Role in Cadmium Stress Tolerance in Rice, Revealed by the Functional Characterization of a Novel Serotonin N-Acetyltransferase 3 (SNAT3) in Rice. *Int. J. Mol. Sci.* **2024**, *25*, 5952. [CrossRef]
9. Li, J.; Zhang, S.; Lei, P.; Guo, L.; Zhao, X.; Meng, F. Physiological and Proteomic Responses of the Tetraploid Robinia Pseudoacacia L. to High CO2 Levels. *Int. J. Mol. Sci.* **2024**, *25*, 5262. [CrossRef]
10. Wu, W.; Yang, J.; Yu, N.; Li, R.; Yuan, Z.; Shi, J.; Chen, J. Evolution of the WRKY Family in Angiosperms and Functional Diversity under Environmental Stress. *Int. J. Mol. Sci.* **2024**, *25*, 3551. [CrossRef] [PubMed]
11. Bernacki, M.J.; Rusaczonek, A.; Gołębiewska, K.; Majewska-Fala, A.B.; Czarnocka, W.; Karpiński, S.M. METACASPASE8 (MC8) Is a Crucial Protein in the LSD1-Dependent Cell Death Pathway in Response to Ultraviolet Stress. *Int. J. Mol. Sci.* **2024**, *25*, 3195. [CrossRef] [PubMed]

12. Lin, Z.; Yi, X.; Ali, M.M.; Zhang, L.; Wang, S.; Tian, S.; Chen, F. RNAi-Mediated Suppression of OsBBTI5 Promotes Salt Stress Tolerance in Rice. *Int. J. Mol. Sci.* **2024**, *25*, 1284. [CrossRef] [PubMed]
13. Engelberth, J. Green Leaf Volatiles: A New Player in the Protection against Abiotic Stresses? *Int. J. Mol. Sci.* **2024**, *25*, 9471. [CrossRef] [PubMed]
14. Boycheva, I.; Bonchev, G.; Manova, V.; Stoilov, L.; Vassileva, V. How Histone Acetyltransferases Shape Plant Photomorphogenesis and UV Response. *Int. J. Mol. Sci.* **2024**, *25*, 7851. [CrossRef] [PubMed]
15. Liu, J.; Wang, X.; Wu, H.; Zhu, Y.; Ahmad, I.; Dong, G.; Zhou, G.; Wu, Y. Association between Reactive Oxygen Species, Transcription Factors, and Candidate Genes in Drought-Resistant Sorghum. *Int. J. Mol. Sci.* **2024**, *25*, 6464. [CrossRef] [PubMed]
16. Corpas, F.J. NO and H_2S Contribute to Crop Resilience against Atmospheric Stressors. *Int. J. Mol. Sci.* **2024**, *25*, 3509. [CrossRef] [PubMed]

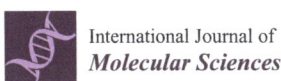

International Journal of
Molecular Sciences

MDPI

Article

Effects of Corm Treatment with Cold Plasma and Electromagnetic Field on Growth and Production of Saffron Metabolites in *Crocus sativus*

Vida Mildažienė [1,*], Rasa Žūkienė [1], Laima Degutytė Fomins [1], Zita Naučienė [1], Rima Minkutė [2], Laurynas Jarukas [3], Iryna Drapak [4], Victoriya Georgiyants [5], Vitalij Novickij [6,7], Kazunori Koga [8,9], Masaharu Shiratani [8] and Olha Mykhailenko [5,10,11,*]

[1] Department of Biochemistry, Faculty of Natural Sciences, Vytautas Magnus University, Studentu Str. 10, LT-53361 Akademija, Lithuania; rasa.zukiene@vdu.lt (R.Ž.); laima.degutyte-fomins@vdu.lt (L.D.F.); zita.nauciene@vdu.lt (Z.N.)
[2] Department of Clinical pharmacy, Lithuanian University of Health Sciences, A. Mickevičiaus g. 9, LT-44307 Kaunas, Lithuania; rima.minkute@kmu.lt
[3] Department of Analytical and Toxicological Chemistry, Lithuanian University of Health Sciences, A. Mickevičiaus g. 9, LT-44307 Kaunas, Lithuania; laurynas.jarukas@lsmuni.lt
[4] Department of General, Bioinorganic, Physical and Colloidal Chemistry, Danylo Halytsky Lviv National Medical University, Pekarska Str. 69, 79010 Lviv, Ukraine; iradrapak@ukr.net
[5] Department of Pharmaceutical Chemistry, National University of Pharmacy, 4-Valentinivska St., 61168 Kharkiv, Ukraine; vgeor@nuph.edu.ua
[6] Institute of High Magnetic Fields, Vilnius Gediminas Technical University, Saulėtekio al. 11, LT-10223 Vilnius, Lithuania; vitalij.novickij@vilniustech.lt
[7] Department of Immunology and Bioelectrochemistry, State Research Institute Centre for Innovative Medicine, Santariškių g. 5, LT-08406 Vilnius, Lithuania
[8] Center of Plasma Nano-interface Engineering, Kyushu University, Fukuoka 819-0395, Japan; koga@ed.kyushu-u.ac.jp (K.K.); siratani@ed.kyushu-u.ac.jp (M.S.)
[9] Center for Novel Science Initiatives, National Institutes of Natural Sciences, Tokyo 105-0001, Japan
[10] Department of Pharmaceutical and Biological Chemistry, Pharmacognosy and Phytotherapy Group, UCL School of Pharmacy, 29-39 Brunswick Square, London WC1N 1AX, UK
[11] Department of Pharmaceutical Biology, Kiel University, 24118 Kiel, Germany
* Correspondence: vida.mildaziene@vdu.lt (V.M.); o.mykhailenko@nuph.edu.ua (O.M.)

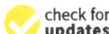
check for updates

Citation: Mildažienė, V.; Žūkienė, R.; Fomins, L.D.; Naučienė, Z.; Minkutė, R.; Jarukas, L.; Drapak, I.; Georgiyants, V.; Novickij, V.; Koga, K.; et al. Effects of Corm Treatment with Cold Plasma and Electromagnetic Field on Growth and Production of Saffron Metabolites in *Crocus sativus. Int. J. Mol. Sci.* **2024**, 25, 10412. https://doi.org/10.3390/ijms251910412

Academic Editors: Philippe Jeandet and Mateusz Labudda

Received: 26 July 2024
Revised: 9 September 2024
Accepted: 24 September 2024
Published: 27 September 2024

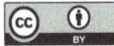
Abstract: *Crocus sativus* L. is a widely cultivated traditional plant for obtaining dried red stigmas known as "saffron," the most expensive spice in the world. The response of *C. sativus* to pre-sowing processing of corms with cold plasma (CP, 3 and 5 min), vacuum (3 min), and electromagnetic field (EMF, 5 min) was assessed to verify how such treatments affect plant performance and the quality and yield of herbal raw materials. The results show that applied physical stressors did not affect the viability of corms but caused stressor-dependent changes in the kinetics of sprouting, growth parameters, leaf trichome density, and secondary metabolite content in stigmas. The effect of CP treatment on plant growth and metabolite content was negative, but all stressors significantly (by 42–74%) increased the number of leaf trichomes. CP3 treatment significantly decreased the length and dry weight of flowers by 43% and 60%, respectively, while EMF treatment increased the length of flowers by 27%. However, longer CP treatment (5 min) delayed germination. Vacuum treatment improved the uniformity of germination by 28% but caused smaller changes in the content of stigma compounds compared with CP and EMF. Twenty-six compounds were identified in total in *Crocus* stigma samples by the HPLC-DAD method, including 23 crocins, rutin, picrocrocin, and safranal. Processing of *Crocus* corms with EMF showed the greatest efficiency in increasing the production of secondary metabolites in saffron. EMF increased the content of marker compounds in stigmas (crocin 4: from 8.95 to 431.17 mg/g; crocin 3: from 6.27 to 164.86 mg/g; picrocrocin: from 0.4 to 1.0 mg/g), although the observed effects on growth were neutral or slightly positive. The obtained findings indicate that treatment of *C. sativus* corms with EMF has the potential application for increasing the quality of saffron by enhancing the amounts of biologically active compounds.

Int. J. Mol. Sci. **2024**, *25*, 10412

Keywords: cold plasma; crocin; electromagnetic field; HPLC; picrocrocin; safranal; saffron

1. Introduction

Pre-sowing treatment of seeds or other planting material with physical stressors is a modern method of plant growth stimulation via triggering numerous physiological and biochemical changes, including an increase in the content of valuable secondary metabolites [1–5]. The application of physical stressors in pre-sowing treatment to corm plants, including *Crocus sativus*, has not been studied before.

The dried red stigmas of *Crocus sativus* L. (Iridaceae) are used as saffron, one of the oldest and most expensive spices in the world, due to the laborious way it is harvested and processed. Saffron is used in Mediterranean and Asian cuisines to improve food taste, flavor, and color and is cultivated in various parts of the world, mostly in Iran, India, Spain, Greece, and Turkey [6]. The growing interest in cultivating and using saffron in Ukraine [7] and different EU countries may increase agricultural production revenues.

Saffron gains its special value due to its chemical composition. It contains significant amounts of unique compounds: apocarotenoids, crocins, as well as picrocrocin and safranal, which are formed by zeaxanthin cleavage followed by specific glycosylation steps [8]. Crocin determines the color of saffron, picrocrocin provides a bitter taste, and safranal gives a specific aroma [8]. Besides apocarotenoids, a wide variety of other biologically active compounds have been isolated from *Crocus* stigmas. More than 150 components, including lipophilic and hydrophilic carbohydrates, proteins, amino acids, minerals, mucilage, starch, gums, vitamins (such as riboflavin and thiamine), pigments, alkaloids, and saponins, have been found in different parts of *C. sativus* [9]. Due to the biological activity of secondary metabolites, saffron extracts have numerous therapeutically relevant effects, including anticatarrhal, anticancer, anti-inflammatory, antimicrobial, antioxidant, laxative, eupeptic, antispasmodic, antidepressant, respiratory decongestant, nerve sedative, stomachic, expectorant, carminative, diaphoretic, anodyne, gingival sedative, galactogogue, and effects against amenorrhea, dysmenorrhea, and others [9]. Therefore, the growing demand for saffron production is driven by pharmacological applications [7].

The typical low yield of saffron is attributed partly to primitive agronomic practices. The quality of saffron is related to the concentration of secondary metabolites and determined according to the international ISO 3632 standards [10], the European Medicines Agency, Food and Drug Administration, and European Pharmacopeia on the international trading market. Saffron yield and quality are influenced by cultivation methods and the environment [11]. It also depends on the methods used for its processing, such as drying, extraction, separation, storage, and quantification stages [12]. The traditional ways for increasing productivity through breeding are restrained because *C. sativus* is a perennial sterile plant characterized by vegetative reproduction using corms. Several attempts to develop superior varieties of saffron via inducing genetic variability have been carried out using tissue culture and hybridization [13,14]. However, propagation through corms offers none or very few genetic variations. Considering the high price and low production yield of valuable saffron components, innovative technologies to increase the production of saffron marker compounds are in high demand. This study aimed to test the hypothesis that pre-sowing corm processing with physical stressors induces stress, leading to increased amounts of secondary metabolites in saffron. The idea is based on similar effects observed in medicinal plants after seed treatment with cold plasma (CP) or electromagnetic field (EMF).

It has been recognized recently that pre-sowing seed treatment with CP or EMF may result in stimulation of plant growth as well as in numerous physiological and biochemical changes, including an increase in the amounts of valuable secondary metabolites [1–5]. For example, irradiation of *Echinacea purpurea* seeds with low-pressure CP and radiofrequency (RF) EMF induced a strong increase in the content of vitamin C and phenolic acids in the leaves of seedlings 3 months after sowing [15]. Changes in the secondary metabolite amounts after seed treatments with CP and EMF were also observed in red clover [16,17], common buckwheat [18], and other plants [13]. CP has been applied for seed treatment in a wide variety of plant species (see reviews [10–13]), but only one study [19] has reported results on planting material of geophyte plants [20], which are propagated through underground storage organs such as bulbs, tubers, corms, or rhizomes. In several recent studies, CP was used to irradiate dried saffron, revealing its potential for microbial decontamination and for increasing color intensity while maintaining the primary quality properties of saffron [20–22].

As an extension of previous studies and taking into account the important pharmaco-logical properties of saffron secondary metabolites, this experiment studied the effect of corm treatment with several physical stressors on plant germination parameters and the composition of saffron metabolites.

2. Results

2.1. Effects on Sprouting Kinetics, Seedling Growth, and Number of Leaf Trichomes

The control and treated corms of *C. sativus* were planted in field experimental plots 4 days after treatment. Corms started sprouting on the 17th day after planting (DAP), and their sprouting dynamics were observed and registered every other day until the 49th DAP (Figure 1).

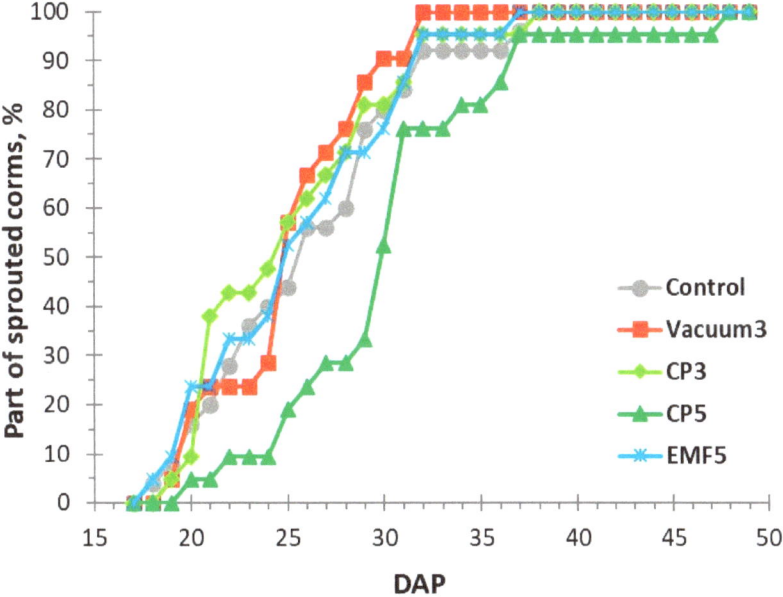

Figure 1. Kinetic curves of *Crocus sativus* corm sprouting following treatments with physical stressors: cold plasma for 3 and 5 min (CP3 and CP5, respectively), vacuum for 3 min (Vacuum3), and electromagnetic field for 5 min (EMF5), along with untreated controls. DAP—days after planting.

Richards plots [15,23] were used to quantify the main indices of sprouting kinetics, and the results are presented in Table 1. Treatments did not affect the maximal sprouting percentage, indicating that corms were equally viable in all groups. CP5 treatment reduced sprouting (increased the median sprouting half-time) by 15% so that 50% of the corms sprouted with a 4-day delay compared with the control. The uniformity of corm sprouting was increased in the Vacuum3-treated group, as indicated by a 28% decrease in Qu compared with the control.

Table 1. Indices of *C. sativus* sprouting kinetics after planting in field plots.

Indice/Treatment Group	Control	Vacuum3	CP3	CP5	EMF5
Vi (%)	100.0 ± 0.0	100.0 ± 0.0	100.0 ± 0.0	100.0 ± 0.0	100.0 ± 0.0
Me (days)	25.6 ± 0.5	25.1 ± 0.4	24.5 ± 1.1	$29.5 \pm 0.5\,{}^{*}$	25.3 ± 1.1
Qu (days)	3.6 ± 0.3	$2.6 \pm 0.1\,{}^{*}$	3.3 ± 0.2	3.0 ± 0.1	3.2 ± 0.4

Vi, the maximal sprouting percentage; Me, the median sprouting half-time; Qu, the quartile deviation. Mean values $\pm$ standard error are presented (8 corms used in each of three replicates, n = 24 corms in one group); *, significantly different from the control group ($p < 0.05$).

The height of the aerial part of the seedling did not differ among groups in the early stages of sprout growth (Figure 2). Seedling growth in the period of 56 DAP was similar in the Vacuum3, CP3, and EMF5 groups compared with the control, except for a 15% reduction in height observed in the EMF5 seedlings on 50th DAP. However, the CP5 group showed a significant reduction in seedling height during the 50–56 DAP interval, with 19% and 28% smaller heights, respectively, compared with the control, and 17% and 13% smaller, respectively, compared with the Vacuum3 group.

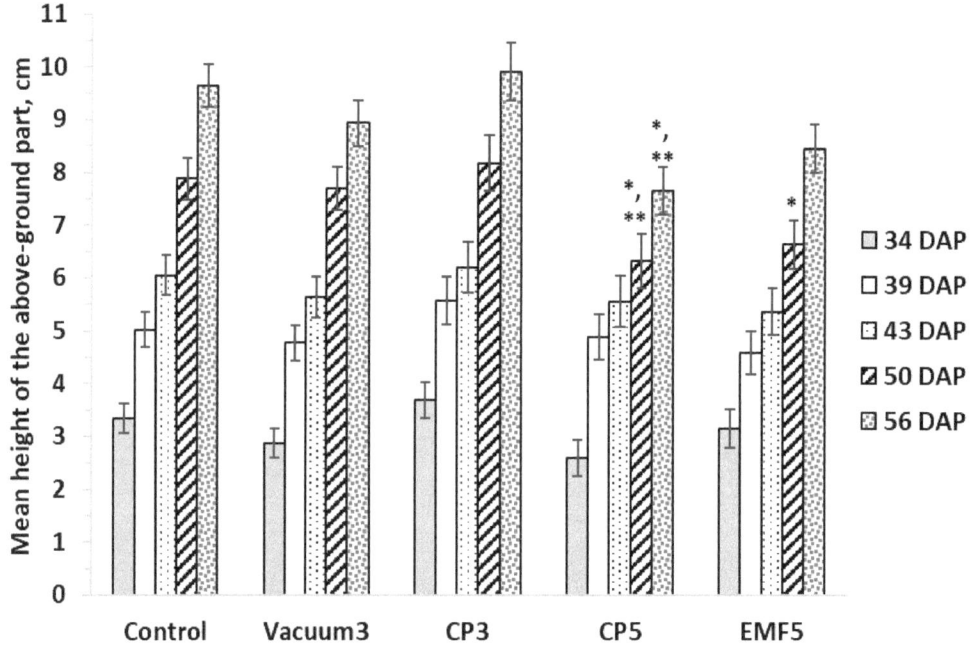

Figure 2. The dynamics of seedling growth estimated by sprout height. Mean values $\pm$ standard error are presented (n = 24); *, significantly different from the control group ($p < 0.05$); **, significantly different from the Vacuum3 group ($p < 0.05$). DAP—days after planting.

The relative number of sprouted buds per corm in the experimental groups is presented in Table 2. A larger variation and an increased number of buds per corm were observed in the Vacuum3 group, while the bud profile in the EMF5 corms was the most similar to the control (with prevailing three buds per corm). The largest proportion of corms with two buds per corm was found in the CP-treated groups, with a stronger shift to a smaller number of buds observed after the CP5 treatment.

Table 2. The percentage of sprouted buds per corm at the 56th DAP.

Bud Number per Corm	Control	Vacuum3	CP3	CP5	EMF5
1	16.0	9.5	14.3	33.3	9.5
2	12.0	23.8	38.1	33.3	28.6
3	36.0	19.0	23.8	28.6	38.1
4	28.0	28.6	14.3	4.8	19.0
5	4.0	9.5	9.5	0.0	4.8
6	4.0	4.8	0.0	0.0	0.0
7	0.0	4.8	0.0	0.0	0.0

Results are presented as percent of corms with the indicated number of buds (n = 24 corms).

The mean number of leaves developed per bud was counted starting from the 34th DAP till the 56th DAP (Figure 3). The number of leaves in the Vacuum3 and CP5 groups was not different from the control, while CP3 and EMF5 treatments increased the mean number of leaves per bud by approximately 10%.

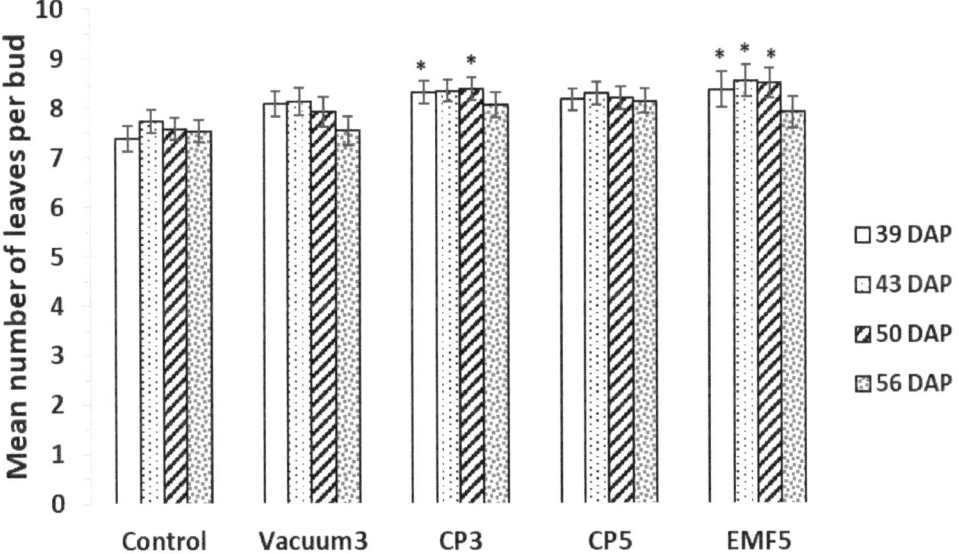

Figure 3. The mean number of leaves per bud in seedlings. Mean values ± standard error are presented (n = 24); *, significantly different from the control group ($p < 0.05$). DAP—days after planting.

Microscopic analysis of leaf trichomes [23,24] was performed on 56th DAP corms. Simple unicellular trichomes of different sizes were found on the abaxial surface of the crypts (Figure 4). Treatments of *C. sativus* corms with all stressors resulted in an increased density of leaf trichomes (Figure 5). The largest effect (74%) was observed in the CP-treated groups (CP3 and CP5), while Vacuum3 and EMF5 treatments were slightly less effective (43 and 63%, respectively). The density of trichomes in both of the CP-treated groups was 23% higher than in the Vacuum3 group. In addition, the size of trichomes was larger in all treated groups compared with the control, as seen in Figure 4.

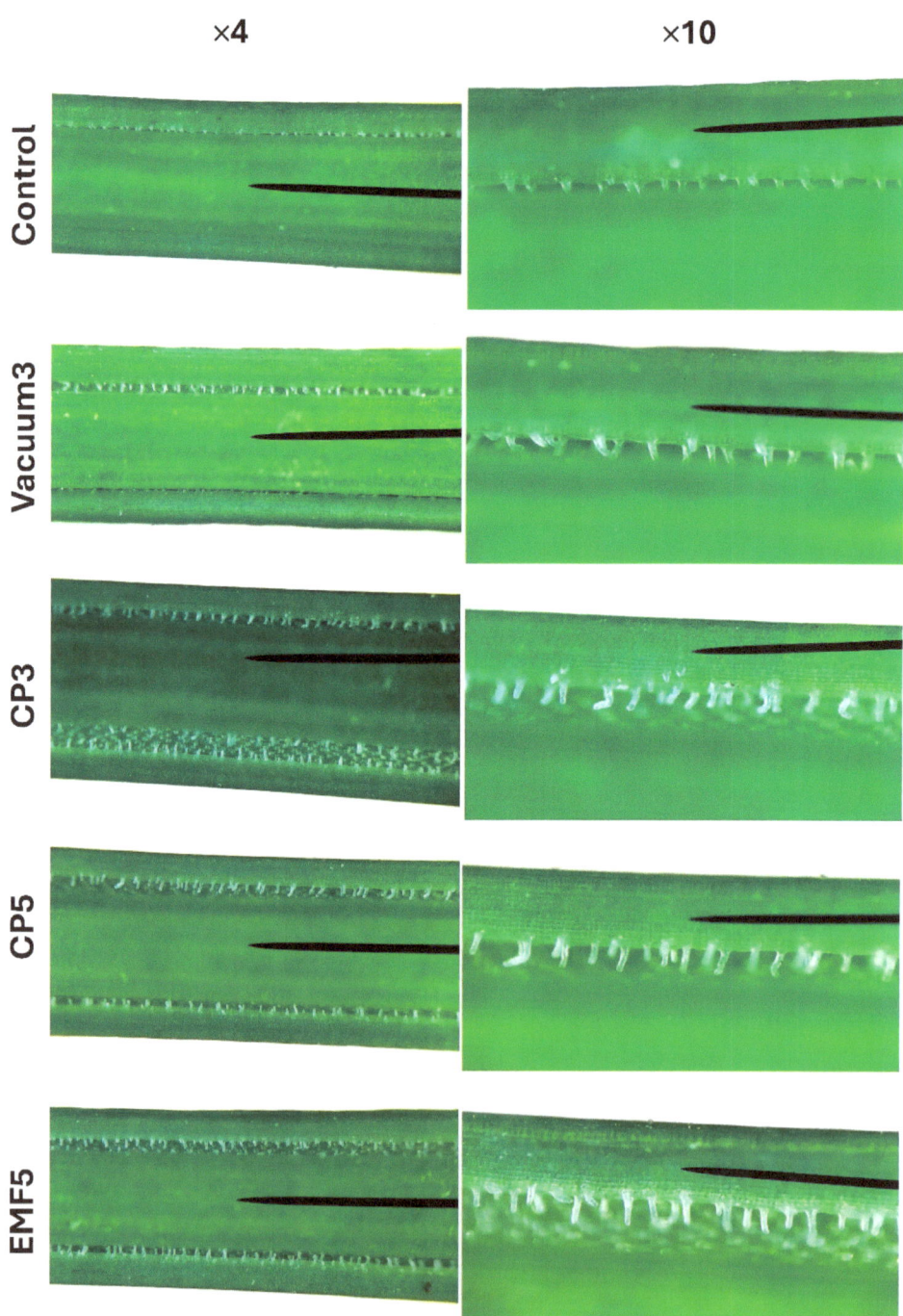

Figure 4. Trichomes in *C. sativus* leaves on the abaxial surface of crypt aperture (the position at the distance between 8 and 9 cm from the tip of a leaf was used for the image). ×4, ×10—magnification four and ten times, respectively.

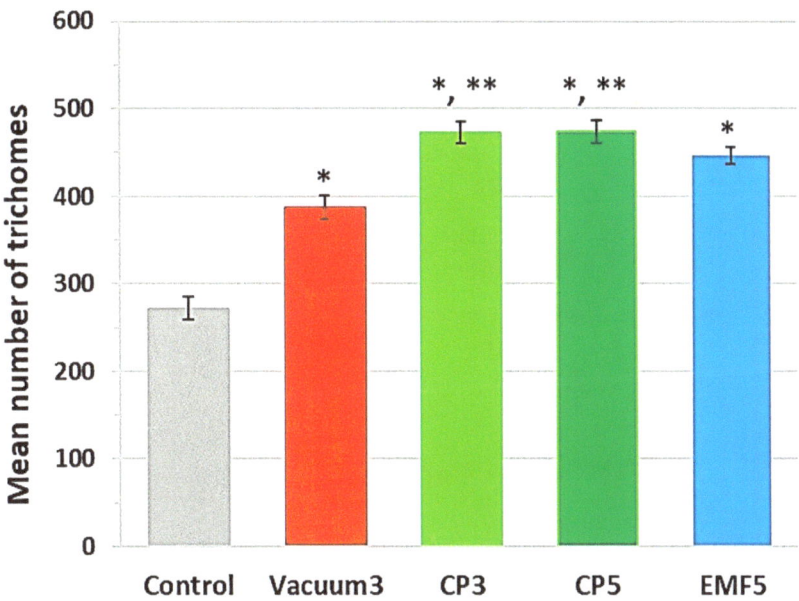

Figure 5. The number of trichomes in a 1 cm long section located between 8 and 9 cm from the tip of the leaf. Mean values ± standard error are presented (n = 24); *, significantly different from the control group ($p < 0.05$); **, significantly different from the Vacuum3 group ($p < 0.05$).

Flowers were collected from November 6th until December 3rd, the day the experiment was concluded due to winter cold. CP5 group did not flower at all during the first year after planting corms. Morphometric parameters of flowers collected from the other treatment groups and the control are presented in Table 3.

Table 3. The morphometric parameters of the collected flowers.

Morphometric Parameter	Control (6)	Vacuum3 (6)	CP3 (4)	EMF5 (7)
Flower length, cm	7.90 ± 0.00	8.00 ± 0.50	4.50 ± 0.50 *	10.00 ± 0.00 *
Flower fresh weight, g	0.43 ± 0.05	0.46 ± 0.05	0.22 ± 0.03	0.52 ± 0.07
Flower dry weight, g	0.05 ± 0.002	0.05 ± 0.003	0.02 ± 0.001 *	0.07 ± 0.01
Pistil length, cm	4.10 ± 0.20	4.07 ± 0.23	3.80 ± 0.18	3.87 ± 0.19
Pistil fresh weight, g	0.03 ± 0.003	0.03 ± 0.003	0.02 ± 0.002	0.03 ± 0.009
Pistil dry weight, g	0.004 ± 0.0005	0.007 ± 0.002	0.004 ± 0.0007	0.004 ± 0.0003

Mean values ± standard error are presented (the number of flowers indicated in parenthesis); *, significantly different from the control group ($p < 0.05$).

The results demonstrate that corm processing with CP3 significantly reduced the length and dry weight (43 and 60%, respectively) of the flowers. This indicates a negative effect of CP on flowering, which intensified with the duration of treatment. Consequently, plants from the CP5 group did not develop flowers. EMF5 treatment had a positive effect on flowering and increased flower length by 27% compared with the control. No statistically significant differences between experimental groups in the morphometric parameters of the stigmas were observed.

2.2. Effects on Amounts of Secondary Metabolites in the Stigma of C. sativus

The amounts of secondary metabolites in dried stigma extracts were quantified by HPLC analysis [25,26]. The typical chromatogram is shown in Figure 6, and the chromatographic characteristics of the identified esters: crocetin, safranal, picrocrocin, and rutin, their retention time (t_R) at 440 nm, and UV-visible spectra are presented in Table 4. In total, 26 compound peaks were identified in the HPLC chromatograms of *Crocus* stigma extracts. However, six compounds were not identified. Of the 17 different derivatives of crocetin, 15 compounds have been identified. The content of pricrocrocin, rutin, and safranal was estimated.

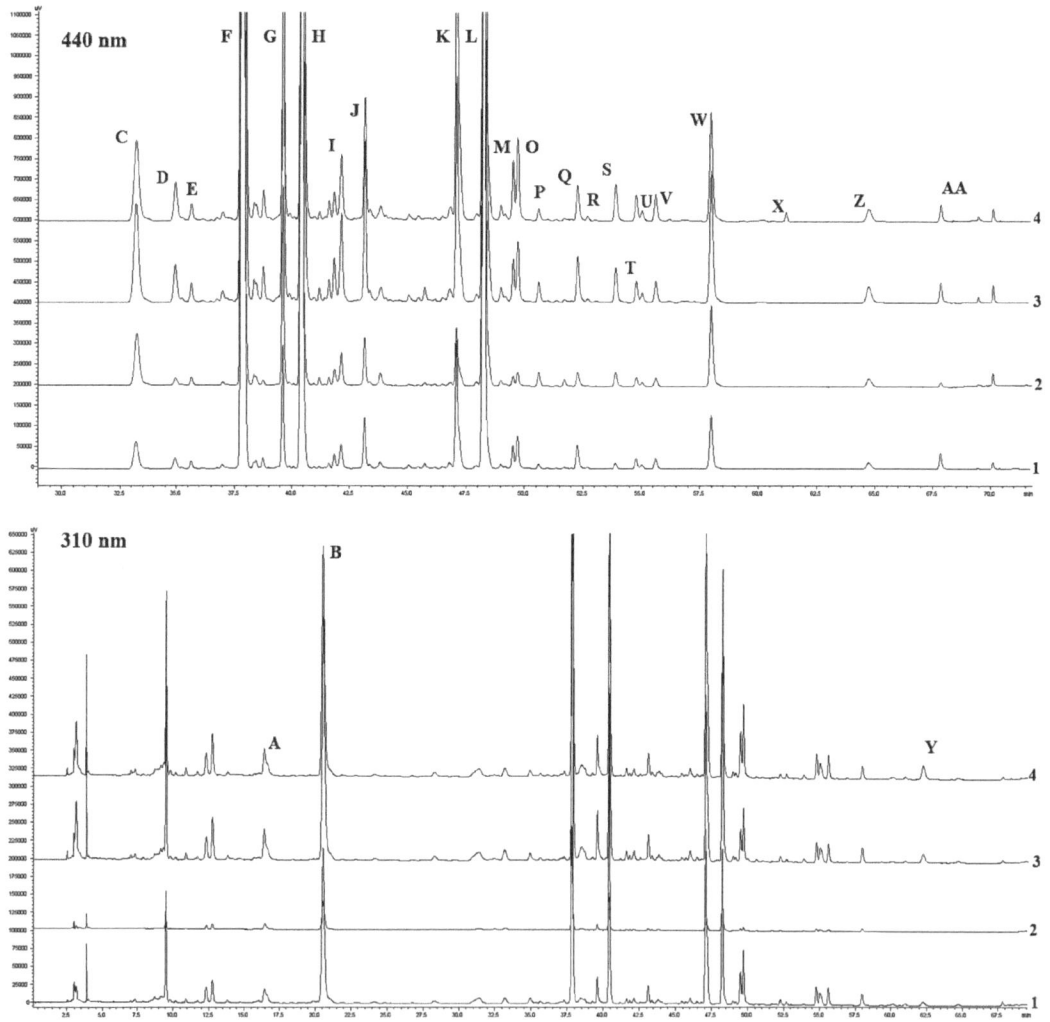

Figure 6. HPLC chromatogram of *C. sativus* stigma methanol extracts. Detection wavelength—440 nm and 310 nm.

Table 4. Peak number, retention time (t_R), and content of each chromatographic peak corresponding to crocetin esters (crocins) tentative identification * in *C. sativus* stigma extract.

Compound	No Glucose Moieties	Abbreviation **	t_R (min)	UV/Vis, λmax, nm	MW, g·mol^{-1}	MolFor
trans-crocetin (tri-β-D-glucosyl)(β-D-gentiobiosyl) ester	Crocin 5	t-5tG	33.190	262, 332sh, 443, 468	1138	$C_{50}H_{74}O_{29}$
trans-crocetin (β-D-neapolitanosyl)(β-D-gentiobiosyl) ester	-	t-5nG	34.928	234, 300sh, 418, 439	1138	$C_{50}H_{74}O_{29}$
trans-crocetin (β-D-neapolitanosyl)(β-D-glucosyl) ester	-	t-4ng	35.630	263, 441, 466	976	$C_{44}H_{64}O_{24}$
trans-crocetin di(β-D-gentiobiosyl)ester	Crocin 4	t-4GG	37.825	261, 331sh, 440, 466	976	$C_{44}H_{64}O_{24}$
trans-crocetin (β-D-gentiobiosyl)(β-D-glucosyl) ester	Crocin 3	t-3Gg	39.608	261, 327sh, 440, 466	814	$C_{38}H_{54}O_{19}$
trans-crocetin mono(β-D-gentiobiosyl) ester	Crocin 2	t-2G	40.424	261, 331sh, 440, 466	652	$C_{33}H_{44}O_{14}$
cis-crocetin (β-D-neapolitanosyl)(β-D-gentiobiosyl) ester	-	c-5nG	42.119	242, 260, 414, 436	1139	$C_{50}H_{74}O_{29}$
trans-crocetin di(β-D-glucosyl) ester	Crocin 2′	t-2gg	43.147	261, 322, 439, 465	652	$C_{33}H_{44}O_{14}$
cis-crocetin di(β-D-gentiobiosyl)ester	*cis*-Crocin 4	c-4GG	47.084	262, 326, 435, 457	976	$C_{44}H_{64}O_{24}$
cis-crocetin (β-D-gentiobiosyl)(β-D-glucosyl) ester	*cis*-Crocin 3	c-3Gg	48.252	258, 325, 435, 460	814	$C_{38}H_{54}O_{19}$
cis-crocetin mono(β-D-gentiobiosyl) ester	*cis*-Crocin 2	c-2G	49.511	262, 327, 433, 456	652	$C_{33}H_{44}O_{14}$
cis-crocetin di(β-D-glucosyl) ester	cis-Crocin 2′	c-2gg	49.711	262, 326, 434, 456sh	652	$C_{33}H_{44}O_{14}$
trans-crocetin mono(β-D-glucosyl) ester	Crocin 1	t-1g	50.592	258, 434, 459	490	$C_{26}H_{34}O_{9}$
Crocin derivative	-	-	52.256	258, 434, 459	479~	$C_{44}H_{64}O_{24}$
Crocin derivative	-	-	52.685	258, 327, 434	479~	$C_{44}H_{64}O_{24}$
cis-crocetin (tri-β-D-glucosyl)(β-D-gentiobiosyl) ester	*cis*-Crocin 5	c-5tG	53.893	263, 332sh, 445, 469	1138	$C_{50}H_{74}O_{29}$
Crocin derivative	-	-	54.780	259, 323, 428, 452	479~	$C_{44}H_{64}O_{24}$
Crocin derivative	-	-	55.140	245sh, 332, 431, 454	479~	$C_{44}H_{64}O_{24}$
cis-crocetin mono(β-D-glucosyl) ester	*cis*-Crocin 1	c-1g	55.614	259, 323, 428, 452	490	$C_{26}H_{34}O_{9}$
Crocin derivative	-	-	57.965	258, 324sh, 434, 460	479~	$C_{44}H_{64}O_{24}$
Crocin derivative	-	-	61.007	249, 326, 430, 453	479~	$C_{44}H_{64}O_{24}$
trans-crocetin	-	*t*-crocetin	64.716	258, 434, 459	328	$C_{20}H_{24}O_{4}$
cis-crocetin	-	c-crocetin	67.827	255, 318sh, 427, 453	328	$C_{20}H_{24}O_{4}$

*—tentative detected according to [7,25–27]. **—Meaning of each letter in the abbreviation of the name of each crocetin ester: number (5, 4, 3, 2)—number of glucose molecules attached to the molecule of crocetin; t—triglucose; G—gentiobiose; g—glucose; n—neapolitanose.

The compounds of the crocetin group dominated stigma extracts in the control, with *trans*-crocetin di(β-D-gentiobiosyl) ester, *trans*-crocetin mono(β-D-gentiobiosyl) ester, *cis*-crocetin di(β-D-gentiobiosyl) ester, and *cis*-crocetin (β-D-gentiobiosyl)(β-D-glucosyl) ester present in amounts as high as 114.3 mg/g, 49.0 mg/g, 25.4 mg/g, and 23.9 mg/g of dry weight, respectively (Table 5). The chemical structures of crocetin derivatives are presented in Figure 7.

Table 5. Content of identified secondary metabolites in *C. sativus* stigma (µg/g dry weight).

Code [1]	Compound	Rt. min	Control	Vacuum3	CP3	EMF5
A	Picrocrocin	16.49	720.6 ± 88.4	965.6 ± 9.2 *	395.4 ± 2.4 *	847.3 ± 6.2 *
B	Rutin	20.81	889.0 ± 147.2	762.6 ± 21.0	171.0 ± 2.0 *	750.0 ± 33.1
C	*trans*-crocetin (*tri*-β-D-glucosyl) (β-D-gentiobiosyl) ester	33.19	2180.6 ± 19.4	2085.0 ± 130.1	591.2 ± 3.2 *	18,898.4 ± 17,021.5 **
D	*trans*-crocetin (β-D-neapolitanosyl) (β-D-gentiobiosyl) ester	34.93	867.2 ± 90.4	786.6 ± 6.5	76.4 ± 1.6 *	6356.2 ± 251.4 **
E	*trans*-crocetin (β-D-neapolitanosyl) (β-D-glucosyl) ester	35.63	357.0 ± 83.0	-	-	2034.7 ± 692.2 **
F	*trans*-crocetin di(β-D-gentiobiosyl)ester *	37.83	114,319.0 ± 513.6	124,350.4 ± 996.2	8949.1 ± 38.2 *	431,173.0 ± 965.0 *
G	*trans*-crocetin (β-D-gentiobiosyl) (β-D-glucosyl) ester	39.61	1714.2 ± 90.6	4225.0 ± 71.9 *	886.8 ± 9.2 *	37,187.7 ± 144.9 *
H	*trans*-crocetin mono(β-D-gentiobiosyl) ester	40.42	49,042.2 ± 1983.0	42,026.4 ± 251.0 *	6399.4 ± 101.8 *	188,232.6 ± 1415.9 **
I	*cis*-crocetin (β-D-neapolitanosyl) (β-D-gentiobiosyl) ester	42.12	1200.8 ± 24.6	575.0 ± 49.6 *	131.6 ± 14.8 *	781.9 ± 13.9 *
J	*trans*-crocetin di(β-D-glucosyl) ester	43.15	1735.6 ± 127.6	1363.8 ± 90.5 *	207.0 ± 1.4 *	1197.8 ± 34.7 *
K	*cis*-crocetin di(β-D-gentiobiosyl)ester	47.08	25,398.0 ± 195.0	12,675.6 ± 87.6	1899.8 ± 30.6 *	20,536.6 ± 74.9 *
L	*cis*-crocetin (β-D-gentiobiosyl) (β-D-glucosyl) ester	48.25	23,894.2 ± 137.8	21,464.2 ± 285.2 *	6270.6 ± 43.0 *	164,859.6 ± 14,739.5 **
M	*cis*-crocetin mono(β-D-gentiobiosyl) ester	49.51	3594.4 ± 162.4	1878.0 ± 19.0 *	192.2 ± 30.4 *	2530.7 ± 3.5 *
O	*cis*-crocetin di(β-D-glucosyl) ester	49.71	5529.8 ± 296.0	2812.1 ± 39.8 *	309.4 ± 19.2 *	17,151.2 ± 123.7 **
P	*trans*-crocetin mono(β-D-glucosyl) ester	50.59	-	257.9 ± 14.9 *	78.6 ± 5.8 *	1446.8 ± 124.9 *
Q	Crocin derivative	52.26	792.6 ± 56.6	400.5 ± 7.1 *	69.0 ± 0.18 *	4345.0 ± 401.2 **
R	Crocin derivative	52.69	-	-	61.6 ± 1.8	511.5 ± 33.4
S	*cis*-crocetin (*tri*-β-D-glucosyl) (β-D-gentiobiosyl) ester	53.89	251.4 ± 12.2	458.2 ± 11.8 *	95.6 ± 2.8 *	4876.2 ± 404.6 *
T	Crocin derivative	54.78	1289.6 ± 36.6	734.4 ± 3.0 *	171.8 ± 7.6 *	3238.4 ± 328.5 *
U	Crocin derivative	55.14	-	-	-	1531.6 ± 84.3
V	*cis*-crocetin mono (β-D-glucosyl) ester	55.61	1297.2 ± 16.0	737.6 ± 6.4 *	167.4 ± 9.2 *	3810.5 ± 157.4 **
W	Crocin derivative	57.97	1528.4 ± 85.6	1115.2 ± 55.7 *	144.6 ± 33.0 *	1374.1 ± 18.1 *
X	Crocin derivative	61.01	-	-	-	200.4 ± 23.6
Y	Safranal	62.28	8.4 ± 1.8	10.3 ± 0.5	1.60 ± 0.04 *	16.3 ± 0.2 **
Z	*trans*-crocetin	64.72	-	-	197.7 ± 1.2 *	225.4 ± 9.1 *
AA	*cis*-crocetin	67.83	-	-	-	204.6 ± 8.2

[1]—The code numbering of compounds in the chromatogram (Figure 6) and Table 5 is the same. Mean values ± SD are presented (n = 3). *, significantly different from the control group ($p < 0.05$); **, statistically significant difference compared to the control ($p \leq 0.001$).

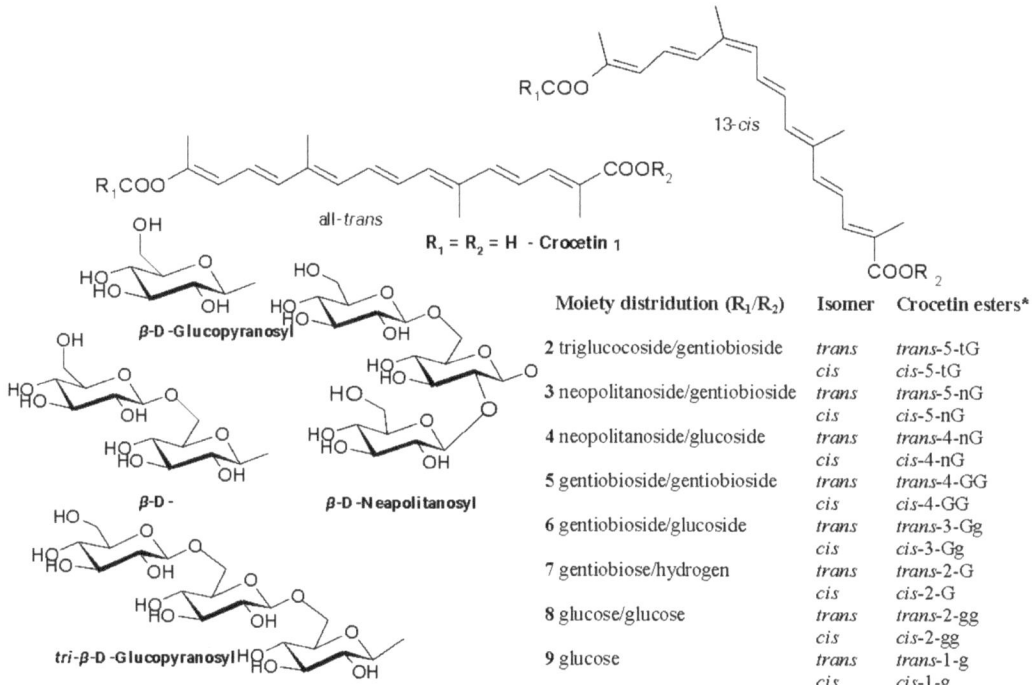

Moiety distridution (R₁/R₂)	Isomer	Crocetin esters*
2 triglucocoside/gentiobioside	*trans*	*trans*-5-tG
	cis	*cis*-5-tG
3 neopolitanoside/gentiobioside	*trans*	*trans*-5-nG
	cis	*cis*-5-nG
4 neopolitanoside/glucoside	*trans*	*trans*-4-nG
	cis	*cis*-4-nG
5 gentiobioside/gentiobioside	*trans*	*trans*-4-GG
	cis	*cis*-4-GG
6 gentiobioside/glucoside	*trans*	*trans*-3-Gg
	cis	*cis*-3-Gg
7 gentiobiose/hydrogen	*trans*	*trans*-2-G
	cis	*cis*-2-G
8 glucose/glucose	*trans*	*trans*-2-gg
	cis	*cis*-2-gg
9 glucose	*trans*	*trans*-1-g
	cis	*cis*-1-g

Figure 7. Structural formulas of esters of *trans*- and *cis*-crocetin and substituents at R1 and R2. Nomenclature according to [27]. Note: * Meaning of each letter in the abbreviation of the name of each crocetin ester: Number (5, 4, 3, 2)—number of glucose molecules attached to the molecule of crocetin; t—triglucose; G—gentiobiose; g—glucose; n—neapolitanose.

The results showed that treatment of corms with CP, vacuum, and EMF induced significant changes in the content of secondary metabolites in *Crocus* stigma, and the change strongly depended on the nature of the stressor (Figure 8). The changes induced by Vacuum3 treatment were smaller compared with those induced by CP3 and EMF5. Vacuum3 had no effect on the amount of certain metabolites (e.g., B, C, D, F, etc.), increased the amount of some (A, G, S), and decreased the amount of other metabolites (H-O, Q, V, W). CP3 treatment had a strong negative effect on the content of secondary metabolites. It significantly reduced the amount of all metabolites, including more than 10 times of some of them (e.g., F, L, M.O). On the contrary, EML5 had a significant positive effect on the accumulation of many secondary metabolites in *Crocus* stigma. For example, EMF5 increased the amount of G and S twenty-two and nineteen times, C and L nine and seven times, and F and H four times. On the other hand, EMF5 did not change the amount of rutin and reduced the amounts of I, J, K, and M metabolites in the stigma. The amount of picrocrocin was increased by the exposure to Vacuum3 and EMF (34 and 18%) and strongly reduced (45%) by CP3. Vacuum3 did not change the amount of safranal, while CP3 reduced it five times, in contrast to EML5, which induced a two-fold increase. Certain compounds that were not present in the control group (e.g., P, U, X, AA) were only identified in the stigma after EMF5 treatment, while R and Z synthesis was induced by both CP3 and EMF5, with a stronger effect observed with the latter treatment.

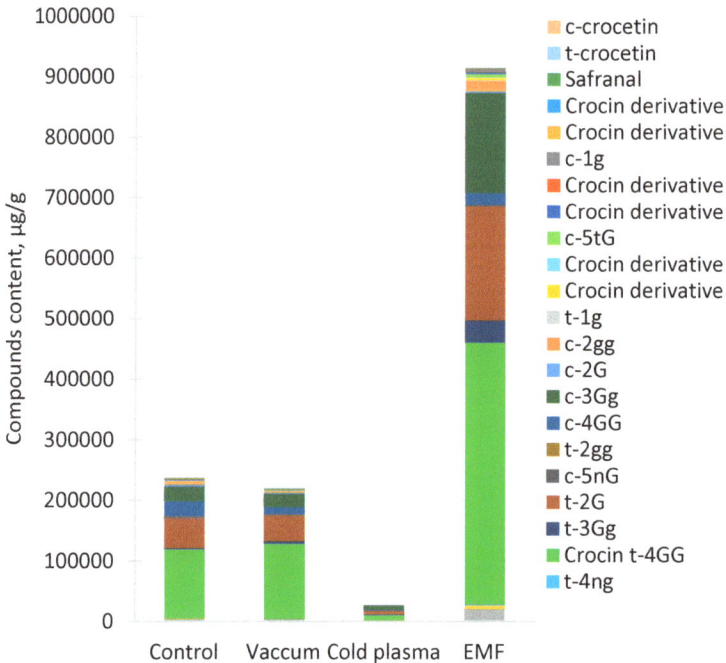

Figure 8. Distribution of the compounds in *C. sativus* stigma depending on the pre-sowing treatment method.

3. Discussion

The experimental study on the effects of corm treatment with CP, vacuum, and EMF on sprouting, plant growth, and secondary metabolite content in the stigma was performed to estimate the potential of such treatments to improve saffron production yield and quality. Our hypothesis was based on numerous reports about the positive effects of pre-sowing seed treatment on the growth and metabolite content of medicinal plants, including those used as herbal supplements, such as purple coneflower [15], red clover [16,17], industrial hemp [28], and Norway spruce [29]. However, similar research on the planting material of geophyte plants is limited by a single report [19]. In the said study, low-pressure radio frequency oxygen plasma was applied for 60 s on peeled garlic cloves of a spring-planted Slovenian autochthonous cultivar "Ptujski spomladanski". This resulted in increased water uptake during germination as well as early seedling growth stimulation under laboratory conditions. However, treatments did not have an effect on garlic yield after 4 months of cultivation in a field experiment. The effects of treatments on the amounts of secondary metabolites in garlic tissues were not assessed in this study [19]. The results of our study revealed that a strong impact on secondary metabolite content may not be associated with the obvious effects on plant seedling growth.

Increased generation of the protective secondary metabolites is a common hallmark of plant stress response controlled by a complex network of regulatory molecules, including phytohormones [30]. The main phytohormones responsible for stress-induced enhancement of secondary metabolite synthesis are salicylic acid and jasmonates [31]. Synthesis of carotenoids (including crocins) in plants is also under the tight control of phytohormone signaling [32,33]. It was experimentally demonstrated that treatment with cold plasma and electromagnetic field induces a rapid shift in the balance of phytohormones in dry seeds [34–38]. According to the suggested hypothesis [4], seed treatment-induced changes in seed phytohormone composition are further retained in growing plants, entailing the modified patterns in phytohormonal networks and generating a multitude of changes in gene expression, resulting in numerous effects on plant biochemical and physiological processes, including the activity of biosynthetic pathways of secondary metabolites. Such explanation is based on the reported examples of enhanced activity of the enzymes in the secondary metabolite biosynthesis pathways induced by seed treatment with CP in hemp [39], pink periwinkle [40], and blue sage [41], as well as activity of two key enzymes of the pathway of carotenoid biosynthesis, phytoene-synthase and phytoene desaturase, in bitter melon [42]. The results of our study show that processing of *C. sativus* corms with CP has only an adverse impact on the biosynthesis of crocins, in contrast to strong positive effects elicited by EMF treatment. We suggest that changes in the balance of phytohormones and signal transduction pathways in corms and growing seedlings are dependent on the nature of the stressor.

The main reason why CP (or vacuum) has been widely applied for seed treatment but not for planting material of geophytes is the much smaller size and low water content of orthodox seeds, which undergo desiccation during maturation and the moisture content in the anhydrobiotic state decreases to less than 10 percent [43,44]. The anhydrobiotic state is crucially important for seed adaptability to environmental changes, stress resistance, and longevity. In contrast, moisture content in the planting material of geophytes is much higher; for example, 72–74% of water was detected in *C. sativus* corms [45]. Numerous chemical products are formed during the interaction of aggressive particles from the CP gaseous phase with water in the plasma target interphase, giving rise to damaging factors such as nitric acids or a rapid pH drop [46]. In addition, water evaporates rapidly under high vacuum conditions, and that can cause a structural disruption and collapse of biological structures [47]. Assumptions about the potential damage have possibly held researchers back from testing the effects of CP (or vacuum) on botanical samples other than anhydrobiotic seeds. In this respect, EMF seems to be a more acceptable stressor for corms or bulbs containing relatively high amounts of moisture.

Nevertheless, the results obtained in this study provide evidence that the short duration of CP or vacuum treatment did not reduce the viability of *C. sativus* corms, although CP did not stimulate sprouting like it was reported earlier for garlic cloves [19]. However, numerous negative effects of CP treatment were observed in the later stages of seedling development, including reduced height, percentage of sprouted buds per corm, length, and number of developed flowers (adverse effects were much stronger in the CP5 group). Vacuum3 treatment did not have obvious effects on plant growth but increased uniformity of sprouting and the number of sprouted buds per corm, possibly indicating stimulation of secondary buds. EMF treatment exerted no negative effects, did not change corm sprouting kinetics or plant height, but increased the mean number of leaves per bud and the length of flowers, which was associated with a strong positive effect of EMF on the content of secondary metabolites in the dried stigma of *C. sativus*. At the same time, the adverse effects of the CP treatment were related to a drastic decrease in the secondary metabolite content. The effects of Vacuum3 on secondary metabolite content were less pronounced; the concentrations of certain compounds were increased, while the amounts of other metabolites were decreased.

Interestingly, despite the different effects of CP, vacuum, and EMF on plant growth and secondary metabolites in stigma, corm treatment with all stressors strongly increased the density and size of leaf trichomes. Trichomes, the outgrowths of epidermal cells present on the aerial parts of most plant tissues, have an enormous variety in terms of morphology and perform a range of protective and other functions [24]. One of the main functions of trichomes is the synthesis and accumulation of secondary metabolites and defensive proteins [24], but the impact of the different types of stress on amounts of trichomes is poorly understood [48,49]. Our results support the hypothesis that corm exposure to abiotic stress leads to an increase in the density of leaf trichomes, although these effects do not correlate with the changes in secondary metabolite amounts in dried stigma.

At least two studies have been published on the application of cold plasma technology on *Crocus* stigmas to increase the content of key compounds, such as crocin and safranal [50,51]. Unfortunately, a decrease in marker compounds, namely crocin esters and safranal, was observed after the treatments, and no trans-2G, cis-4GG, or cis-3Gg compounds were observed at all in the samples after cold plasma treatment with Ar/10% O_2 at 12 kV [52]. However, these treatments were applied to the stigma itself, not to the corms. Cold plasma technology generates reactive species that can interact with plant tissues, potentially enhancing the production of secondary metabolites at the plant germination level.

In summary, our study demonstrated that corm treatment with CP, vacuum, and EMF does not have an effect on corm viability, and the effects on secondary metabolite amount in stigma are much stronger compared with the effects observed on plant growth and development. The most interesting finding was the obvious potential of corm treatment with EMF to increase the amounts of valuable biologically active compounds in saffron.

4. Materials and Methods

4.1. Plant Material and Seedling Cultivation

Corms of *Crocus sativus* L. were obtained from a Ukrainian manufacturer ("Shafran Lyubimovske" farm, Lyubimovka village, Kherson region, Ukraine). Raw material was collected and identified by Dr. Mykhailenko, and samples were deposited at the Herbarium of Botany Department of the National University of Pharmacy, Kharkiv, Ukraine (voucher specimen No. 20198).

The field experiment was carried out in the experimental plots at Vytautas Magnus University Botanical Garden (Kaunas, Lithuania, coordinates 54.868567, 23.911813). Four days before planting, corms were treated with physical stressors: low-pressure cold plasma for 3 and 5 min, further denoted as CP3 and CP5; vacuum for 3 min (as an additional control for CP), denoted as Vacuum3; and electromagnetic field for 5 min, denoted as EMF5. The control and treated corms (24 corms per treatment group) were planted in half-shaded, well-cultivated loam soil in 3 rows (replicates) at the beginning of autumn in 2020. Corms were planted at a depth of 10 cm, keeping a distance of 20 cm between corms, 20 cm between rows of the same treatment group, and 45 cm spacing between different treatment groups. The experimental plots were irrigated manually two times in the first two weeks after planting to reduce the impact of summer drought. No fertilization was applied.

4.2. Corm Treatment by CP, Vacuum, and EMF

Corms were irradiated with CP using a low-pressure not-thermal plasma device constructed by Prof. Koga and Prof. M. Shiratani (Kyushu University, Japan). The hermetic chamber (length 152 mm, diameter 102 mm) of the CP generator was made of stainless steel (SUS-304). To generate the discharge, a helical power electrode-antenna (20 mm long and 15 mm in diameter) installed at the top of the chamber was switched to a high-frequency voltage of 430 MHz by a radio transmitter (the power supply was 45 W). The reactor chamber performed the function of the other electrode. Three corms were placed at the bottom of the chamber per treatment. The distance between the upper electrode and the corms adjusted with additional glass stands was 8 cm. Atmospheric air was used as a gaseous phase, and a vacuum (100 Pa) was created before the discharge by pumping out air with a pump system. The same chamber was used to treat the corms with a vacuum (100 Pa) for 3 min as an additional control for the CP treatment.

Corms were treated with radiofrequency (RF) EMF using a pulsed magnetic field generator (peak parameters 100 kHz, 0–10 mT) designed at Vilnius Gediminas Technical University by Prof. Vitalij Novickij. The treatment was performed for 5 min (the treatment is further abbreviated as EMF5) using 100 kHz, 400 ± 50 µT oscillating magnetic field at atmospheric pressure and room temperature. Three corms were treated at one time, keeping them at a 3 cm distance above the center of the induction coil.

4.3. Analysis of Sprouting and Plant Morphometric Parameters

Sprouting dynamics of *Crocus* corms were observed and registered every other day for 32 days after the first sprout appeared. Richards plots were constructed [15,23] to quantify the main indices of plant sprouting kinetics: Vi (%)—the maximal sprouting percentage indicating corm viability, Me (days)—the median sprouting time ($t_{50\%}$) indicating halftime of corm sprouting rate, Qu (days)—the quartile deviation indicating the dispersion of sprouting time or sprouting uniformity.

Morphometric parameters were measured two weeks after the first sprout appeared. The height of the above-ground plant part was measured, and the mean number of sprouted buds per corm, as well as the mean number of leaves per bud, were counted starting from the 34th till the 56th DAP.

Trichomes were counted on the abaxial side of a leaf to estimate the possible response of growing seedlings to stress induced by corm treatments. A light microscope was used to quantify trichomes, and the size of the microscopic view was calibrated using a Motic calibration slide. Simple unicellular trichomes on the crypt aperture were counted on both edges of the crypt at 1 cm, approximately in the middle of a leaf (in the distance between the 8th and the 9th centimeters from the tip of a mature leaf).

C. sativus flowers were collected manually, and after morphometric measurements, their stigmas were separated and dried for 2–3 h at 50 °C under forced air. Dried stigmas were stored in dark glass jars at 4 °C.

4.4. Sample Preparation and HPLC-DAD Analysis

Saffron samples (0.1 g each) were ground and extracted with methanol/water (85:15 v/v, 10 mL). The extractions were performed in an ultrasonic bath (Wise Clean WUC-A06H, Witeg Labortechnik GmbH, Wertheim, Germany) with a working frequency of 33 kHz. The samples were sonicated at room temperature for 30 min, and the resulting solutions were filtered through a membrane filter (0.45 μm) and analyzed.

Acetonitrile and methanol of HPLC grade were purchased from Roth GmbH (Karlsruhe, Germany), while water was purified through a Milli-Q system (Millipore, Bedford, MA, USA). Standards compounds crocin (CAS number 42553-65-1) and safranal (CAS number 116-26-7) with a purity of >90% were purchased from Sigma-Aldrich (St. Louis, MO, USA).

Crocin, safranal, and picrocrocin were identified and quantified using a Shimadzu Nexera X2 LC-30AD high-performance liquid chromatography system (HPLC, Shimadzu, Kyoto, Japan) composed of a quaternary pump, an online degasser, a column temperature controller, the SIL-30AC autosampler (Shimadzu, Japan), the CTO-20AC thermostat (Shimadzu, Japan), and SPD-M20A diode array detector (DAD). All data processing was carried out using LabSolutions Analysis Data System (Shimadzu Corporation) as described earlier [38]. Chromatographic separation was performed with an ACE C18 column (250 mm × 4.6 mm, 5.0 μm; Radnor, PA, USA). Elution was performed at a flow rate of 1 mL/min. The binary solvent system of the mobile phase consisted of solvent A (0.1% acetic acid in water) and solvent B (acetonitrile). All solvents were filtered through a 0.22 μm membrane filter after ultrasonic degassing. Following that, a linear elution gradient was applied: 0–8 min, 5–15% B; 8–30 min, 15–20% B; 30–48 min, 20–40% B; 48–58 min, 40–50% B; 58–65 min, 50% B; 65–66 min, 50–95% B. Column temperature was constant at 25 °C. The injection volume of the sample solution was 10 μL. The DAD detector was set at 260, 310, and 440 nm wavelengths for picrocrocin, safranal, and crocin, respectively. Standard solutions, including crocin and safranal, were used for calibration of a standard curve using an external standard method. Analyses were performed in duplicate. Identifications of crocin were carried out using the UV–Vis spectrum, the retention time of the crocin standard at 440 nm according to the HPLC-DAD method. Picrocrocin content in the extracts was recalculated as a safranal equivalent. Safranal identification was carried out using the UV–Vis spectrum and the retention time of the safranal standard at 310 nm according to the HPLC-DAD. The calibration curve for safranal and crocin was constructed by plotting the chromatogram peak area at absorption maxima versus the known concentration of the standard solution.

4.5. Statistical Analysis

Means of various parameters between the control and treatment groups were compared using Student's *t*-tests for independent samples. Differences were considered to be statistically significant at $p \leq 0.05$. The number of measured plants in the control and treatment groups was 24 (analysis of morphometric parameters), or 8 plants for one replicate. Three extract samples were analyzed via the HPLC-DAD method. Data are presented as means of 3 independent repetitions $\pm$ standard error of the mean.

5. Conclusions

Treatment of *Crocus sativus* corms with CP, vacuum, and EMF did not reduce their viability; the final sprouting in all groups was 100% under field experiment conditions. However, the longer duration of the CP treatment (5 min) reduced sprouting, while more uniform sprouting of corms was observed in the vacuum-treated group.

The effects of three different stressors in the later stages of plant growth strongly depend on the nature of the stressor. The adverse effects of the CP treatment on plant height, number of sprouted buds, length, and number of flowers increased with the treatment duration. The vacuum had a minor positive impact on sprouting, while EMF treatment had a positive effect, e.g., increased the number of *Crocus* leaves per bud and the length of flowers. Treatment with all stressors significantly increased the density of leaf trichomes.

Corm processing with EMF presents a promising application for enhancing saffron production, improving the quality, and increasing the content of its bioactive compounds. The obtained results indicate that corm exposure to EMF can stimulate growth, increase biomass, and improve the yield of saffron stigmas, which are the primary source of valuable compounds like crocin, picrocrocin, and safranal. Additionally, EMF treatments may enhance the synthesis and accumulation of these key metabolites, leading to higher-quality saffron with greater medicinal and culinary value. Overall, integrating EMF treatment into saffron cultivation could be a sustainable and innovative approach to boosting both yield and quality, providing significant economic benefits to saffron producers. However, the reproducibility and persistence of this effect have to be studied further to optimize corm treatment conditions.

Author Contributions: Conceptualization, V.M., V.G. and O.M.; methodology, V.N., K.K., M.S. and R.M.; validation, L.J., O.M. and V.G.; investigation, R.Ž., L.D.F. and O.M.; resources, O.M. and I.D.; data curation, V.M.; writing—original draft preparation, V.M.; writing—review and editing, V.M., O.M., V.G., V.N. and K.K.; visualization, Z.N. and L.J.; supervision, V.M. and O.M. All authors have read and agreed to the published version of the manuscript.

Funding: This research received no external funding.

Institutional Review Board Statement: Not applicable.

Informed Consent Statement: Not applicable.

Data Availability Statement: Data are contained within the article.

Acknowledgments: We are grateful to VMU Botanical Garden for technical help and the possibility to perform the study in the experimental field. All authors also sincerely thank the Armed Forces of Ukraine for the opportunity to continue research.

Conflicts of Interest: The authors declare no conflicts of interest.

References

1. Attri, P.; Ishikawa, K.; Okumura, T.; Koga, K.; Shiratani, M. Plasma agriculture from laboratory to farm: A review. *Processes* **2020**, *8*, 1002. [CrossRef]
2. Adhikari, B.; Adhikari, M.; Park, G. The effects of plasma on plant growth, development, and sustainability. *Appl. Sci.* **2020**, *10*, 6045. [CrossRef]
3. Waskow, A.; Howling, A.; Furno, I. Mechanisms of plasma-seed treatments as a potential seed processing technology. *Front. Phys.* **2021**, *9*, 617345. [CrossRef]
4. Mildaziene, V.; Ivankov, A.; Sera, B.; Baniulis, D. Biochemical and Physiological Plant Processes Affected by Seed Treatment with Non-Thermal Plasma. *Plants* **2022**, *11*, 856. [CrossRef]
5. Kaur, S.; Vian, A.; Chandel, S.; Singh, H.P.; Batish, D.R.; Kohli, R.K. Sensitivity of plants to high frequency electromagnetic radiation: Cellular mechanisms and morphological changes. *Rev. Environ. Sci. Biotechnol.* **2021**, *20*, 55–74. [CrossRef]
6. Bukhari, S.I.; Manzoor, M.; Dhar, M.K. A comprehensive review of the pharmacological potential of *Crocus sativus* and its bioactive apocarotenoids. *Biomed. Pharmacother.* **2018**, *98*, 733–745. [CrossRef]
7. Mykhailenko, O.; Desenko, V.; Ivanauskas, L.; Georgiyants, V. Standard operating procedure of Ukrainian saffron cultivation according with Good Agricultural and Collection Practices to assure quality and traceability. *Ind. Crops Prod.* **2020**, *151*, 112376–112387. [CrossRef]
8. Ashraf, N.; Jain, D.; Vishwakarma, R.A. Identification, cloning and characterization of an ultrapetala transcription factor CsULT1 from *Crocus*: A novel regulator of apocarotenoid biosynthesis. *BMC Plant Biol.* **2015**, *15*, 25. [CrossRef]
9. Butnariu, M.; Quispe, C.; Herrera-Bravo, J.; Sharifi-Rad, J.; Singh, L.; Aborehab, N.M.; Bouyahya, A.; Venditti, A.; Sen, S.; Acharya, K.; et al. The pharmacological activities of *Crocus sativus* L.: A review based on the mechanisms and therapeutic opportunities of its phytoconstituents. *Oxid. Med. Cell. Longev.* **2022**, *2022*, 8214821. [CrossRef]
10. ISO 3632-1:2011; Spices—Saffron (*Crocus sativus* L.). Specification (Edition 2, 2011). International Organization for Standardization: Genève, Switzerland, 2011; 6p.
11. Brinckmann, J.A. Geographical indications for medicinal plants: Globalization, climate change, quality and market implications for geo-authentic botanicals. *World J. Tradit. Chin. Med.* **2015**, *1*, 16–23. [CrossRef]
12. D'Archivio, A.A.; Giannitto, A.; Maggi, M.A.; Ruggieri, F. Geographical classification of Italian saffron (*Crocus sativus* L.) based on chemical constituents determined by high-performance liquid-chromatography and by using linear discriminant analysis. *Food Chem.* **2016**, *212*, 110–116. [CrossRef]
13. Rubio-Moraga, A.; Ahrazem, O.; Pérez-Clemente, R.M.; Gómez-Cadenas, A.; Yoneyama, K.; López-Ráez, J.A.; Molina, R.V.; Gómez-Gómez., L. Apical dominance in saffron and the involvement of the branching enzymes CCD7 and CCD8 in the control of bud sprouting. *BMC Plant Biol.* **2014**, *14*, 171. [CrossRef] [PubMed]
14. Mir, J.I.; Ahmed, N.; Singh, D.B.; Khan, M.H.; Zffer, S.; Shafi, W. Breeding and biotechnological opportunities in saffron crop improvement. *Afri. J. Agri. Res.* **2015**, *10*, 1970–1974.
15. Mildažiene, V.; Paužaite, G.; Nauciene, Z.; Malakauskiene, A.; Žukiene, R.; Januškaitiene, I.; Jakštas, V.; Ivanauskas, L.; Filatova, I.; Lyushkevich, V. Pre-sowing seed treatment with cold plasma and electromagnetic field increases secondary metabolite content in purple coneflower (*Echinacea purpurea*) leaves. *Plasma Process. Polym.* **2018**, *14*, 1700059. [CrossRef]
16. Mildaziene, V.; Pauzaite, G.; Nauciene, Z.; Zukiene, R.; Malakauskiene, A.; Norkeviciene, E.; Stukonis, V.; Slepetiene, A.; Olsauskaite, V.; Padarauskas, A.; et al. Effect of seed treatment with cold plasma and electromagnetic field on red clover germination, growth and content of major isoflavones. *J. Phys. D Appl. Phys.* **2020**, *53*, 26. [CrossRef]
17. Mildaziene, V.; Ivankov, A.; Pauzaite, G.; Nauciene, Z.; Zukiene, R.; Degutyte-Fomins, L.; Pukalskas, A.; Venskutonis, P.R.; Filatova, I.; Lyuskevich, V. Seed treatment with cold plasma and electromagnetic field induces changes in red clover root growth dynamics, flavonoid exudation, and activates nodulation. *Plasma Proc. Polym.* **2020**, *18*, 2000160. [CrossRef]
18. Ivankov, A.; Nauciene, Z.; Degutyte-Fomins, L.; Zukiene, R.; Januskaitiene, I.; Malakauskiene, A.; Jakstas, V.; Ivanauskas, L.; Romanovskaja, D.; Slepetiene, A.; et al. Changes in agricultural performance of common buckwheat induced by seed treatment with cold plasma and electromagnetic field. *Appl. Sci.* **2021**, *11*, 4391. [CrossRef]
19. Holc, M.; Primc, G.; Iskra, J.; Titan, P.; Kovač, J.; Mozetič, M.; Junkar, I. Effect of Oxygen Plasma on Sprout and Root Growth, Surface Morphology and Yield of Garlic. *Plants* **2019**, *8*, 462. [CrossRef]
20. Simpson, M.G. Plant Morphology. In *Plant Systematics*, 2nd ed.; Elsevier Inc.: Oxford, UK, 2010; pp. 451–513.
21. Akbarian, M.; Shahidi, F.; Varidi, M.J.; Koocheki, A.; Roshanak, S. Effect of cold plasma on microbial and chemical properties of saffron. *Saffron Agron. Technol.* **2019**, *7*, 425–439.
22. Luque de Castroa, M.D.; Quiles-Zafra, R. Appropriate use of analytical terminology – examples drawn from research on saffron. *Talanta Open* **2020**, *2*, 100005. [CrossRef]
23. Richards, F.J.A. Flexible Growth Function for Empirical Use. *J. Exp. Bot.* **1959**, *10*, 290–300. [CrossRef]
24. Muravnik, L.E. The structural peculiarities of the leaf glandular Trichomes: A review. In *Plant Cell and Tissue Differentiation and Secondary Metabolites: Fundamentals and Applications*; Ramawat, K.G., Ekiert, H.M., Goyal, S., Eds.; Springer International Publishing: Cham, Switzerland, 2021; pp. 63–97.
25. Zarinkamar, F.; Tajik, S.; Soleimanpour, S. Effects of altitude on anatomy and concentration of crocin, picrocrocin and safranal in *Crocus sativus* L. *Aust. J. Crop Sci.* **2011**, *5*, 831–838.

26. Mykhailenko, O.; Bezruk, I.; Ivanauskas, L.; Georgiyants, V. Comparative Analysis of the Major Metabolites of Ukrainian Saffron Samples by HPLC. *Plant Foods Hum. Nutr.* **2021**, *76*, 394–396. [CrossRef]
27. Sánchez, A.M.; Carmona, M.; Ordoudi, S.A.; Tsimidou, M.Z.; Alonso, G.L. Kinetics of individual crocetin ester degradation in aqueous extracts of saffron (*Crocus sativus* L.) upon thermal treatment in the dark. *J. Agric. Food Chem.* **2008**, *56*, 1627–1637. [CrossRef] [PubMed]
28. Ivankov, A.; Nauciene, Z.; Zukiene, R.; Degutyte-Fomins, L.; Malakauskiene, A.; Kraujalis, P.; Venskutonis, P.R.; Filatova, I.; Lyushkevich, V.; Mildaziene, V. Changes in growth and production of non-psychotropic cannabinoids induced by pre-sowing treatment of hemp seeds with cold plasma, vacuum and electromagnetic field. *Appl. Sci.* **2020**, *10*, 8519. [CrossRef]
29. Sirgedaitė-Šėžienė, V.; Lučinskaitė, I.; Mildažienė, V.; Ivankov, A.; Koga, K.; Shiratani, M.; Laužikė, K.; Baliuckas, V. Changes in Content of Bioactive Compounds and Antioxidant Activity Induced in Needles of Different Half-Sib Families of Norway Spruce (*Picea abies* (L.) H. Karst) by Seed Treatment with Cold Plasma. *Antioxidants* **2022**, *11*, 1558. [CrossRef]
30. Gasperini, D.; Howe, G.A. Phytohormones in a universe of regulatory metabolites: Lessons from jasmonate. *Plant Physiol.* **2024**, *195*, 135–154. [CrossRef]
31. Lacchini, E.; Goossens, A. Combinatorial control of plant specialized metabolism: Mechanisms, functions, and consequences. *Annu. Rev. Cell Dev. Biol.* **2020**, *36*, 291–313. [CrossRef]
32. Cazzonelli, C.I.; Pogson, B.J. Source to sink: Regulation of carotenoid biosynthesis in plants. *Trends Plant Sci.* **2010**, *15*, 266–274. [CrossRef] [PubMed]
33. Sun, T.; Rao, S.; Zhou, X.; Li, L. Plant carotenoids: Recent advances and future perspectives. *Mol. Hortic.* **2022**, *2*, 3. [CrossRef] [PubMed]
34. Pérez-Pizá, M.C.; Prevosto, L.; Zilli, C.; Cejas, E.; Kelly, H.; Balestrasse, K. Effects of non–thermal plasmas on seed-borne Diaporthe/Phomopsis complex and germination parameters of soybean seeds. *Innov. Food Sci. Emerg.* **2018**, *49*, 82–91. [CrossRef]
35. Mildažiene, V.; Aleknaviciute, V.; Žukiene, R.; Paužaite, G.; Nauciene, Z.; Filatova, I.; Lyushkevich, V.; Haimi, P.; Tamošiune, I.; Baniulis, D. Treatment of Common sunflower (*Helianthus annus* L.) seeds with radio-frequency electromagnetic field and cold plasma induces changes in seed phytohormone balance, seedling development and leaf protein expression. *Sci. Rep.* **2019**, *9*, 6437. [CrossRef]
36. Degutyte-Fomins, L.; Paužaite, G.; Žukiene, R.; Mildažiene, V.; Koga, K.; Shiratani, M. Relationship between cold plasma treatment-induced changes in radish seed germination and phytohormone balance. *Jpn. J. Appl. Phys.* **2020**, *59*, SH1001. [CrossRef]
37. Attri, P.; Ishikawa, K.; Okumura, T.; Koga, K.; Shiratani, M.; Mildaziene, M. Impact of seed color and storage time on the radish seed germination and sprout growth in plasma agriculture. *Sci. Rep.* **2021**, *11*, 2539. [CrossRef]
38. Šerá, B.; Vanková, R.; Roháček, K.; Šerý, M. Gliding arc plasma treatment of maize (*Zea mays* L.) grains promotes seed germination and early growth, affecting hormone pools, but not significantly photosynthetic parameters. *Agronomy* **2021**, *11*, 2066. [CrossRef]
39. Iranbakhsh, A.; Ardebili, Z.O.; Molaei, H.; Ardebili, N.O.; Amini, M. Cold plasma up-regulated expressions of WRKY1 transcription factor and genes involved in biosynthesis of cannabinoids in hemp (*Cannabis sativa* L.). *Plasma Chem. Plasma Process.* **2020**, *40*, 527–537. [CrossRef]
40. Ghasempour, M.; Iranbakhsh, A.; Ebadi, M.; Oraghi Ardebili, Z. Seed priming with cold plasma improved seedling performance, secondary metabolism, and expression of deacetylvindoline O-acetyltransferase gene in *Catharanthus roseus*. *Contrib. Plasm. Phys.* **2020**, *60*, e201900159. [CrossRef]
41. Ghaemi, M.; Majd, A.; Iranbakhsh, A. Transcriptional responses following seed priming with cold plasma and electromagnetic field in *Salvia nemorosa* L. *J. Theor. Appl. Phys.* **2020**, *14*, 323–328. [CrossRef]
42. Seddighinia, F.S.; Iranbakhsh, A.; Ardebili, Z.O.; Soleimanpour, S. Seed-priming with cold plasma and supplementation of nutrient solution with carbon nanotube enhanced carotenoid contents and the expression of psy and pds in Bitter melon (*Momordica charantia*). *J. Appl. Bot. Food Qual.* **2021**, *94*, 7–14.
43. Leprince, O.; Pellizzaro, A.; Berriri, S.; Buitink, J. Late seed maturation: Drying without dying. *J. Exp. Bot.* **2016**, *68*, 827–841. [CrossRef]
44. Sano, N.; Rajjou, L.; North, H.M.; Debeaujon, I.; Marion-Poll, A.; Seo, M. Staying alive: Molecular aspects of seed longevity. *Plant Cell Physiol.* **2016**, *57*, 660–674. [CrossRef] [PubMed]
45. Renau-Morata, B.; Nebauer, S.G.; Sánchez, M.; Molina, R.V. Effect of corm size, water stress and cultivation conditions on photosynthesis and biomass partitioning during the vegetative growth of saffron (*Crocus sativus* L.). *Ind. Crops Prod.* **2012**, *39*, 40–46. [CrossRef]
46. Barjasteh, A.; Lamichhane, P.; Dehghani, Z.; Kaushik, N.; Gupta, R.; Choi, E.H.; Kaushik, N.K. Recent Progress of Non-thermal Atmospheric Pressure Plasma for Seed Germination and Plant Development: Current Scenario and Future Landscape. *J. Plant Growth Regul.* **2023**, *42*, 5417–5432. [CrossRef]
47. Takaku, Y.; Suzuki, H.; Ohta, I.; Tsutsui, T.; Matsumoto, H.; Shimomura, M.; Hariyama, T. A 'NanoSuit' surface shield successfully protects organisms in high vacuum: Observations on living organisms in an FE-SEM. *Proc. R. Soc. B* **2015**, *282*, 20142857. [CrossRef]
48. Zhang, H.; Ma, X.; Li, W.; Niu, D.; Wang, Z.; Yan, X.; Yang, X.; Yang, Y.; Cui, H. Genome-wide characterization of NtHD-ZIP IV: Different roles in abiotic stress response and glandular Trichome induction. *BMC Plant Biol.* **2019**, *19*, 444. [CrossRef] [PubMed]

49. Kjær, A.; Grevsen, K.; Jensen, M. Effect of external stress on density and size of glandular trichomes in full-grown *Artemisia annua*, the source of anti-malarial artemisinin. *AoB Plants* **2012**, *2012*, pls018. [CrossRef]
50. Amini, M.; Ghoranneviss, M.; Abdijadid, S. Effect of cold plasma on crocin esters and volatile compounds of saffron. *Food Chem.* **2017**, *235*, 290–293. [CrossRef]
51. Darvish, H.; Ramezan, Y.; Khani, M.R.; Kamkari, A. Effect of low-pressure cold plasma processing on decontamination and quality attributes of Saffron (*Crocus sativus* L.). *Food Sci. Nutr.* **2022**, *10*, 1082–2090. [CrossRef]
52. Mykhailenko, O.; Petrikaitė, V.; Korinek, M.; El-Shazly, M.; Chen, B.-H.; Yen, C.-H.; Hsieh, C.-F.; Bezruk, I.; Dabrišiūtė, A.; Ivanauskas, L.; et al. Bio-guided bioactive profiling and HPLC-DAD fingerprinting of Ukrainian saffron (*Crocus sativus* stigma): Moving from Correlation toward Causation. *BMC Complement. Med. Ther.* **2021**, *21*, 203–218. [CrossRef]

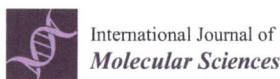

International Journal of
Molecular Sciences

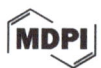

Review

Green Leaf Volatiles: A New Player in the Protection against Abiotic Stresses?

Jurgen Engelberth

Department of Integrative Biology, The University of Texas at San Antonio, San Antonio, TX 78247, USA; jurgen.engelberth@utsa.edu; Tel.: +1-210-458-7831

Abstract: To date, the role of green leaf volatiles (GLVs) has been mainly constrained to protecting plants against pests and pathogens. However, increasing evidence suggests that among the stresses that can significantly harm plants, GLVs can also provide significant protection against heat, cold, drought, light, and salinity stress. But while the molecular basis for this protection is still largely unknown, it seems obvious that a common theme in the way GLVs work is that most, if not all, of these stresses are associated with physical damage to the plants, which, in turn, is the major event responsible for the production of GLVs. Here, I summarize the current state of knowledge on GLVs and abiotic stresses and provide a model explaining the multifunctionality of these compounds.

Keywords: abiotic stress; airborne signal; green leaf volatiles; GLV; plant damage; plant protection; structural integrity; volatile organic compounds

1. Introduction

Green leaf volatiles (GLVs) are a group of plant compounds that are typically associated with damage. Most people have experienced these molecules when mowing their lawns and recognize them as the typical "green" smell of plants. For more than 20 years now, GLVs have come to our attention as volatile signals within and between plants that communicate damage, usually caused by insect herbivores, but also by microbial infections [1]. In doing so, GLVs have been found to not only provide immediate protection by activating defensive measures, but also to prepare or prime receiver plants against the threat of impending damage [2,3]. Generally, priming may initially trigger only a minor part of a defense response, which then leads to an increase in the plant's ability to defend itself against future antagonists (for example, herbivores or pathogens), resulting in a faster, stronger, or more enduring response when actually being attacked [4]. Fittingly, GLVs have their own defense-related biological activity, which is, however, considered to be rather weak when compared to responses signaled, for example, by jasmonic acid, which is the major defense hormone that regulates responses to herbivory and necrotrophic pathogens. Nonetheless, defense priming by GLVs appears to be strongly connected to the jasmonate pathway in that signaling through it becomes more intense [2,3]. Still, little is known about how defense priming actually works. It seems clear that some memory is conserved after the first exposure to a priming agent, including the accumulation of mitogen-activated protein kinases (MAPKs) that remain inactive until triggered by a threat, or epigenetic changes [4]. However, with regard to priming by GLVs, no such mechanisms have been reported with sufficient evidence to accept them as possible regulators of priming.

While most reports on GLVs in the past have focused on their role in mediating biotic interactions, GLVs have more recently been found to provide protection to receiver plants against abiotic stresses, either directly or by priming for them. This includes protection against various stresses, including cold, drought, salt, and light. Still, very little is known about the mechanisms by which GLVs act in mediating abiotic stress protection. In this review, I will therefore summarize GLV-induced protective activities related to abiotic

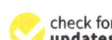

check for updates

Citation: Engelberth, J. Green Leaf Volatiles: A New Player in the Protection against Abiotic Stresses? *Int. J. Mol. Sci.* **2024**, *25*, 9471. https://doi.org/10.3390/ijms25179471

Academic Editor: Hunseung Kang

Received: 5 August 2024
Revised: 29 August 2024
Accepted: 29 August 2024
Published: 30 August 2024

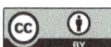

stresses that are signaled by this group of compounds and provide some insight into the potential mechanisms by which they may achieve this.

2. Green Leaf Volatiles and Abiotic Stress

2.1. The Biosynthesis of Green Leaf Volatiles

The biosynthesis of GLVs is rather straight-forward, starting mainly with linolenic acid, either in its free form or as part of typical membrane lipids (Figure 1) [5,6]. In the first step, a lipoxygenase (LOX) inserts molecular oxygen at position 13 of the fatty acid. A hydroperoxide lyase (HPL) then cleaves the fatty acid into a 6-carbon compound, Z-3-hexenal (Z3al), and a 12-carbon unit, which, after a minor conversion, results in traumatin, a molecule that has been recognized as a wound hormone capable of inducing callus formation [7]. The six-carbon unit Z3al is then reduced to its corresponding alcohol (Z-3-hexenol (Z3ol)), which can then be further modified into various esters, mostly into Z-3-hexenyl acetate (Z3ac). Additionally, some plants also have an isomerase that can quickly convert Z3al into E-2-hexenal (E2al) [8,9], which can also be transformed into the corresponding E-2- alcohol and esters. While LOX and HPL are commonly localized in chloroplasts, all other enzymes, including the isomerase, are cytoplasmic. However, upon damage, LOX and HPL become activated, resulting in the rapid production of Z3al. If cells contain an isomerase, it will also become highly active in the damaged tissue and almost instantly transforms Z3al into E2al. In contrast to these initial steps of GLV biosynthesis, all other reactions require intact cells, which take up the aldehydes and transform them into the corresponding alcohols and esters [10].

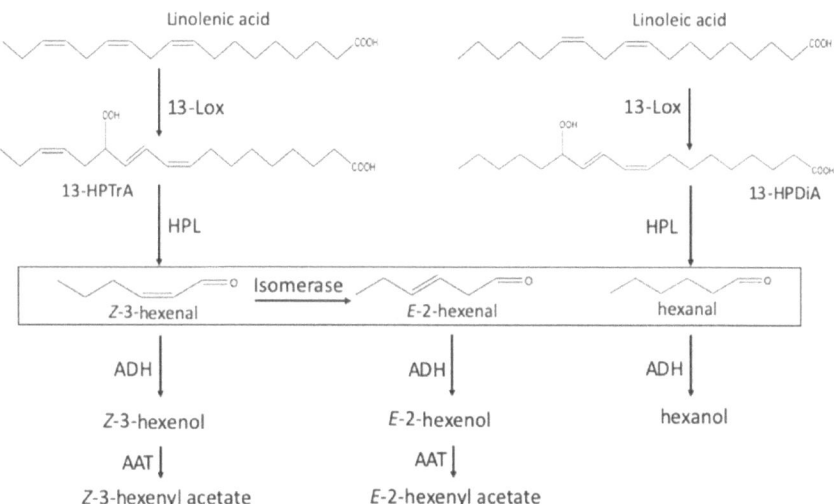

Figure 1. Biosynthetic pathways leading to the production of green leaf volatiles (GLVs) (taken from [11]). A lipoxygenase catalyzes the addition of molecular oxygen at position 13 in linolenic acid or linoleic acid, resulting in 13-hydroperoxy octadecatrienoic (13-HPTrA) or 13-hydroperoxy octadecadienoic acid (13-HPDiA). The oxygenated fatty acids are then cleaved by a hydroperoxide lyase (HPL) into either Z-3-hexenal or hexanal. The remaining 12-cabon unit is further processed into traumatin (not shown). An isomerase can convert Z-3-hexenal into E-2-hexenal. Both aldehydes can be further processed by an alcohol dehydrogenase (ADH), resulting in the respective alcohol. Further modifications by an alcohol acyltransferase (AAT) can convert the alcohols into the corresponding hexenyl acetates. The boxed compounds are those GLVs produced mainly by damaged plant tissue, while alcohols and their esters require intact cells for biosynthesis.

Plants can produce significant quantities of GLVs within seconds to minutes after damage, some up to almost 100 µg per gram of fresh weight [1,11]. This substantial and rapid production makes them ideal volatile signaling molecules for either distant parts of the same plant or other plants in the vicinity. While little is known about how exactly Z3al is made in damaged tissue and what regulates the process, we found that even at temperatures far below 0 °C, damaged plant tissues can still produce significant amounts of Z3al under those conditions [12], while the alcohols and esters are barely detectable, mainly because most cells under these conditions have died and can no longer produce these compounds. However, while basically all plants produce GLVs in various quantities and qualities upon damage and other treatments, most experiments to date have been conducted by using pure chemicals that are commercially available, which allows for a more controlled application of these volatile compounds. The experimental risk here is that the concentrations used may not correlate with what can be found in nature and may produce artifacts. Often, nano- to low micromolar concentrations have been found to sufficiently signal GLV activities. Yet, plants may also experience much higher concentrations upon damage, particularly in the immediate vicinity of the damaged tissue [2,10]. It is therefore often impossible to assess the biological activities of these compounds in contexts with high concentrations being experienced locally but low concentrations serving as a volatile signal over relatively long distances.

Nonetheless, signaling pathways related to GLV activities are currently being elucidated at various levels. Exposure to GLVs, for example, can cause rapid changes in membrane potentials and cytosolic Ca^{2+} concentrations [13,14]. It has been argued that GLVs themselves cause this depolarization directly due to their hydrophobic character and potential interaction with membranes. However, the distinct set of genes that are induced by GLVs and the specificity of the primed responses argues for a more regulated signaling pathway. However, since no receptor has been identified to date, neither mechanism can be excluded.

It further appears that Z3ol is the major biologically active form of GLVs [15]. In a series of experiments performed by Cofer et al., it was shown that after mutating several enzymes involved in the hydrolyzation of GLV esters like Z3ac, the overall activity of these compounds was dramatically reduced, clearly pointing towards Z3ol as the main active molecule. Furthermore, certain GLVs seem to activate a MAP kinase signaling pathway in tomato plants [16]. Interestingly, the same MAP kinase pathway is normally used after pathogen infection. In support of these findings, we found in a microarray study that determined that one MAP kinase was significantly induced in maize plants treated with Z3ol, suggesting that it might be a GLV-specific response [17]. Yet, it is still unclear if this is a common signaling pathway that is recruited by GLV or what other signaling pathways might be involved in regulating responses to these compounds. The activation of the MAP kinase pathway could, however, provide a link to the priming responses and the associated memory effects, as described above [4]; however, this is a hypothesis that still needs to be tested.

2.2. Green Leaf Volatiles in the Atmosphere

As mentioned before, the bioactive roles of GLVs have mostly been studied in the context of plant–insect and plant–pathogen interactions, both of which were also shown to cause the release of significant quantities of GLVs not only from the damaged tissues, but also from undamaged parts of the same plant [1,2,18]. It was further found that the treatment of plants with GLVs often prepared or primed them against the impending threat, resulting in a stronger and/or faster response when actually attacked [2,3,19–22]. This led to the assumption that GLVs mainly have a role in the defense against biotic threats. However, in recent years, several reports have shown the potential for GLVs also being involved in regulating abiotic stresses. Initial reports came from studies investigating the composition of volatile organic compounds, which comprise all volatiles regardless of their origin, in the lower atmosphere of the Earth. There, large quantities of so-called biogenic compounds (compounds that are emitted from organisms) were detected and their effects on the chemistry of the atmosphere studied [23,24]. While the majority of these biogenic volatile compounds were found to be isoprene-related, which are usually emitted in large quantities under heat and light stress, where they provide cooling as well as helping in the recovery of photosynthetic performance, significant amounts of GLVs were also detected. Since it is unlikely that herbivory or pathogen infections are the sole cause of the presence of GLVs in the atmosphere, other factors like grass harvesting for hay in agriculture as well as abiotic stresses need to be taken into consideration. Proof of the latter came, for example, from studies by Karl et al. [25] and Jardine et al. [26]. Karl et al. [25] found increased GLV levels in frost-damaged meadows in the alps, with Z3al being the major compound. Jardine et al. [26] analyzed the composition of the air surrounding the canopy region of rainforests in South America. The authors not only detected large quantities of GLVs, but also found a clear correlation between the amount of GLVs and abiotic stresses like drought and heat, and concluded that atmospheric GLVs could be used as a chemical stress sensor. Similar results were provided by Turan et al. [27] when they investigated the effects of heat on tobacco leaves. When plants were exposed to 52 °C, they produced large quantities of E2al and Z3ol, but very few terpenes. This production of GLVs under heat stress indicates that some kind of membrane damage or at least disturbance occurs resulting in the activation of enzymes in their biosynthetic pathway. Since Z3ol was among the detected compounds, it can also be concluded that even at those high temperatures, intact cells are still abundant and can convert aldehydes into the alcohols. Based on these clear correlations between abiotic stresses and GLV release, it can be assumed that there should also be a functional connection. However, at the time, little was known about how GLVs might contribute to protection against these stresses.

2.3. Green Leaf Volatiles and Cold Stress

Cold stress poses a serious threat to plants. While it is often a seasonal issue, it can still affect plants in regions closer to the poles or at higher altitudes, even during the summer. However, the highest risk of plants experiencing cold stress usually occurs during spring time in temperate climates, when they germinate, and in the fall, when they are usually harvested. Cold stress can cause significant changes in the general physiology of plants. Cold stress may generally reduce enzyme activities, can cause cell membrane damage through altered membrane fluidity and lipid composition, decreases water potential, reduced ATP supply, and may bring about imbalanced ion distribution and solute leakage (Theocharis et al. [28]). This does often result in reduced growth and yield. It is therefore important for plants to have mechanisms in place that help to prevent severe consequences of this stress.

Karl et al. [25], as described above, provided the first insight that GLVs might be a part of such a strategy, since cold-damaged plants emitted significant quantities of these compounds. Likewise, Copolovici et al. [29] found that cold stress caused the release of large quantities of GLVs in cold-stressed, but also in heat-stressed, tomato (*Solanum lycopersicum*) plants. Similar to Jardine et al. [26], the authors proposed the use of these volatile organic compounds as indicators to characterize the severity of the stress. Yet again, no studies have been performed that would test for a protective role of GLVs under these conditions.

In 2013, we published a microarray study on the effects of Z3ol, in particular, on general gene expression in maize [17]. We focused on early events and identified distinct expression patterns, many of which were likely related to defense reactions to insect herbivores. Unfortunately, at the time, many genes on the microarray were still unknown or mislabeled (about 40%). Later, we identified several genes that were typically associated with water stress in plants, including dehydrins, low-temperature-inducible protein, and several others [30]. This pointed towards a potential role of GLVs in protecting cellular integrity, since these types of proteins are usually involved in stabilizing cell structures, including membranes. Upon further analyzing the effects of GLVs on cold stress protection, we found not only that the expression of the identified protective genes was induced by GLVs, but also that their expression levels were primed when they were placed in the cold about 2 h after GLV treatment. This resulted in significantly reduced ion leakage [12,31], less damage, and a growth spurt in the days after the cold stress treatment. Aside from providing immediate protection, this also indicated an effect of GLVs on the general physiology of the plant, which allowed it to compensate for a loss of growth during cold stress. We also found that maize plants do still produce GLVs, in particular, Z3al, at temperatures well below 0 °C [12]. Furthermore, Z3al was able to increase the transcript accumulation of those protective genes even when applied during cold stress [12]. This proved that GLVs can protect plants against cold stress even when perceived during a cold episode and also provides a potential mechanism by which this might be achieved, i.e., the activation of cell-protective proteins, and thus, the maintenance of cellular integrity. This is essential since it allows cells to continue to function properly even under potentially damaging stress conditions.

2.4. Green Leaf Volatiles and Drought Stress

Drought is defined as an absence of water (https://www.ncei.noaa.gov/access/monitoring/dyk/drought-definition (accessed on 28 August 2024)). However, an absence or shortage of water can also be the result of high salt concentrations or an abundance of other water-capturing chemicals, all of which result in a dramatic change in the water potential of plants. While the early effects of drought and salt stress are very similar, both stresses act through distinct signaling pathways. Additionally, salt may also have a toxic ion effect and can lead to nutritional imbalances in plants [32,33]. This makes it more difficult for the plant to maintain a constant transpirational stream, which can lead to the overheating of leaves, but also to the reduced uptake of nutrients. Consequently, plants exposed to drought grow less and provide much lower yields. Water scarcity is therefore one of the most pressing issues when growing plants in a natural environment or in an agricultural setting.

The potential role of GLVs in drought stress responses was initially provided by Jardine et al. [26] through their analysis of the atmosphere of the forest canopy in the rainforest, in which they found a clear correlation between drought, temperature, and GLVs. This was the first clear indication that GLVs may play a role in the regulation of drought and heat stress in a natural system. However, at the time, it was unclear if there might also be a protective role that GLVs play in this context, since studies in a natural system are difficult to perform due to the myriad of other environmental factors that may interfere. In a related study by Catola et al. [34], it was further shown that drought stress affects the capacity to produce GLVs in the leaves of the pomegranate plant (*Punica granatum* L.), further supporting the involvement of GLVs in the response to drought stress. Yet again, no further studies have been performed to evaluate the potential protective role of GLVs.

However, evidence for GLVs playing an active part in protection against drought-related stresses came from a study by Yamauchi et al. [35]. By investigating the potential for activating gene expression, they tested an array of reactive leaf volatiles in a microarray assay on Arabidopsis. While the focus of the study was on reactive α, β-unsaturated carbonyls, they identified E2al as a particularly effective inducer of typical abiotic stress-related genes, including those that protect against drought and salt, but also heat and cold. At the same time, Z3al appeared to be quite inactive and did not show any significant induction of abiotic stress-related gene expression, which could, however, be a species-specific result. While this did not answer the question of whether or not GLVs do actually provide protection against drought, and salt stress in particular, a study by Tian et al. [36] showed that priming with Z-3-hexenyl acetate enhanced salinity stress tolerance in peanut plants (*Arachis hypogaea* L.). As a result, they found positive effects on photosynthesis, higher water content, increased growth, and increased activity of antioxidant proteins. While this broad spectrum of protectionist measures may be surprising, it actually fits into the overall picture of activities provided by GLVs that have been shown for biotic stress responses [3].

A similar study investigated the effects of Z3ol on hyperosmotic stress tolerance in *Camellia sinensis* [37]. As described above, a multitude of effects were found, ranging from regulating stomatal conductance, decreasing malonyl dialdehyde as an indicator of lipid peroxidation, the accumulation of abscisic acid and proline, and typical stress-related gene expression. The activation of ABA and proline, in particular, is interesting, since both are essential responses to hyperosmotic stress: ABA by acting as the major regulator of water stresses [38], and proline by functioning as an important protector of cellular integrity [39]. The involvement of ABA as a mediator of Z3ol-induced protection against drought and cold was further confirmed by Jin et al. [40] in *Camellia sinensis*. They showed that Z3ol activated the glycosylation of ABA through the expression of a specific glycosyl transferase. This allows ABA–glucose conjugates to be stored in the vacuole, from where they can be easily reactivated upon cold and drought stress by a glucosidase. While this provides an elegant system that helps to explain some of the biological activities of GLVs (here: Z3ol), it still needs to be confirmed in other plants. Furthermore, while Z3ol was shown to be the active compound in this study, other GLVs—in particular, Z3al, as the one compound that is instantly produced by damage, including cold—also need to be tested for their specific activity towards the activation of ABA-mediated signaling as a key element in this process.

Altogether, these results clearly show that GLVs are not only released upon drought stress in significant quantities, but can also provide significant protection. Furthermore, these experimental results provide a potential mechanism by which GLVs may activate these processes with ABA, the major regulatory plant hormone for water stresses, being a central target.

2.5. Green Leaf Volatiles and Photosynthesis

Light is a determining factor in the life of plants. It is the predominant energy source that is used by plants and other photosynthetically active organisms, which transform light from a physical power into energy-rich molecules that are essential for the vast majority of living things on Earth. For plants, light also serves as a signal that has a significant impact on growth as plants make an effort to obtain a perfect position for light harvesting. However, light can also be too powerful and under these conditions, and plants may sustain damage due to the high energy levels that are contained in the radiation. This is, among other consequences, extremely challenging for the actual photosynthesis reaction, in particular, the events that occur in photosystem II (PSII). There, the photolysis of water represents one of the main events during photosynthesis, resulting in the production of electrons, protons, and eventually oxygen. Under normal light conditions this is a well-controlled process. But when light intensities increase, oxygen radicals are produced, which can cause significant harm to the whole photosystem, but also other parts of the chloroplast. And it is this process in which GLVs appear to interfere by regulating the status of PSII in particular.

First indications to support a role of GLVs in photosynthesis came from a study by Charron et al. [41]. They found that an increase in the photosynthetic photon flux and the length of the photoperiod would cause an increase in GLV production and release in lettuce. While this was mainly put in the context of growing plants in controlled environments, it nonetheless pointed towards GLVs being directly linked to light stress. Further proof came from a study on bacterial photosynthesis. Mimuro et al. [42] investigated the effects of 1-hexanol on the optical properties of the base plate and energy transfer in *Chloroflexus aurantiacus*. In this system, it was found that adding 1-hexanol caused the suppressed flux of energy from the baseplate of the chlorosome to the photosynthetic elements located in the adhering plasma membrane section. While it is still unclear whether or not bacteria can produce GLVs, the results nonetheless provided evidence that these compounds can have an effect on photosynthetic reactions. Furthermore, considering that this kind of photosynthetic microbe might represent an ancestorial type of what may have eventually ended up as a chloroplast in plants, mechanisms to protect or at least alter the system may also have been already abundant.

Negative alterations of photosynthesis were further investigated by Matsui et al. [10]. While studying the metabolism of GLVs, they identified key mechanisms of the biochemical pathway. As described above, aldehydes are mainly produced in damaged tissue, whereas the corresponding alcohols and esters require intact cells to be made. Aside from identifying these mechanisms, they further investigated the toxicity of various GLVs, including Z3al, E2al, and Z3ol, and found that plants exposed to the compounds as pure chemicals showed a significant impact on photosynthesis, with the aldehydes being much more active than the corresponding alcohol. Similar results were obtained by Tanaka et al. [43]. Together, this led to the conclusion that plant cells have an intrinsic ability to detoxify the much more reactive aldehyde GLVs into less harmful alcohols and esters, which, in turn, appear to serve as the actual signaling molecules that regulate all processes attributed to GLVs [15]. At the same time, plants avoid the toxic effects of the aldehydes. However, new light was shed on this issue when Savchenko et al. [44] studied the effect of GLVs on photosynthesis. By using HPL-overexpressing lines in Arabidopsis, they discovered that GLVs play a major role in the protection of PSII under increased light conditions by observing lower rate constants of PSII photoinhibition and higher rate constants of recovery. Furthermore, the degradation of proteins (in particular, D1, but also others) during photoinhibition was significantly reduced, allowing for a more speedy recovery. Further experiments on isolated thylakoid membranes confirmed these results. In contrast to GLVs, the application of other oxylipins, including linolenic acid, phytodienoic acid, and jasmonates, had the opposite effect, further solidifying the specificity of GLVs' effects on PSII. This important feature of GLVs may also explain why this biochemical system is localized in chloroplasts, more specifically, in the thylakoids. Reducing the uncontrolled production of reactive oxygen species (ROS) may be key in the protection of plant cells under extreme light conditions and may explain why GLVs have a negative impact on photosynthesis, which, while considered toxic in the past, actually help to avoid damage in leaf cells.

However, little is known about the actual mechanisms that are activated by GLVs to protect against light stress. Further studies in the area of light stress protection in particular are needed to identify these mechanisms, which may, in turn, further help to explain the diverse and complex roles GLVs play in plants.

3. Future Perspectives

The definition of GLVs as a plant's multifunctional weapon [3] was created at a time when mainly its defensive functions were recognized. This view has now been expanded by adding a multitude of abiotic stresses that are also covered by GLVs, as described herein. A summary of these findings is presented in Figure 2.

This extreme multifunctionality raises the question of how these compounds can be utilized to better plant protection against biotic and abiotic stresses. A summary of approaches towards protection against biotic stresses by volatile organic compounds in general was provided by Wang et al. [45]. Two major paths were outlined, one using intercropping with sentinel plants, and the other using pure chemicals to help to protect plants. These approaches could also be chosen for using GLVs as protectors against abiotic stresses. Intercropping would require a sentinel plant that is more sensitive to certain abiotic stresses, in particular, drought and cold, and that produces GLVs upon being exposed to these stresses in sufficient quantities to protect the main crop. At the same time, these sentinel plants should not take away too many of the nutrients and, ideally, should continue to grow even after suffering damage to allow for longer-term protection. Alternatively, pure chemicals like Z3ol or Z3ac could be deployed over fields at critical times to assist in protection against relevant abiotic stresses. However, there are several issues here that need to be addressed. One is costs, which could be significant. Another issue lies in the fact that these compounds are volatile and may dissipate very quickly, making it necessary to repeat the application regularly. At this time, we do not know how long a protective or priming effect against certain stresses remains active within a certain plant species, but this is necessary information that would determine how often such a treatment would have to be repeated to be effective. One solution could be the development of a slow-release mechanism for GLVs or to produce a conjugate that can be taken up by the plant without dissipating as a volatile into the atmosphere. Another issue is that while GLVs can protect against a variety of biotic stresses, they may very well interfere with alternative defense signaling pathways. As mentioned before, GLVs appear to act through the jasmonate signaling pathway, and in doing so, protect against many insect herbivores and necrotrophic pathogens. However, this does, for example, allow biotrophic pathogens to infect plants and thrive. For biotrophic pathogens, salicylic acid is the major defense regulator. However, its activity is down-regulated by the jasmonate pathway and vice versa [46]. These interactions need to be fully understood before treatments that activate one or the other pathway can be deployed. It also necessitates more studies on how GLVs may interfere with other signaling pathways to avoid any negative side effects with significant impacts on growth and yield. To date, no such study has been performed in the area of GLVs and abiotic stress responses.

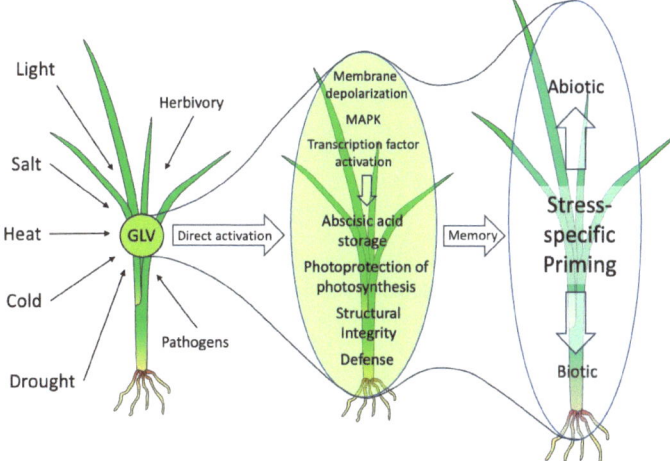

Figure 2. Green leaf volatiles and abiotic stress responses. Green leaf volatiles (GLV) are produced by many plants under various abiotic stress conditions. As volatiles, they move as a plume through the air and can reach neighboring plants, where they can activate various protective measures directly through specific signaling pathways, resulting in abscisic acid storage, the photoprotection of photosynthesis, increased structural integrity, and defense activation. Aside from these more direct measures, GLVs may prepare or prime plants against impending stresses through a yet-to-be-identified memory effect, which allows them to respond faster and/or more strongly when actually threatened. These primed responses are specific towards the actual threat and are likely a consequence of the direct activation of protective measures by GLVs. The direction of the activation from left to right in this figure represents a time scale and not the distance between plants. The green background shows more direct effects, while the blue background represents priming.

Another path forward could lie in the molecular manipulation of GLV production and sensing. While we know most of the genes involved in their biosynthesis [5–9], we are still at the beginning of understanding how GLVs are sensed. But even with biosynthesis, we only have a limited understanding of the regulation of the initial steps, in particular, after tissue damage, but also regarding the release of GLVs from intact tissues. In this context, an interesting finding is the release of a burst of GLVs at the onset of darkness. This has been described for some plant species [47,48], but it is yet unknown why plants do this. Also, this GLV burst seems to require a rather quick transition from light to dark.

However, exploring and eventually exploiting this phenomenon of potentially self-priming may provide a starting point for future manipulations, resulting in the better protection of plants.

We still know very little about how plants perceive GLVs as signals and exactly how they transduce them into a physiological response. Is it just the physical perturbation of membranes, or are specific receptors involved? These are questions for which we do not have any answers at this time. Once resolved, this information could provide more targeted approaches for manipulation. Increasing the sensitivity of plants to GLVs might be one promising line of exploitation. Overexpressing key enzymes might be one way, but also, providing the substrates for the reaction (i.e., poly-unsaturated fatty acids) may help to boost the production of these compounds. However, as mentioned above, manipulating one signaling pathway may have severe consequences for others, and this must therefore be carefully studied with consideration of the whole plant's physiology. For example, only a few studies so far have looked into the costs of GLV-activated responses [49–51]. Surprisingly, the application of these compounds has often resulted in an increase in growth [12,31,49–51]. Should this be confirmed for other plant species and stresses, it might very well justify more thorough investigations into the feasibility of using GLVs as an almost universal protection system that would not have negative effects on other physiological responses.

However, our knowledge regarding GLV regulation is still very limited, not only with regard to the enzymes involved, but also when it comes to how different plant species regulate the process of producing and sensing these compounds. This becomes extremely clear when we look at the number of plants that have been used to provide the results presented herein. Aside from Arabidopsis, fewer than 10 different plant species have been used to study the effects of GLVs on abiotic stress protection. Furthermore, the experimental approaches are very different depending on the goal of the study. I believe that a more comprehensive and coordinated approach is indeed necessary to better understand how GLVs affect plants on a global scale. A summary of current findings regarding the protective roles of GLVs against abiotic stresses is shown in Table 1.

Table 1. Protective effects of green leaf volatiles in different plant species.

Stress	Organism	Active Compound	Responses	Citation
Cold stress	*Zea mays*	Z-3-hexenal Z-3-hexenol	Abiotic stress genes Reduced ion leakage Reduced damage	[12,31]
Drought	*Arabidopsis thaliana*	E-2-hexenal	Abiotic stress genes	[35]
	Arachis hypogaea	Z-3-hexenyl acetate	Photosynthesis Increased water content Growth Antioxidant proteins	[36]
	Camellia sinensis	Z-3-hexenol	Stomatal conductance Reduced lipid peroxidation ABA accumulation Proline accumulation Stress gene expression	[37]
	Camellia sinensis	Z-3-hexenol	ABA glycosyl transferase ABA storage	[40]
Photosynthesis	*Chloroflexus auratiacus*	1-hexanal	Reduced energy flux	[42]
	Arabidopsis thaliana	E-2-hexenal Z-3-hexenal E-2-hexenol	Reduction in photosynthetic activity	[10,43]
	Arabidopsis thaliana	E-2-hexenal Z-3-hexenal Z-3-hexenyl acetate	Protection of PSII Recovery Reduced protein degradation	[44]

4. Summary and Conclusions

While the number of publications on the topic of GLVs and abiotic stress protection is far exceeded by those on GLVs and biotic stresses, it cannot be denied that GLVs can provide significant protection through yet-to-be-identified signaling pathways. But even with the limited number of publications on the topic, it is astounding how GLVs can protect against such a broad variety of abiotic stresses. If we compare this with other plant signaling compounds, including hormones like jasmonic acid, abscisic acid, salicylic acid, and many others, it becomes obvious how limited these are in the regulation of protective functions when compared to GLVs. This broad protection makes GLVs somewhat unique within the regulatory network of plant stress responses.

To best describe the protective roles of GLVs, one has to look at what is causing damage to plants. Damage in most instances is physical, and thus directly linked to water loss, which may lay at the core of GLV activity. But it clearly goes beyond that when they also protect against herbivores, pathogens, drought, cold, intense light, salt, and other damaging stresses. Also, while they protect against those stresses, they are also often released by the same stresses they protect against, thereby potentially providing protection to other parts of the same plant or even other plants nearby, either by directly activating protective responses or by priming for them. This will result in a faster and/or stronger reaction should the stress actually occur. Surprisingly, all this is carried out with minor investments, making this a very low-cost investment on the plant's side.

GLVs have been labeled 'the plants multifunctional weapon" in the past based on their multifaceted biological activities against biotic stresses in particular [3]. It is, however, obvious from the findings summarized herein that we have to expand this characterization to include protection against abiotic stresses as well. I would therefore also not describe GLVs as new players in this context, but rather, as very old ones that just need to be further studied to reveal their full potential in regulating a multitude of stress responses in plants.

To conclude, the role of GLVs seems to lie in in the protection of plants against all those stresses, biotic and abiotic, that can cause damage in the widest meaning of this word. However, how these complex activities are regulated by these compounds is mostly still unknown. But the potential of GLVs in protecting plants on such a broad scale is definitely worthy of further investigation.

Funding: This research was funded in part by the USDA, NIFA, grant number 2020-65114-30767, to JE.

Institutional Review Board Statement: Not applicable.

Data Availability Statement: Not applicable.

Conflicts of Interest: The author declares no conflicts of interest.

References

1. Ameye, M.; Allmann, S.; Verwaeren, J.; Smagghe, G.; Haesaert, G.; Schuurink, R.C.; Audenaert, K. Green leaf volatile production by plants: A meta-analysis. *New Phytol.* **2018**, *220*, 666–683. [CrossRef] [PubMed]
2. Matsui, K.; Engelberth, J. Green leaf volatiles-the forefront of plant responses against biotic attack. *Plant Cell Physiol.* **2022**, *63*, 1378–1390. [CrossRef] [PubMed]
3. Scala, A.; Allmann, S.; Mirabella, R.; Haring, M.A.; Schuurink, R.C. Green leaf volatiles: A plant's multifunctional weapon against herbivores and pathogens. *Int. J. Mol. Sci.* **2013**, *14*, 17781–17811. [CrossRef]
4. Westman, S.M.; Kloth, K.J.; Hanson, J.; Kloth, K.J.; Hanson, J.; Ohlsson, A.B.; Albrectsen, B.R. Defence priming in Arabidopsis—A Meta-Analysis. *Sci. Rep.* **2019**, *9*, 13309. [CrossRef]
5. Hatanaka, A. The biogeneration of green odour by green leaves. *Phytochemistry* **1993**, *34*, 1201–1218. [CrossRef]
6. Matsui, K. Green leaf volatiles: Hydroperoxide lyase pathway of oxylipin metabolism. *Curr. Opin. Plant Biol.* **2006**, *9*, 274–280. [CrossRef]
7. Zimmerman, D.C.; Coudron, C.A. Identification of traumatin, a wound hormone, as 12-oxo-trans-10-dodecenoic acid. *Plant Physiol.* **1979**, *63*, 536–541. [CrossRef]
8. Kunishima, M.; Yamauchi, Y.; Mizutani, M.; Kuse, M.; Takikawa, H.; Sugimoto, Y. Identification of (Z)-3:(E)-2-hexenal isomerases essential to the production of the leaf aldehyde in plants. *J. Biol. Chem.* **2016**, *291*, 14023–14033. [CrossRef]

9. Spyropoulou, E.A.; Dekker, H.L.; Steemers, L.; van Maarseveen, J.H.; de Koster, C.G.; Haring, M.A.; Schuurink, R.C.; Allmann, S. Identification and characterization of (3Z):(2E)-hexenal isomerases from cucumber. *Front. Plant Sci.* **2017**, *8*, 1342. [CrossRef]

10. Matsui, K.; Sugimoto, K.; Mano, J.; Ozawa, R.; Takabayashi, J. Differential metabolism of green leaf volatiles in injured and intact parts of a wounded leaf meet distinct ecophysiological requirements. *PLoS ONE* **2012**, *7*, e36433. [CrossRef] [PubMed]

11. Engelberth, J.; Engelberth, M. Variability in the capacity to produce damage-induced aldehyde green leaf volatiles among different plant species provides novel insights into biosynthetic diversity. *Plants* **2020**, *9*, 213. [CrossRef] [PubMed]

12. Engelberth, M.; Selman, S.M.; Engelberth, J. In-cold exposure to Z-3-hexenal provides protection against ongoing cold stress in *Zea mays*. *Plants* **2019**, *8*, 165. [CrossRef] [PubMed]

13. Zebelo, S.A.; Matsui, K.; Ozawa, R.; Maffei, M.E. Plasma membrane potential depolarization and cytosolic calcium flux are early events involved in tomato (*Solanum lycopersicon*) plant-to-plant communication. *Plant Sci.* **2012**, *196*, 93–100. [CrossRef]

14. Aratani, Y.; Uemura, T.; Hagihara, T.; Matsui, K.; Toyota, M. Green leaf volatile sensory calcium transduction in Arabidopsis. *Nat. Commun.* **2023**, *14*, 6236. [CrossRef]

15. Cofer, T.M.; Erb, M.; Tumlinson, J.H. The *Arabidopsis thaliana* carboxylesterase AtCXE12 converts volatile (Z)-3-hexenyl acetate to (Z)-3-hexenol. *bioRxiv* **2023**. [CrossRef]

16. Tanarsuwongkul, S.; Fisher, K.W.; Mullis, B.T.; Negi, H.; Roberts, J.; Tomlin, F.; Wang, Q.; Stratmann, J.W. Green leaf volatiles co-opt proteins involved in molecular pattern signalling in plant cells. *Plant Cell Environ.* **2024**, *47*, 928–946. [CrossRef]

17. Engelberth, J.; Contreras, C.F.; Dalvi, C.; Li, T.; Engelberth, M. Early Transcriptome Analyses of Z-3-Hexenol-Treated *Zea mays* Revealed Distinct Transcriptional Networks and Anti-Herbivore Defense Potential of Green Leaf Volatiles. *PLoS ONE* **2012**, *8*, e77465. [CrossRef]

18. Röse, U.S.R.; Tumlinson, J.H. Systemic induction of volatile release in cotton: How specific is the signal to herbivory? *Planta* **2005**, *222*, 327–335. [CrossRef]

19. Engelberth, J.; Alborn, H.T.; Schmelz, E.A.; Tumlinson, J.H. Airborne signals prime plants against herbivore attack. *Proc. Natl. Acad. Sci. USA* **2004**, *101*, 1781–1785. [CrossRef]

20. Kessler, A.; Halitschke, R.; Diezel, C.; Baldwin, I.T. Priming of plant defense responses in nature by airborne signaling between *Artemisia tridentata* and *Nicotiana attenuata*. *Oecologia* **2006**, *148*, 280–292. [CrossRef]

21. Heil, M.; Bueno, J.C. Within-plant signaling by volatiles leads to induction and priming of an indirect plant defense in nature. *Proc. Natl. Acad. Sci. USA* **2007**, *104*, 5467–5472. [CrossRef]

22. Frost, C.J.; Mescher, M.C.; Dervinis, C.; Davis, J.M.; Carlson, J.E.; De Moraes, C.M. Priming defense genes and metabolites in hybrid poplar by the green leaf volatile cis-3-hexenyl acetate. *New Phytol.* **2008**, *180*, 722–734. [CrossRef]

23. Laothawornkitkul, J.; Taylor, J.E.; Paul, N.D.; Hewitt, C.N. Biogenic volatiles organic compounds in the earth system. *New Phytol.* **2009**, *183*, 27–51. [CrossRef] [PubMed]

24. Sarang, K.; Rudziński, K.J.; Szmigielski, R. Green Leaf Volatiles in the Atmosphere—Properties, Transformation, and Significance. *Atmosphere* **2021**, *12*, 1655. [CrossRef]

25. Karl, T.; Fall, R.; Crutzent, P.J.; Jordan, A.; Lindinger, W. High concentrations of reactive biogenic VOCs at a high altitude in late autumn. *Geophys. Res. Lett.* **2001**, *28*, 507–510. [CrossRef]

26. Jardine, K.J.; Chambers, J.Q.; Holm, J.; Jardine, A.B.; Fontes, C.G.; Zorzanelli, R.F.; Meyers, K.T.; Fernandez de Souza, V.; Garcia, S.; Giminez, B.O.; et al. Green leaf volatile emissions during high temperature and drought stress in a Central Amazon rainforest. *Plants* **2015**, *4*, 678–690. [CrossRef]

27. Turan, S.; Kask, K.; Kanagendran, A.; Li, S.; Anni, R.; Talts, E.; Rasulov, B.; Kannaste, A.; Niinements, U. Lethal heat stress-dependent volatile emissions from tobacco leaves: What happens beyond the thermal edge? *J. Exp. Bot.* **2019**, *70*, 5017–5030. [CrossRef] [PubMed]

28. Theocharis, A.; Clement, C.; Barka, E.A. Physiological and molecular changes in plant growth at low temperatures. *Planta* **2012**, *235*, 1091–1105. [CrossRef] [PubMed]

29. Copolovici, L.; Kannaste, A.; Pazouki, L.; Niinemets, U. Emissions of green leaf volatiles and terpenoids from *Solanum lycopersicum* are quantitatively related to the severity of cold and heat shock treatments. *J. Plant Physiol.* **2012**, *169*, 664–672. [CrossRef] [PubMed]

30. Bray, E.A.; Bailey-Serres, J.; Weretilnyk, E. Response to abiotic stresses. In *Biochemistry and Molecular Biology of Plants*; Gruissem, W., Buchanan, B.B., Jones, R., Eds.; American Society of Plant Physiologists: Rockville, MA, USA, 2000; pp. 1158–1249.

31. Cofer, T.M.; Engelberth, M.J.; Engelberth, J. Green leaf volatiles protect maize (*Zea mays*) seedlings against damage from cold stress. *Plant Cell Environ.* **2018**, *41*, 1673–1682. [CrossRef]

32. Zhu, J.-K. Salt and drought stress signal transduction in plants. *Annu. Rev. Plant Biol.* **2002**, *53*, 247–273. [CrossRef]

33. Cao, H.; Ding, R.; Kang, S.; Du, T.; Tong, L.; Zhang, Y.; Chen, J.; Shukla, M.K. Chapter 3—Drought, salt, and combined stresses in plants: Effects, tolerance mechanisms, and strategies. *Adv. Agron.* **2023**, *178*, 107–163.

34. Catola, S.; Marino, G.; Emiliani, G.; Huseynova, T.; Musayev, M.; Akparov, Z.; Maserti, B.E. Physiological and metabolomic analysis of *Punica granatum* (L.) under drought stress. *Planta* **2016**, *243*, 441–449. [CrossRef] [PubMed]

35. Yamauchi, Y.; Kunishima, M.; Mizutani, M.; Sugimotot, Y. Reactive short-chain leaf volatiles act as powerful inducers of abiotic stress-related gene expression. *Sci. Rep.* **2015**, *5*, 8030. [CrossRef]

36. Tian, S.; Guo, R.; Zou, X.; Zhang, X.; Yu, X.; Zhan, Y.; Ci, D.; Wang, M.; Wang, Y.; Si, T. Priming with the green leaf volatile (Z)-3-hexeny-1-yl acetate enhances salinity stress tolerance in peanut (*Arachis hypogaea* L.) seedlings. *Front. Plant Sci.* **2019**, *10*, 785. [CrossRef] [PubMed]

37. Hu, S.; Chen, Q.; Guo, F.; Wang, M.; Zhao, H.; Wang, Y.; Ni, D.; Wang, P. (Z)-3-hexen-1-ol accumulation enhances hyperosmotic stress tolerance in *Camellia sinensis*. *Plant Mol. Biol.* **2020**, *103*, 287–302. [CrossRef] [PubMed]

38. Chen, K.; Li, G.-J.; Bressan, R.A.; Song, C.-P.; Zhu, J.-K.; Zhao, Y. Abscisic acid dynamics, signaling, and functions in plants. *J. Int. Plant Biol.* **2020**, *62*, 25–54. [CrossRef] [PubMed]

39. Hayat, S.; Hayat, Q.; Alyemeni, M.N.; Wani, A.S.; Pichtel, J.; Ahmad, A. Role of proline under changing environments. *Plant Signal. Behav.* **2012**, *7*, 1456–1466. [CrossRef]

40. Jin, J.; Zhao, M.; Jing, T.; Wang, J.; Lu, M.; Pan, Y.; Du, W.; Zhao, C.; Bao, Z.; Zhao, W.; et al. (Z)-3-hexenol integrates drought and cold stress signaling by activating abscisic acid glucosylation in tea plants. *Plant Physiol.* **2023**, *193*, 1491–1507. [CrossRef]

41. Charron, C.S.; Cantliffe, D.J.; Wheeler, R.M.; Manukian, A.; Heath, R.R. Photosynthetic photon flux, photoperiod, and temperature effects on emissions of (Z)-3-hexenal, (Z)-3-hexenol, and (Z)-3-hexenyl acetate from lettuce. *J. Am. Soc. Hortic. Sci.* **1996**, *121*, 488–494. [CrossRef]

42. Mimuro, M.; Nishimura, Y.; Yamazaki, I.; Kobayashi, M.; Wang, Z.Y.; Nozawa, T.; Shimada, K.; Matsuura, K. Excitation energy transfer in the green photosynthetic bacterium *Chloroflexus aurantiacus*: A specific effect of 1-hexenol on the optical properties of baseplate and energy transfer processes. *Photosynth. Res.* **1996**, *48*, 263–270. [CrossRef] [PubMed]

43. Tanaka, T.; Ikeda, A.; Shiojiri, K.; Ozawa, R.; Shiki, K.; Nagai-Kunihiro, N.; Fujita, K.; Sugimoto, K.; Yamato, K.T.; Dohra, H.; et al. Identification of a hexenal reductase that modulates the composition of green leaf volatiles. *Plant Physiol.* **2018**, *178*, 552–564. [CrossRef]

44. Savchenko, T.; Yanykin, D.; Khorobrykh, A.; Terentyev, V.; Klimov, V.; Dehesh, K. The hydroperoxide lyase branch of the oxylipin pathway protects against photoinhibition of photosynthesis. *Planta* **2017**, *245*, 1179–1192. [CrossRef]

45. Wang, M.H.; Rodriguez-Saona, C.; Lavoir, A.-V.; Ninkovic, V.; Shiojiri, K.; Takabayashi, J.; Han, P. Leveraging air-borne VOC-mediated plant defense priming to optimize Integrated Pest Management. *J. Pest. Sci.* **2024**. [CrossRef]

46. Hou, S.; Tsuda, K. Salicylic acid and jasmonic acid crosstalk in plants. *Essays Biochem.* **2022**, *66*, 647–656. [PubMed]

47. Chamberlain, K.; Khan, Z.R.; Pickett, J.A.; Toshova, T.; Wadhams, L.J. Diel periodicity in the production of green leaf volatiles by wild and cultivated host plants of stemborer moths, *Chilo partellus* and *Busseola fusca*. *J. Chem. Ecol.* **2006**, *32*, 565–577. [CrossRef]

48. Jardine, K.; Barron-Gafford, G.A.; Norman, J.P.; Abrell, L.; Monson, R.K.; Meyers, K.T.; Pavao-Zuckerman, M.; Dontsova, K.; Kleist, E.; Werner, C.; et al. Green leaf volatiles and oxygenated metabolite emission bursts from mesquite branches following light-dark transitions. *Photosynth. Res.* **2012**, *113*, 321–333. [CrossRef]

49. Maurya, A.K.; Pazouki, L.; Frost, C.J. Primed seeds with indole and (Z)-3-hexenyl acetate enhances resistance against herbivores and stimulates growth. *J. Chem. Ecol.* **2022**, *48*, 441–454. [CrossRef]

50. Engelberth, J.; Engelberth, M. The costs of green leaf volatile-induced defense priming: Temporal diversity in growth response to mechanical wounding and insect herbivory. *Plants* **2019**, *8*, 23. [CrossRef]

51. Engelberth, J. Primed to growth: A new role for green leaf volatiles in plant stress responses. *Plant Signal. Behav.* **2020**, *15*, 1701240. [CrossRef]

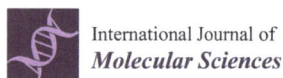

International Journal of
Molecular Sciences

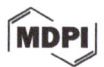

Communication

Singlet-Oxygen-Mediated Regulation of Photosynthesis-Specific Genes: A Role for Reactive Electrophiles in Signal Transduction

Tina Pancheri, Theresa Baur and Thomas Roach *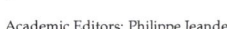

Department of Botany, Faculty of Biology, University of Innsbruck, 6020 Innsbruck, Austria
* Correspondence: thomas.roach@uibk.ac.at

Abstract: During photosynthesis, reactive oxygen species (ROS) are formed, including hydrogen peroxide (H_2O_2) and singlet oxygen ($^1O_2$), which have putative roles in signalling, but their involvement in photosynthetic acclimation is unclear. Due to extreme reactivity and a short lifetime, $^1O_2$ signalling occurs via its reaction products, such as oxidised poly-unsaturated fatty acids in thylakoid membranes. The resulting lipid peroxides decay to various aldehydes and reactive electrophile species (RES). Here, we investigated the role of ROS in the signal transduction of high light (HL), focusing on GreenCut2 genes unique to photosynthetic organisms. Using RNA seq. data, the transcriptional responses of *Chlamydomonas reinhardtii* to 2 h HL were compared with responses under low light to exogenous RES (acrolein; 4-hydroxynonenal), β-cyclocitral, a β-carotene oxidation product, as well as Rose Bengal, a $^1O_2$-producing photosensitiser, and H_2O_2. HL induced significant ($p < 0.05$) up- and down-regulation of 108 and 23 GreenCut2 genes, respectively. Of all HL up-regulated genes, over half were also up-regulated by RES, including *RBCS1* (ribulose bisphosphate carboxylase small subunit), NPQ-related *PSBS1* and *LHCSR1*. Furthermore, 96% of the genes down-regulated by HL were also down-regulated by $^1O_2$ or RES, including *CAO1* (chlorophyllide-*a* oxygnease), *MDH2* (NADP-malate dehydrogenase) and *PGM4* (phosphoglycerate mutase) for glycolysis. In comparison, only 0–4% of HL-affected GreenCut2 genes were similarly affected by H_2O_2 or β-cyclocitral. Overall, $^1O_2$ plays a significant role in signalling during the initial acclimation of *C. reinhardtii* to HL by up-regulating photo-protection and carbon assimilation and down-regulating specific primary metabolic pathways. Our data support that this pathway involves RES.

Keywords: lipid peroxidation; acrolein; 4-hydroxynonenal; Rose Bengal; reactive carbonyl species; non-photochemical quenching; algae; stress metabolism

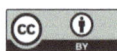

check for
updates

Citation: Pancheri, T.; Baur, T.; Roach, T. Singlet-Oxygen-Mediated Regulation of Photosynthesis-Specific Genes: A Role for Reactive Electrophiles in Signal Transduction. *Int. J. Mol. Sci.* **2024**, *25*, 8458. https://doi.org/10.3390/ijms25158458

Academic Editors: Philippe Jeandet and Mateusz Labudda

Received: 14 June 2024
Revised: 11 July 2024
Accepted: 22 July 2024
Published: 2 August 2024

1. Introduction

Solar energy drives photosynthesis, which is fundamental for sustaining almost all life on earth. Photosynthesis starts with the capture of light energy by pigments in the protein complexes of thylakoid membranes and its transfer to chlorophyll in the reaction centres of photosystems (PS) for initiating photochemistry. Photosynthetic activity requires a variety of unique processes not found in non-photosynthetic organisms (heterotrophs). In total, 597 nucleus-encoded proteins have been identified in green lineage organisms, but not, or poorly conserved, in heterotrophs, which have collectively been grouped as GreenCut2 [1]. About 30% of GreenCut2 genes are of prokaryotic origin, with about half having an unknown function and most encoding proteins predicted to be localized to the chloroplast [2]. Rational for inclusion in GreenCut2 was a putative protein orthologue in the green lineage eukaryotes (Viridiplantae), including the algae *Chlamydomonas reinhardtii* and *Ostreococcus taurii*, the moss *Physcomitrella patens*, and the vascular plant *Arabidopsis thaliana*, not found in heterotrophs (e.g., *Pseudomonas aeruginosa*, *Sulfolobus solfataricus*, *Caenorhabditis elegans*, *Homo sapiens*, etc.) [1].

Molecular oxygen, a product of oxygenic photosynthesis, can form unstable intermediates called reactive oxygen species (ROS). It is well established that across the diversity of life, the many signalling networks functioning in development, or sensing physiological state and environmental change, integrate redox components involving ROS [3,4]. Organelles, including mitochondria, chloroplasts and peroxisomes, are major sites of ROS production in plant cells, which can invoke responses not only locally, but also in the nucleus by activating or suppressing transcription. Here, it is important to distinguish the species of ROS, since they can have significantly different chemical properties. For example, hydrogen peroxide (H_2O_2) signalling filters through catalytic sites of peroxiredoxins, thioredoxins and glutaredoxins to trigger target thiol/disulfide redox 'switches' [5]. In contrast, singlet oxygen ($^1O_2$) is short-lived, and the associated signalling is largely in response to the oxidation of, for example, carotenoids (e.g., β-carotene), proteins (e.g., EXECUTER1) or cellular components (e.g., membranes) [6]. Increases in H_2O_2 and $^1O_2$ production of *C. reinhardtii* have been observed in response to a 5-fold increase in light intensity [7,8], and could be involved in acclimation to high light (HL) by affecting the transcription of GreenCut2 genes.

In response to HL, photosynthetic organisms activate non-photochemical quenching (NPQ), which can safely dissipate excess light energy to heat [9]. However, NPQ has limits and ROS formation is an unavoidable part of photosynthesis. In particular, $^1O_2$, formed by charge recombination in PSII, is considered the most damaging ROS produced under excess light [10,11]. It has become apparent that $^1O_2$ likely has a role in HL signal transduction [6,12–17]. One of the most important components of thylakoid membranes that house photosynthetic complexes are galactolipids, of which a significant fraction is composed of the poly-unsaturated fatty acid (PUFA) linolenic acid [18]. The three electron-rich C=C bonds of linolenic acid are prone to non-enzymatic oxidation by $^1O_2$, thereby forming lipid peroxides [19]. These can spontaneously dissociate, releasing a variety of carbonyls, including short-chain α,β-unsaturated aldehydes called reactive electrophile species (RES), including acrolein and 4-hydroxynonenal (HNE), which may play a role in HL signalling.

Chlamydomonas reinhardtii was the first Chlorophyte (green alga) to have its genome sequenced [20] and has since become a model organism for investigating HL stress acclimation [17]. In the model angiosperm *Arabidopsis thaliana*, β-cyclocitral from the oxidation of β-carotene has emerged as part of the $^1O_2$ stress response via the zinc finger protein *methylene blue-sensitive 1* (MBS1) protein [21]. However, despite possessing an MBS1 signalling pathway [22], β-cyclocitral has a minor role in $^1O_2$ signalling in *C. reinhardtii* [23]. In contrast, the exogenous treatment of low light (LL)-treated *C. reinhardtii* with the RES acrolein was able to lead to a remarkably similar differential expression of genes (DEG) compared with the response to the photosensitizer Rose Bengal, which can be used to mimic HL-induced $^1O_2$ production [15].

Here, using an RNA seq. approach with *C. reinhardtii*, we investigated the involvement of various ROS-mediated signal-transduction pathways in the HL acclimation of photosynthesis by focusing specifically on the GreenCut2 gene cluster. Comparisons were drawn between the influence of HL and cells treated under LL with H_2O_2 or Rose Bengal, the latter of which induced a similar level of lipid peroxidation as occurred under the HL treatment [24]. To investigate potential intermediates in ROS signalling, the response of cells under LL to acrolein, HNE and β-cyclocitral were included.

2. Results

2.1. Differential Expression of GreenCut2 Genes in Response to HL

In total, 532 GreenCut2 genes (89% of the total) were identified among the RNA seq. data (Table S1). Of these, 2 h HL of LL-acclimated cells caused a significant ($p < 0.05$) up-regulation of 86 (Table 1) or 108 genes (Table 2), with or without a false discovery rate (FDR), respectively.

Int. J. Mol. Sci. **2024**, *25*, 8458

Table 1. GreenCut2 genes significantly affected by 2 h HL. Significance was considered by $p < 0.05$ with FDR and >2-fold change (FC) relative to LL conditions, i.e., >1 or <-1 after $log2$ transformation. Red and blue shading of FC values denotes up- and down-regulation, respectively. When known, the gene name, protein description and putative or likely function are provided.

JGI v5.5 ID	FC ($log2$)	Gene	Description	Function
Cre01.g016750	10.5	-	Photosystem II 22 kDa protein (psbS) (1 of 2)	NPQ (likely)
Cre01.g016600	6.5	PSBS1	Chloroplast PSII-associated 22 kDa protein	NPQ
Cre09.g394325	4.3	ELI3	Early-light-inducible protein	High light stress response
Cre12.g510400	4.2	RBD4	Putative rubredoxin-like protein	
Cre03.g166650	4.1	-	DEAD/DEAH-box DNA/RNA helicase	
Cre12.g554103	3.8	CGL74	-	
Cre03.g145567	3.6	CGL18	-	
Cre12.g558550	3.4	-	Hydrolase, alpha/beta fold family protein	
Cre06.g272850	3.4	PRPL10	Plastid ribosomal protein L10	Plastid protein synthesis
Cre03.g145587	3.4	CPLD1	Putative thiol-disulphide oxidoreductase DCC	PSII assembly (likely)
Cre12.g508300	3.3	-	Protein of unknown function (DUF493)	
Cre12.g556050	3.3	PRPL9	Plastid ribosomal protein L9	Plastid protein synthesis
Cre13.g562750	3.2	-	Domain of unknown function (DUF4336)	
Cre12.g519300	3.2	TEF9	-	
Cre02.g088500	3.2		Conserved expressed protein	
Cre06.g265800	3.2	PRPL28	Plastid ribosomal protein L28	Plastid protein synthesis
Cre13.g580300	3.2	-	ABC transporter family protein	
Cre02.g109950	3.1	HLIP	Single-helix LHC light protein	High light stress response
Cre13.g579550	3.1	CGL27	-	
Cre12.g509650	3.1	PDS1	Phytoene desaturase	Carotenoid biosynthesis
Cre12.g498550	3.0	CHLM	Magnesium protoporphyrin O-methyltransferase	Chlorophyll biosynthesis
Cre03.g199535	3.0	-	Low-molecular-mass early-light-induced protein	Chlorophyll biosynthesis
Cre01.g049000	3.0	-	Pterin dehydratase	
Cre05.g242000	3.0	CHLD	Magnesium chelatase subunit D	Chlorophyll biosynthesis
Cre12.g494750	3.0	PRPS20	Plastid ribosomal protein S20	Plastid protein synthesis
Cre01.g004450	2.9	CPLD42	Membrane protein	
Cre02.g145000	2.9	-	K02834 ribosome-binding factor A (rbfA)	
Cre09.g411200	2.8	TEF5	Rieske [2Fe-2S] domain-containing protein	Stability of PSII–LHCII
Cre17.g721700	2.7	CPLD44	Thylakoid luminal protein	
Cre07.g334600	2.7	CGL20	-	
Cre02.g120100	2.6	RBCS1	RuBisCO small subunit 1	CO_2 assimilation
Cre12.g541777	2.6	-	Ribosomal n-lysine methyltransferase 3	CO_2 assimilation
Cre05.g246800	2.6	GUN4	Tetrapyrrole-binding protein	Chlorophyll biosynthesis
Cre03.g150350	2.6	-	KOG1803—DNA helicase	
Cre03.g195200	2.5	-	Haloalkane dehalogenase-like hydrolase	
Cre18.g748397	2.5	-	-	
Cre12.g490500	2.5	CGL78	-	
Cre10.g440450	2.5	PSB28	Photosystem II subunit 28	PSII biogenesis (likely)
Cre12.g510850	2.5	CGL73	-	
Cre03.g175200	2.3	TOC75	Translocon; outer envelope membrane of chloroplasts	
Cre13.g562850	2.3	THF1	Thylakoid formation protein	
Cre10.g466850	2.3	FKB18	Peptidyl-prolyl cis-trans isomerase, FKBP-type	
Cre08.g372000	2.2	CGLD11	-	ATP synthesis
Cre07.g328200	2.2	PSBP6	Lumen-targeted protein	
Cre03.g151200	2.2	CGLD16	-	
Cre03.g176350	2.2	PLP5	Plastid-lipid-associated protein	Acyl-lipid metabolism (likely)

Table 1. *Cont.*

JGI v5.5 ID	FC (*log*2)	Gene	Description	Function
Cre14.g629650	2.1	NIK1	Nickel transporter	
Cre06.g252200	2.1	TOC34	Translocon; outer envelope membrane of chloroplasts	
Cre09.g398700	2.1	CFA2	Cyclopropane-fatty-acyl-phospholipid synthase	
Cre03.g165000	2.1	LPA1	Translation elongation factor EFG/EF2	PSII assembly
Cre12.g537850	2.1	CCB2	Protein required for cyt b6 assembly	Cytochrome b6 assembly
Cre02.g082300	2.0	-	Surfeit locus protein 6	
Cre01.g015950	2.0	CPL11	Translation factor	Plastid protein synthesis
Cre03.g145207	2.0	CPLD33	-	
Cre06.g251150	2.0	OHP1	Low-CO_2 and stress-induced one-helix protein	PSII assembly
Cre12.g530300	2.0	-	Peptidyl-prolyl cis-trans isomerase, FKBP-type	
Cre13.g578650	2.0	HCF173	Similar to complex I intermediate-associated protein 30	PSII assembly (likely)
Cre16.g670950	2.0	CYC4	Chloroplast cytochrome c	Redox
Cre16.g679300	2.0	-	-	
Cre01.g042800	1.9	DVR1	3,8-divinyl protochlorophyllide a 8-vinyl reductase	Chlorophyll biosynthesis
Cre13.g566850	1.9	SOUL2	SOUL heme-binding protein	Heme binding
Cre13.g570350	1.9	AKC4	ABC1-like kinase	
Cre10.g438550	1.9	TAT1	TatA-like sec-independent protein translocator	Protein transport
Cre06.g261500	1.9	-	Thioredoxin family protein	Redox
Cre16.g673550	1.9	-	S-methyl-5-thio-D-ribose-1-phosphate isomerase	Methionine metabolism
Cre01.g002250	1.9	-	Acyl-CoA n-Acyltransferase domain-containing	
Cre06.g294750	1.9	CHLG	Chlorophyll synthetase	Chlorophyll biosynthesis
Cre03.g157800	1.8	-	Thioredoxin-like protein	Redox
Cre07.g315150	1.7	RBD1	Rubredoxin	PSII assembly
Cre07.g329000	1.7	CPLD47	Predicted membrane protein	PSII assembly
Cre12.g500650	1.7	RNB2	3-5 exoribonuclease II	RNA processing
Cre16.g666050	1.7	-	Saccharopine dehydrogenase	Cyt. b_6f assembly
Cre01.g000850	1.6	CPLD38	-	Stability of Cyt. b_6f
Cre12.g498700	1.6	CPLD13	-	
Cre09.g416200	1.6	MBB1	PsbB mRNA maturation factor, chloroplastic	PSII assembly
Cre06.g278236	1.6	-	Ubiquinone/menaquinone methyltransferase	
Cre01.g021600	1.6	-	RNA helicase//subfamily not named	
Cre06.g269300	1.6	-	PF07103 —protein of unknown function (DUF1365)	
Cre17.g720050	1.6	FHL2	FtsH-like membrane ATPase/metalloprotease	
Cre02.g095097	1.6	-	Peptidyl-prolyl cis-trans isomerase, FKBP-type	
Cre16.g661150	1.5	CGL5	-	Carotenoid modification
Cre03.g182150	1.5	TEF8	-	PSII assembly (likely)
Cre06.g296250	1.5	-	Lysyl-tRNA synthetase	
Cre01.g052050	1.5	-	Ubiquinol-cytochrome C chaperone	Cyt. b assembly
Cre03.g184550	1.5	CPLD28	-	PSII assembly (likely)
Cre16.g665250	1.4	APE1	Thykaloid-associated protein	Acclimation to variable light
Cre02.g114750	−1.4	-	MAP kinase-activated protein kinase 5	Protein phosphorylation
Cre05.g248000	−1.5	CGL29	-	
Cre12.g540500	−1.6	-	Peroxisomal membrane protein pmp27	
Cre12.g543000	−1.7	-	-	
Cre08.g379350	−1.7	TPT1	Triose phosphate transporter	Sugar transporter

Table 1. *Cont.*

JGI v5.5 ID	FC (*log2*)	Gene	Description	Function
Cre06.g268501	−1.8	-	2-5 RNA ligase superfamily	
Cre17.g712100	−1.8	MDAR1	Pyridine nucleotide–disulphide oxidoreductase	Redox
Cre06.g272300	−2.0	-	Phosphoglycerate mutase family protein	Glycolysis (potential)
Cre06.g268550	−2.1	-	Glucomannan 4-beta-mannosyltransferase	
Cre01.g043350	−2.1	CAO1	Chlorophyllide a oxygenase	Chlorophyll *b* synthesis
Cre06.g303300	−2.5	CYN37	Putative peptidyl-prolyl cis-trans isomerase	
Cre04.g225800	−2.5	-	Ankyrin repeat protein	
Cre07.g320350	−2.8	CDJ5	Chloroplast DnaJ-like protein	
Cre09.g410700	−3.0	MDH5	NADP-dependent malate dehydrogenase	Organic acid metabolism
Cre05.g232550	−3.0	PGM4	Phosphoglycerate mutase	Glycolysis
Cre10.g466500	−3.4	-	Glyoxylase I family protein	Glycolysis (potential)
Cre10.g460150	−4.3	ERM9	ERD4-related membrane protein	
Cre10.g439700	−5.6	CGL28	RNA-binding protein	

Table 2. Number of differentially expressed GreenCut2 genes and the % shared amongst treatments. Numbers below the arrows indicate total up-(↑) and down-(↓)regulated GreenCut2 genes in response to treatments listed above ($p < 0.05$ without FDR). Numbers in the table indicate % of the total ↑ or ↓ DEG listed on top that were also ↑ or ↓ regulated, respectively, by the treatments listed vertical–left. HL: high light, $^1O_2$: Rose Bengal, HNE: 4-hydroxynonenal, β-CC: β-cyclocitral, H_2O_2: hydrogen peroxide.

Total DEG	HL		$^1O_2$		Acrolein		HNE		β-CC		H_2O_2	
	↑ 108	↓ 23	↑ 140	↓ 180	↑ 138	↓ 144	↑ 53	↓ 114	↑ 2	↓ 14	↑ 32	↓ 31
HL	-	-	19	10	28	8	34	12	0	7	9	3
$^1O_2$	24	78	-	-	59	57	55	71	50	43	59	61
Acrolein	36	48	58	46	-	-	72	59	50	50	56	52
HNE	16	61	21	45	28	47	-	-	0	43	25	52
β-CC	0	4	1	3	1	5	0	5	-	-	3	19
H_2O_2	3	4	14	11	13	11	15	14	50	43	-	-

Four HL-up-regulated genes (Cre01.g016750, Cre01.g016600, Cre10.g440450 and Cre05.g243800) encode four potential PSII subunits (*PSBS*, *PSBS1*, *PSB28* and *PSB27/CPLD45*), and many others have roles in PSII assembly (Table 1). Furthermore, six genes were also upregulated towards chlorophyll synthesis (Cre12.g510050, Cre06.g294750, Cre05.g242000, Cre12.g498550, Cre05.g246800 and Cre01.g042800, encoding *CTH1*, *CHLG*, *CHLD*, *CHLM*, *GUN4* and *DVR1*, respectively; Table S1), while Cre01.g043350 encoding for *CAO1* for the synthesis of chlorophyll *b* was down-regulated (Table 1). A further HL-up-regulated gene, Cre03.g199535, encoding a low-molecular-mass early light-induced protein (Table 1), is also likely involved in chlorophyll biosynthesis [25]. Indeed, 'porphyrin and chlorophyll metabolism' was the only KEGG pathway up-regulated by HL that contained more than three genes (Table S2). No HL-down-regulated KEGG pathway contained more than one gene (Table S3).

HL was the only treatment assessed that induced more up- than down-regulation of GreenCut2 genes (Table 2). More total GreenCut2 genes were up-regulated by Rose Bengal ($n = 140$) and acrolein ($n = 138$), but an even greater number were also down-regulated ($n = 180$ and $n = 114$, respectively, Table 2). β-cyclocitral and H_2O_2 (from [26]) led to an up-regulation of 2 and 32 GreenCut2 genes, respectively, but <4% overlapped with the response to HL (Table 2).

2.2. Shared Genes

When considering significantly affected genes at $p < 0.05$ without FDR, the number of up- and down-regulated genes in response to 2 h HL increased to 108 and 23, respectively (Table 2). Many of these were also similarly regulated by exogenous treatment with Rose Bengal, or the RES acrolein and HNE (Table 2 and Table S1).

A significant positive correlation ($r^2 = 0.32$) was found when correlating the $log2$FC values of these treatments with HL for all 98 shared significantly affected genes (Figure 1), whereas for H_2O_2, the overall relationship with HL was negative (Figure S1), although only 16 genes were shared. However, it was also obvious that a proportion of genes up-regulated by HL was down-regulated by RES or Rose Bengal (Figure 1). We could not find a KEGG pathway represented by more than two genes within these 29 genes (Table S4). A very close relationship in the regulation of significantly affected GreenCut2 genes was found when correlating $log2$FC values in response to Rose Bengal and either acrolein ($r^2 = 0.67$; 179 genes) or HNE ($r^2 = 0.78$; 108 genes) or H_2O_2 ($r^2 = 0.60$; 46 genes), and in response to HNE and either acrolein ($r^2 = 0.71$; 104 genes) or H_2O_2 ($r^2 = 0.62$; 28 genes) (Figure S1).

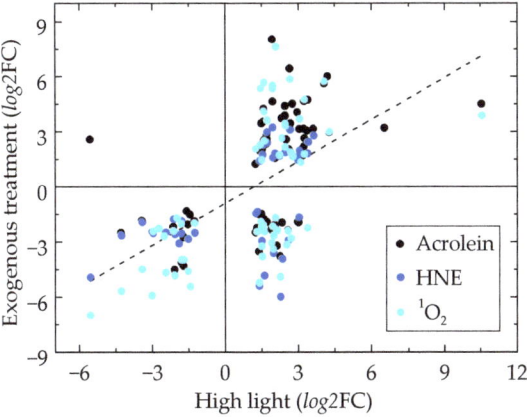

Figure 1. Correlation of the expression levels of GreenCut2 genes significantly affected by high light (HL) and singlet oxygen ($^1O_2$)-related treatments under low light. Data are separated along the *x*-axis by a $log2$-fold change ($log2$FC) in response to HL and along the *y*-axis by $log2$FC in response to exogenous treatments (acrolein; black, HNE; dark blue, Rose Bengal ($^1O_2$); turquoise). The line of best fit is of all data.

Considering only the 15 most down-regulated genes under HL, 13, 11, 5, 1 and 0 were also significantly down-regulated by Rose Bengal, 4-hydroxynonenal, acrolein, β-cyclocitral and H_2O_2, respectively (Figure 2). Focusing on the 15 most up-regulated genes by HL, 10, 4, 3, 0 and 0 were significantly up-regulated by acrolein, Rose Bengal, 4-hydroxynonenal, β-cyclocitral and H_2O_2, respectively (Figure 1).

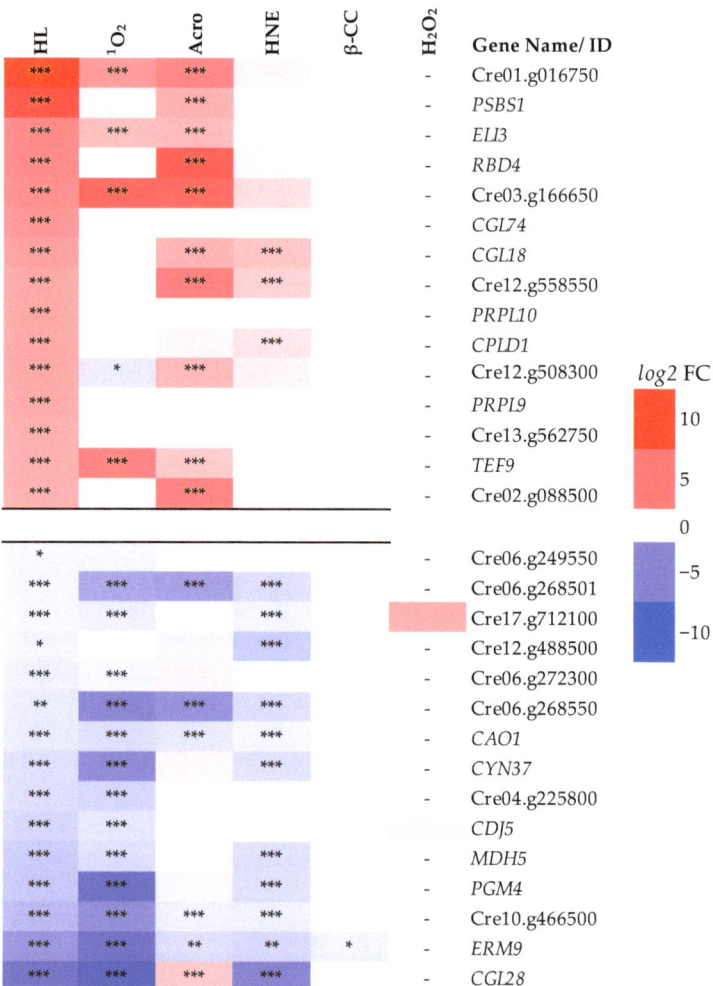

Figure 2. Fold-change (FC) of the 15 most up- and down-regulated GreenCut2 genes in response to high light (HL) and exogenous treatments under low light. Red and blue indicate up- and down-regulation, respectively on a $log2FC$ scale shown on the right. When known, the gene names are given, otherwise the gene ID is denoted. HL: high light, $^1O_2$: Rose Bengal, Acro: acrolein, HNE: 4-hydroxynonenal, β-CC: β-cyclocitral, H_2O_2: hydrogen peroxide. Significance: $p < 0.05$, $p < 0.05$ + FDR and $p < 0.01$ + FDR are denoted by *, ** and ***, respectively. Dash (-): insignificant [26].

3. Discussion

3.1. A Role for $^1O_2$ but Not H_2O_2 in Affecting the Gene Expression of GreenCut2 under HL

To investigate how ROS contribute to the signalling of photosynthesis-specific genes during HL acclimation, we compared the differential expression of GreenCut2 genes in response to 2 h HL with 2 h treatment in response to exogenous chemicals related to ROS under LL. Previously, physiological as well as molecular responses showed that exogenous molecules (e.g., H_2O_2, RES and β-cyclocitral) at the concentrations investigated here were able to penetrate cells to induce a response, thus be available to act in signalling pathways [8,23,26]. For example, using fluorescent H_2O_2 sensors in *C. reinhardtii*, it was shown that 0.1–1.0 mM exogenous H_2O_2, and chloroplast-derived H_2O_2 under HL leaked into the cytosol [27]. Transcripts encoding the proteins involved in photosynthesis showed a general downward trend after treatment with 1 mM H_2O_2, but mostly insignificantly [26]. By far, the most up-regulated H_2O_2-responsive gene was a heat shock protein, *HSP22A* [26], which, although also highly up-regulated by Rose Bengal, acrolein and HNE, was not up-regulated in response to HL (Table S1). This is less surprising than could be expected considering that the concentrations of H_2O_2 in HL-treated *C. reinhardtii* were measured at low µM [8], similar to measurements in leaves [28] and far from the 1 mM concentration used for the RNA seq. [26]. In contrast, the $^1O_2$ gene marker, *SOUL2* [14], was significantly up-regulated by HL (Table 1) and Rose Bengal (Table S1), supporting that $^1O_2$ was contributing to signalling under the HL treatment. Moreover, of all GreenCut2 genes up- and down-regulated by HL, only 3% and 4%, respectively, were similarly regulated by H_2O_2, whereas 24% and 78%, respectively, were similarly regulated by Rose Bengal (Table 2). Worth mentioning is that the differential expression of GreenCut2 genes in response to 1 mM H_2O_2 was ca. 60% shared with the response to Rose Bengal (Table 1), with the *log*2FC gene expression of these treatments significantly correlating (Figure S1). Therefore, it seems that a high proportion of H_2O_2 signalling under such high H_2O_2 concentrations may pass through the same pathway(s) as $^1O_2$. Since each ROS has distinct chemical properties, this may indicate an involvement of a common oxidative modification in response to both treatments, such as lipid oxidation and derived RES. Of all measured RES, only HNE significantly accumulated in response to 1 mM H_2O_2 (personal observation). However, we concluded that $^1O_2$ has much more influence on the expression of photosynthesis-specific genes during HL acclimation than H_2O_2.

3.2. Intermediates of $^1O_2$ Signalling Likely Include RES

The known targets of $^1O_2$ in *C. reinhardtii* include β-carotene and PUFA, from which oxidation products could be secondary messengers in $^1O_2$ signalling. It was shown by Roach et al. [23] that β-cyclocitral at concentrations used for the treatment (600 ppm same as used for acrolein) were also affecting the bioenergetics of the chloroplast and were thus entering the cells and available to act in chloroplast-to-nucleus signalling. However, like H_2O_2, the shared DEG in response to β-cyclocitral and HL was very limited (Figure 2; Table 2), thus unlikely to play a major role in HL signalling in *C. reinhardtii*. Furthermore, while β-cyclocitral down-regulated porphyrin and chlorophyll synthesis [23], HL up-regulated this pathway (Table 1). As for H_2O_2, the concentrations of potential $^1O_2$-derived molecules formed under HL are also relevant for signalling. In HL-treated photoautotrophic *C. reinhardtii*, the concentration of HNE was about half that of β-cyclocitral, whereas acrolein concentrations were >5 times higher than β-cyclocitral [29]. In our study, we showed that HNE or acrolein can be mediators in $^1O_2$ signalling of GreenCut2 genes, as revealed by the strong correlation of the *log*2FC of gene expression in response to these RES and Rose Bengal (Figure S1), but due to the higher concentration of acrolein in HL-treated *C. reinhardtii*, we expect this RES to be more involved.

There are multiple ways $^1O_2$ signal transduction can occur. The cytosolic phospho-protein Sak1 [14], the zinc finger protein MBS [22], the PSII subunit P-2 (PsbP2) [30] and the ERE-containing bZIP transcription factor Sor1 [31] have all previously been shown to contribute in *C. reinhardtii*. Therefore, $^1O_2$ signalling may pass through several of these pathways. RES-mediated $^1O_2$ signalling was first reported in the biotic stress response of plants to pathogens [32,33]. The $^1O_2$-induced oxidation of thylakoid membranes [11] and derived RES was shown in *C. reinhardtii* to pass through the Sor1 transcription factor [24,31]. Due to the strong positive correlation of GreenCut2 genes in response to Rose Bengal and HNE or acrolein (Figure S1), and all three treatments with HL (Figure 1), RES likely transmit the $^1O_2$ signal from the chloroplast to the nucleus, triggering changes in gene expression under HL.

3.3. Up-Regulation via $^1O_2$ of RuBisCO Activity and Down-Regulation of Glycolysis under HL

Light intensity directly impacts photosynthetic activity and, as can be expected, up-regulated many GreenCut2 genes. Those also up-regulated by HNE, acrolein and Rose

Bengal include Cre02.g120100, encoding *RBCS1* (ribulose-1,5-bisphosphate carboxylase [RuBisC] small subunit 1). Although this small subunit is not catalytic, it is essential for maximal RuBisCO activity [34]. Also upregulated by HL and Rose Bengal was Cre17.g718950, encoding *RCA2* a RuBisCO activase-like protein. Increasing CO_2 assimilation would enhance use of HL for photosynthesis, as well as preventing ROS formation from decreasing excess light absorption. Lowered RuBisCO activity in *C. reinhardtii* mutants led to increased ROS production under HL [35], and our results support a role for $^1O_2$-derived RES in the signalling of increasing RuBisCO activity under HL.

Of all GreenCut2 genes down-regulated by HL, 78% were also down-regulated by RB, indicating a high level of the involvement of $^1O_2$ signalling in lowering the transcription of unbeneficial photosynthetic processes under HL. This group includes Cre05.g232550 and Cre06.g2723, encoding *PGM4* (phosphoglycerate mutase 4) and another putative phosphoglycerate mutase, respectively, which can be involved in glycolysis by catabolising 3-phosphoglycerate (PGA), also an intermediate in the Calvin–Benson cycle. Thus, lowered PGM4 activity would increase PGA availability for inorganic carbon assimilation via RuBisCO. The involvement of $^1O_2$ signalling in this pathway seems independent of RES (Table S1). However, Cre10.g466500 encoding for glyoxylase I family protein was highly down-regulated by HL, as well as by HNE, acrolein and Rose Bengal. The glyoxylase pathway breaks down the products of glycolysis. Also highly down-regulated by HL, Rose Bengal and HNE was Cre09.g410700 encoding *MDH5* (chloroplastic NADP-dependent malate dehydrogenase) that converts malate to oxaloacetate. MDH5 is an oxidoreductase with NADP as a ligand and is exclusively located in chloroplasts [36]. Since MDH activity consumes NADPH [36], more NADPH would potentially be available for RuBisCO activity. Overall, the data indicate that $^1O_2$ signalling is involved in enhancing inorganic carbon assimilation under HL.

A typical response to HL is an increase in chlorophyll *a:b* ratio due to less need for chlorophyll *b*-rich light-harvesting complexes (LHC). The gene Cre01.g043350 encoding *CAO1* (chlorophyllide *a* oxygenase), which plays a role in chlorophyll *b* synthesis, was down-regulated by HL, RB, HNE and acrolein, supporting a role for $^1O_2$-derived RES in this response.

3.4. Photoprotection Was Up-Regulated by Acrolein Without HL

The dissipation of excess light energy to heat via NPQ is a universal strategy of photosynthetic organisms activated by HL [9]. In *C. reinhardtii*, NPQ via LHC-stress-related (LHCSR) proteins protects from $^1O_2$ formation and photoinhibition [23,29]. Of the 15 GreenCut2 genes most up-regulated by HL, 10 were also significantly up-regulated by acrolein, despite acrolein treatments being made under LL (Table 2). Included in this group are Cre01.g016750 encoding a PSBS protein, Cre01.g016600 encoding *PSBS1* (the two most up-regulated GreenCut2 genes), Cre09.g394325 encoding *ELI3* (Early light-inducible protein) and Cre02.g109950 encoding *HLIP* (single-helix LHC light protein). In *A. thaliana*, *ELIP2* (ELI3 homologue in *C. reinhardtii*) was shown to be involved in various stress responses, such as cold and UV-B [37], while *PSBS1* is required for the activation of NPQ, possibly by promoting the conformational changes needed for the activation of LHCSR-dependent quenching in the antenna of PSII [38,39]. Although not a GreenCut2 gene, *LHCSR1* is also strongly up-regulated by HL and acrolein [24]. Overall, acrolein seems to have an important function in the acclimation process against HL by up-regulating photoprotection.

4. Materials and Methods

Material Source and Origin of Data

Chlamydomonas reinhardtii wild-type (WT) strain 4A mt^+ (CC-4051) was used for all analyses. For treatments, axenic cultures were established in TAP (TRIS-acetate-phosphate) media under LL at 50 µmol quanta m^{-2} s^{-1} (sub-saturating), and once in exponential phase, were transferred to photoautotrophic THP media or placed on solid agar TAP media, depending on the treatment. For volatile treatments (acrolein, β-cyclocitral), homogenous algal 'lawns' were initiated on agar by distributing 0.75 mL of liquid TAP culture evenly across 11 cm Petri dishes half-filled with TAP +1.5% agar and left for 0.5 h in a laminar flow bench to evaporate the liquid media in sterile air. The lid was then closed but not sealed, and the cells were cultivated for 4 days at 20 °C under LL before treatment with volatile acrolein or β-cyclocitral (both Sigma-Aldrich, St. Louis, MI, USA). For more details, see [23,24]. For treatments of liquid cultures (HL, Rose Bengal, HNE), TAP cultures were transferred to a photoautotrophic THP medium, whereby the media was pH-adjusted to 7.0 with HCl rather than with acetic acid. The cells were pelleted at $1000\times g$ for 1 min and TAP media was replaced with THP. Liquid THP cultures were bubbled with sterile air, achieved with a 0.2 μM air-filter (Minisart NML Plus cellulose acetate filters; Sartorius, Göttingen, Germany) and cultivated for at least 24 h under LL with a culture rotation at 75 rpm before treatment. The concentration of HNE (>98% pure, Cayman Chemical Co. Ann Arbor, MI, USA) in the culture was 37.5 μM with 14.6 μL of 10 mg/mL ethanol stock solution added to 25 mL culture under LL, which was calculated to be the same concentration as for the volatile acrolein treatment [24]. Cells were treated with 1 μM Rose Bengal dissolved in H_2O (95% pure disodium salt, Sigma-Aldrich) under LL, which provides a tolerable dose of $^1O_2$ [23]. For HL treatment, the light intensity was increased to 750 μmol quanta $m^{-2}\,s^{-1}$ (*ca.* double the saturating light intensity for *C. reinhardtii* [7]). Liquid cultures were at a density of 15 μg chlorophyll ml^{-1} for all samples, and during all treatments, they were rotated, but no longer bubbled with air. For the analysis of differential gene expression, comparisons were either made to the respective non-treated liquid or agar-grown cultures from LL. Three separate cultures were used as replicates for controls and treatments.

Total RNA was extracted with the RNeasy Plant Mini Kit (Qiagen, Hilden, Germany) and additional on-column DNAse treatment (RNAse-free DNAse set, Qiagen) according to the manufacturer's instructions. Briefly, 15 mg of agar culture carefully scraped from the surface or 25 mg of pelleted liquid culture (after centrifugation for 1 min at $1000\times g$) were frozen with three 3 mm RNAse free glass beads in a 2 mL Eppendorf tube and stored at −80 °C. They were then shaken in pre-ice-cooled adaptors for 2 min at 30 Hz (TissueLyzer II, Qiagen) and 450 μL of an RLC buffer with β-mercaptoethanol was added immediately. After extraction, the samples were stored at −80 °C before the poly A enrichment of mRNA. The RNA seq. was performed by the NGS Core Facility of the Vienna Biocenter, Vienna, Austria, with Illumina's HiSeq2500 instrument using single-end sequencing with 50 bp read length. Raw reads were aligned against the *C. reinhardtii* reference genome (JGI v5.5 release) with STAR version 2.5.1b using a 2-pass alignment mode. Three biological replicates were analysed for each treatment and a significant FC was considered at $p < 0.05$ with or without FDR, as calculated with the Limma package [40].

The Algal Functional Annotation Tool was used (http://pathways.mcdb.ucla.edu/algal/index.html, accessed on 4 June 2024) for exploring the KEGG pathways of shared DEGs.

5. Conclusions

Previously, we have shown that $^1O_2$ formation during HL peroxidises PUFA in thylakoid membranes, leading to the release of RES. Here, evidence is provided that RES, such as acrolein and HNE, can be the secondary messengers of $^1O_2$ signalling, up-regulating photo-protection and possibly carbon assimilation, while down-regulating specific primary metabolic pathways towards HL acclimation. In contrast, we found that H_2O_2 and β-cyclocitral most likely do not contribute.

Supplementary Materials: The following supporting information can be downloaded at: https://www.mdpi.com/article/10.3390/ijms25158458/s1.

Author Contributions: Conceptualisation, T.R.; methodology, T.R. and T.B.; data curation, T.P.; writing—original draft preparation, T.P and T.R.; writing—review and editing, T.R.; visualisation, T.P.; supervision, T.R.; funding acquisition, T.R. All authors have read and agreed to the published version of the manuscript.

Funding: This research was funded by the Austrian Research Promotion Agency (FFG), project no. 41863779.

Institutional Review Board Statement: Not applicable.

Informed Consent Statement: Not applicable.

Data Availability Statement: RNA seq. data are available at the Sequencing Read Archive of NCBI project PRJNA1123657 https://www.ncbi.nlm.nih.gov/sra/PRJNA1123657.

Conflicts of Interest: The authors declare no conflicts of interest.

References

1. Karpowicz, S.J.; Prochnik, S.E.; Grossman, A.R.; Merchant, S.S. The GreenCut2 Resource, a phylogenomically derived inventory of proteins specific to the plant lineage. *J. Biol. Chem.* **2011**, *286*, 21427–21439. [CrossRef] [PubMed]
2. Grossman, A.; Sanz-Luque, E.; Yi, H.; Yang, W. Building the GreenCut2 suite of proteins to unmask photosynthetic function and regulation. *Microbiology* **2019**, *165*, 697–718. [CrossRef] [PubMed]
3. Halliwell, B. Reactive species and antioxidants. Redox biology is a fundamental theme of aerobic life. *Plant Physiol.* **2006**, *141*, 312–322. [CrossRef] [PubMed]
4. Schippers, J.H.M.; Nguyen, H.M.; Lu, D.; Schmidt, R.; Mueller-Roeber, B. ROS homeostasis during development: An evolutionary conserved strategy. *Cell. Mol. Life Sci.* **2012**, *69*, 3245–3257. [CrossRef] [PubMed]
5. Dietz, K.-J.; Vogelsang, L. A general concept of quantitative abiotic stress sensing. *Trends Plant Sci.* **2024**, *29*, 319–328. [CrossRef] [PubMed]
6. Dogra, V.; Kim, C. Singlet Oxygen Metabolism: From Genesis to Signaling. *Front. Plant Sci.* **2020**, *10*, 1640. [CrossRef]
7. Roach, T.; Sedoud, A.; Krieger-Liszkay, A. Acetate in mixotrophic growth medium affects photosystem II in *Chlamydomonas reinhardtii* and protects against photoinhibition. *Biochim. Biophys. Acta Bioenerg.* **2013**, *1827*, 1183–1190. [CrossRef]
8. Roach, T.; Na, C.S.; Krieger-Liszkay, A. High light-induced hydrogen peroxide production in *Chlamydomonas reinhardtii* is increased by high CO_2 availability. *Plant J.* **2015**, *81*, 759–766. [CrossRef]
9. Niyogi, K.K.; Truong, T.B. Evolution of flexible non-photochemical quenching mechanisms that regulate light harvesting in oxygenic photosynthesis. *Curr. Opin. Plant Biol.* **2013**, *16*, 307–314. [CrossRef]
10. Gorman, A.A.; Rodgers, M.A.J. New trends in photobiology. Current perspectives of singlet oxygen detection in biological environments. *J. Photochem. Photobiol. B* **1992**, *14*, 159–176. [CrossRef]
11. Triantaphylidès, C.; Krischke, M.; Hoeberichts, F.A.; Ksas, B.; Gresser, G.; Havaux, M.; Van Breusegem, F.; Mueller, M.J. Singlet oxygen is the major reactive oxygen species involved in photooxidative damage to plants. *Plant Physiol.* **2008**, *148*, 960–968. [CrossRef] [PubMed]
12. Fischer, B.B.; Krieger-Liszkay, A.; Hideg, É.; Šnyrychová, I.; Wiesendanger, M.; Eggen, R.I.L. Role of singlet oxygen in chloroplast to nucleus retrograde signaling in *Chlamydomonas reinhardtii*. *FEBS Lett.* **2007**, *581*, 5555–5560. [CrossRef]
13. Roach, T.; Baur, T.; Stöggl, W.; Krieger-Liszkay, A. *Chlamydomonas reinhardtii* responding to high light: A role for 2-propenal (acrolein). *Physiol. Plant.* **2017**, *161*, 75–87. [CrossRef] [PubMed]
14. Wakao, S.; Chin, B.L.; Ledford, H.K.; Dent, R.M.; Casero, D.; Pellegrini, M.; Merchant, S.S.; Niyogi, K.K. Phosphoprotein SAK1 is a regulator of acclimation to singlet oxygen in *Chlamydomonas reinhardtii*. *eLife* **2014**, *3*, e02286. [CrossRef]
15. Ledford, H.K.; Chin, B.L.; Niyogi, K.K. Acclimation to singlet oxygen stress in *Chlamydomonas reinhardtii*. *Eukaryot. Cell* **2007**, *6*, 919–930. [CrossRef]
16. Kim, C.; Apel, K. $^1O_2$-mediated and EXECUTER-dependent retrograde plastid-to-nucleus signaling in norflurazon-treated seedlings of *Arabidopsis thaliana*. *Mol. Plant* **2013**, *6*, 1580–1591. [CrossRef] [PubMed]
17. Erickson, E.; Wakao, S.; Niyogi, K.K. Light stress and photoprotection in *Chlamydomonas reinhardtii*. *Plant J.* **2015**, *82*, 449–465. [CrossRef]
18. Vieler, A.; Wilhelm, C.; Goss, R.; Süß, R.; Schiller, J. The lipid composition of the unicellular green alga *Chlamydomonas reinhardtii* and the diatom *Cyclotella meneghiniana* investigated by MALDI-TOF MS and TLC. *Chem. Phys. Lipids* **2007**, *150*, 143–155. [CrossRef] [PubMed]
19. Farmer, E.E.; Mueller, M.J. ROS-mediated lipid peroxidation and RES-activated signaling. *Annu. Rev. Plant Biol.* **2013**, *64*, 429–450. [CrossRef]
20. Merchant, S.S.; Prochnik, S.E.; Vallon, O.; Harris, E.H.; Karpowicz, S.J.; Witman, G.B.; Terry, A.; Salamov, A.; Fritz-Laylin, L.K.; Maréchal-Drouard, L.; et al. The *Chlamydomonas* Genome Reveals the Evolution of Key Animal and Plant Functions. *Science* **2007**, *318*, 245–250. [CrossRef]
21. Havaux, M. Review β-Cyclocitral and derivatives: Emerging molecular signals serving multiple biological functions. *Plant Physiol. Biochem.* **2020**, *155*, 35–41. [PubMed]
22. Shao, N.; Duan, G.Y.; Bock, R. A mediator of singlet oxygen responses in *Chlamydomonas reinhardtii* and *Arabidopsis* identified by a luciferase-based genetic screen in algal cells. *Plant Cell* **2013**, *25*, 4209–4226. [CrossRef] [PubMed]
23. Roach, T.; Baur, T.; Kranner, I. β-Cyclocitral Does Not Contribute to Singlet Oxygen-Signalling in Algae, but May Down-Regulate Chlorophyll Synthesis. *Plants* **2022**, *11*, 2155. [CrossRef] [PubMed]

24. Roach, T.; Stöggl, W.; Baur, T.; Kranner, I. Distress and eustress of reactive electrophiles and relevance to light stress acclimation via stimulation of thiol/disulphide-based redox defences. *Free Radic. Biol. Med.* **2018**, *122*, 65–73. [CrossRef]
25. Wang, L.; Patena, W.; Van Baalen, K.A.; Xie, Y.; Singer, E.R.; Gavrilenko, S.; Warren-Williams, M.; Han, L.; Harrigan, H.R.; Hartz, L.D.; et al. A chloroplast protein atlas reveals punctate structures and spatial organization of biosynthetic pathways. *Cell* **2023**, *186*, 3499–3518.e14. [CrossRef] [PubMed]
26. Blaby, I.K.; Blaby-Haas, C.E.; Pérez-Pérez, M.E.; Schmollinger, S.; Fitz-Gibbon, S.; Lemaire, S.D.; Merchant, S.S. Genome-wide analysis on *Chlamydomonas reinhardtii* reveals the impact of hydrogen peroxide on protein stress responses and overlap with other stress transcriptomes. *Plant J.* **2015**, *84*, 974–988. [CrossRef] [PubMed]
27. Niemeyer, J.; Scheuring, D.; Oestreicher, J.; Morgan, B.; Schroda, M. Real-time monitoring of subcellular H_2O_2 distribution in *Chlamydomonas reinhardtii*. *Plant Cell* **2021**, *33*, 2935–2949. [CrossRef] [PubMed]
28. Queval, G.; Hager, J.; Gakière, B.; Noctor, G. Why are literature data for H_2O_2 contents so variable? A discussion of potential difficulties in the quantitative assay of leaf extracts. *J. Exp. Bot.* **2008**, *59*, 135–146. [CrossRef]
29. Roach, T.; Na, C.S.; Stöggl, W.; Krieger-Liszkay, A. The non-photochemical quenching protein LHCSR3 prevents oxygen-dependent photoinhibition in *Chlamydomonas reinhardtii*. *J. Exp. Bot.* **2020**, *71*, 2650–2660. [CrossRef]
30. Brzezowski, P.; Wilson, K.E.; Gray, G.R. The PSBP2 protein of *Chlamydomonas reinhardtii* is required for singlet oxygen-dependent signaling. *Planta* **2012**, *236*, 1289–1303. [CrossRef]
31. Fischer, B.B.; Ledford, H.K.; Wakao, S.; Huang, S.G.; Casero, D.; Pellegrini, M.; Merchant, S.S.; Koller, A.; Eggen, R.I.L.; Niyogi, K.K. SINGLET OXYGEN RESISTANT 1 links reactive electrophile signaling to singlet oxygen acclimation in *Chlamydomonas reinhardtii*. *Proc. Natl. Acad. Sci. USA* **2012**, *109*, E1302–E1311. [CrossRef]
32. Bate, N.J.; Rothstein, S.J. C6-volatiles derived from the lipoxygenase pathway induce a subset of defense-related genes. *Plant J.* **1998**, *16*, 561–569. [CrossRef]
33. Améras, E.; Stolz, S.; Vollenweider, S.; Reymond, P.; Mène-Saffrané, L.; Farmer, E.E. Reactive electrophile species activate defense gene expression in *Arabidopsis*. *Plant J.* **2003**, *34*, 205–216. [CrossRef]
34. Taylor, T.C.; Backlund, A.; Bjorhall, K.; Spreitzer, R.J.; Andersson, I. First Crystal Structure of Rubisco from a Green Alga, *Chlamydomonas reinhardtii*. *J. Biol. Chem.* **2001**, *276*, 48159–48164. [CrossRef] [PubMed]
35. Johnson, X. Manipulating RuBisCO accumulation in the green alga, *Chlamydomonas reinhardtii*. *Plant Mol. Biol.* **2011**, *76*, 397–405. [CrossRef] [PubMed]
36. Scheibe, R. NADP$^+$-malate dehydrogenase in C3-plants: Regulation and role of a light-activated enzyme. *Physiol. Plant.* **1987**, *71*, 393–400. [CrossRef]
37. Hayami, N.; Sakai, Y.; Kimura, M.; Saito, T.; Tokizawa, M.; Iuchi, S.; Kurihara, Y.; Matsui, M.; Nomoto, M.; Tada, Y.; et al. The responses of *Arabidopsis* early light-induced protein2 to ultraviolet B, high light, and cold stress are regulated by a transcriptional regulatory unit composed of two elements. *Plant Physiol.* **2015**, *169*, 840–855. [CrossRef] [PubMed]
38. Tibiletti, T.; Auroy, P.; Peltier, G.; Caffarri, S. *Chlamydomonas reinhardtii* PsbS protein is functional and accumulates rapidly and transiently under high light. *Plant Physiol.* **2016**, *171*, 2717–2730. [CrossRef] [PubMed]
39. Correa-Galvis, V.; Redekop, P.; Guan, K.; Griess, A.; Truong, T.B.; Wakao, S.; Niyogi, K.K.; Jahns, P. Photosystem II Subunit PsbS Is involved in the induction of LHCSR Protein-dependent energy dissipation in *Chlamydomonas reinhardtii*. *J. Biol. Chem.* **2016**, *291*, 17478–17487. [CrossRef]
40. Ritchie, M.; Phipson, B.; Wu, D.; Hu, Y.; Law, C.; Shi, W.; Smyth, G. Limma powers differential expression analyses for RNA-sequencing and microarray studies. *Nucleic Acids Res.* **2015**, *43*, e47. [CrossRef]

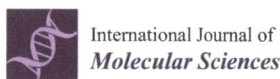

International Journal of
Molecular Sciences

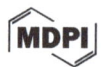

Review

How Histone Acetyltransferases Shape Plant Photomorphogenesis and UV Response

Irina Boycheva 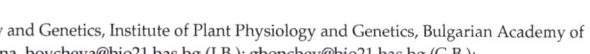, Georgi Bonchev, Vasilissa Manova, Lubomir Stoilov and Valya Vassileva *

Department of Molecular Biology and Genetics, Institute of Plant Physiology and Genetics, Bulgarian Academy of Sciences, 1113 Sofia, Bulgaria; irina_boycheva@bio21.bas.bg (I.B.); gbonchev@bio21.bas.bg (G.B.); vmanova@bas.bg (V.M.); molgen@bas.bg (L.S.)
* Correspondence: valyavassileva@bio21.bas.bg; Tel.: +359-887217112

Abstract: Higher plants have developed complex mechanisms to adapt to fluctuating environmental conditions with light playing a vital role in photosynthesis and influencing various developmental processes, including photomorphogenesis. Exposure to ultraviolet (UV) radiation can cause cellular damage, necessitating effective DNA repair mechanisms. Histone acetyltransferases (HATs) play a crucial role in regulating chromatin structure and gene expression, thereby contributing to the repair mechanisms. HATs facilitate chromatin relaxation, enabling transcriptional activation necessary for plant development and stress responses. The intricate relationship between HATs, light signaling pathways and chromatin dynamics has been increasingly understood, providing valuable insights into plant adaptability. This review explores the role of HATs in plant photomorphogenesis, chromatin remodeling and gene regulation, highlighting the importance of chromatin modifications in plant responses to light and various stressors. It emphasizes the need for further research on individual HAT family members and their interactions with other epigenetic factors. Advanced genomic approaches and genome-editing technologies offer promising avenues for enhancing crop resilience and productivity through targeted manipulation of HAT activities. Understanding these mechanisms is essential for developing strategies to improve plant growth and stress tolerance, contributing to sustainable agriculture in the face of a changing climate.

Keywords: chromatin remodeling; histone acetyltransferases; plant photomorphogenesis; light signaling pathways; UV-B radiation; DNA repair mechanisms

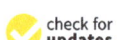

check for
updates

Citation: Boycheva, I.; Bonchev, G.; Manova, V.; Stoilov, L.; Vassileva, V. How Histone Acetyltransferases Shape Plant Photomorphogenesis and UV Response. *Int. J. Mol. Sci.* **2024**, *25*, 7851. https://doi.org/10.3390/ijms25147851

Academic Editors: Philippe Jeandet and Mateusz Labudda

Received: 4 July 2024
Revised: 15 July 2024
Accepted: 16 July 2024
Published: 18 July 2024

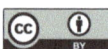
1. Introduction

Higher plants, being immobile, have developed intricate mechanisms to acclimate to changing environmental conditions, optimizing their morphology in response to specific variables. One of the most important adaptations for green plants is to the surrounding light, as it is the primary energy source for photosynthesis [1–4]. Light signals act as informational cues that modulate various development processes, with different wavelengths exerting diverse effects on plant photosynthesis and photomorphogenesis. Green plants are exposed to fluctuating levels of solar ultraviolet B (UV-B) radiation, a potentially harmful factor that can damage cellular components like DNA, proteins, lipids and RNA [5–9]. To counteract these effects, plants have developed specific DNA repair mechanisms that protect them from this damage and ensure normal growth and development [10–13]. The repair mechanisms are closely related to chromatin remodeling events, DNA methylation and histone acetylation, which contribute to the regulation of gene expression and plant stress adaptability. It is important to acknowledge the role of histones, particularly the H2A class, not only in DNA repair processes [14] but also in degradosome formation and subsequent chromatinolysis [15]. The degradosome is essential for chromatin degradation during programmed cell death. In this context, the Apoptosis-Inducing Factor (AIF) collaborates with histone H2AX and cyclophilin A (CypA) to form a DNA–degradosome complex, which is vital for large-scale DNA fragmentation. This complex enhances the affinity of degradosome for DNA, systematically degrading damaged DNA and associated histones, thus preventing the accumulation of compromised chromatin, and promoting cellular recovery and survival [15].

Chromatin-level regulation is closely linked to light signaling and transcriptional control. The relationship between chromatin-based mechanisms and light responses has been recognized for several decades. For instance, elevated transcription resulting from increased histone acetylation and reduced nucleosomal density in the promoter region of the photosynthetic *PetE* gene illustrates this relationship [16]. Another example is the main repressor of photomorphogenesis, DET1 (DE-ETIOLATED 1) [17,18], which binds histone H2B proteins with different affinity depending on their acetylation state [19].

Regulation of chromatin structure and function through histone modifications greatly contributes to plant development and stress responses [20]. These epigenetic modulations are responsible for the precise control of gene expression in response to environmental cues, including light signals [21]. Histone acetyltransferases (HATs) modulate the acetylation of histone proteins, resulting in a more relaxed chromatin state conducive to transcriptional activation. Advances over the past decade in understanding the relationship between HATs and light signaling pathways have revealed the complex regulatory networks that govern plant photomorphogenesis [22]. Investigating the roles of specific HATs in these processes offers a valuable understanding of the mechanisms of plant development and adaptation. Furthermore, elucidating how HATs interact with other epigenetic factors and signaling molecules will provide deeper insights into plant resilience to environmental stressors.

In this review, we explore the current knowledge on HATs as main regulators of plant photomorphogenesis and discuss their roles in chromatin remodeling, regulation of gene expression and interaction with light signaling pathways. By examining the molecular mechanisms underlying HAT-mediated responses, we aim to elucidate the specific roles of HATs in modulating chromatin dynamics and gene expression, focusing on their involvement in light signaling pathways, photomorphogenesis and UV-induced DNA repair mechanisms in higher plants.

2. Chromatin Dynamics and Gene Regulation

2.1. Chromatin Structure as a Natural Barrier to Transcription Factor Access

Chromatin organization is fundamental to all nuclear-based processes, such as DNA replication, transcription, recombination and repair. The proper functioning and efficiency of these mechanisms depend on the correct relaxation and remodeling of chromatin structure [23]. Figure 1A illustrates loosely packed nucleosomes (LPN), where DNA is more accessible to transcription factors (TFs) and other regulatory proteins, and tightly packed nucleosome (TPN) regions, which form a more compact chromatin structure that acts as a barrier to protein access. Close-up views of individual nucleosomes show DNA wrapped around a histone octamer composed of histones H2A, H2B, H3 and H4 (Figure 1B). Loosely packed nucleosomes facilitate the binding of TFs (Figure 1C) supporting critical cellular activities and the expression of DNA repair genes that fix DNA damage (Figure 2). In contrast, the compacted chromatin structure restricts access to regulatory proteins. Chromatin dynamics, therefore, is the major factor regulating chromatin accessibility. This regulation is achieved through three main mechanisms: covalent modification of histones, chromatin remodeling and methylation of DNA cytosines [24–27].

Additionally, the activation of DNA damage response (DDR) pathways plays a crucial role in maintaining genome integrity [28]. When DNA damage occurs, DDR pathways are activated to recognize and repair the damage. This process often involves chromatin remodeling to provide repair machinery access to the damaged sites (Figure 2). The proper functioning of DDR pathways is essential for the efficient repair of DNA and the prevention of mutations.

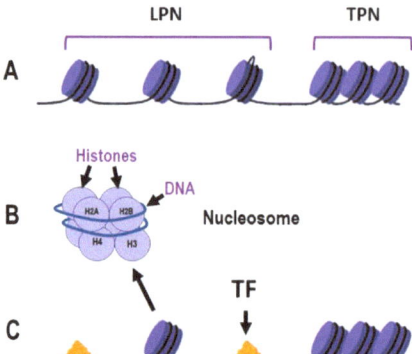

Figure 1. Schematic representation of the dynamics of DNA packaging in nucleosomes. (**A**): Chromatin organization illustrating loosely packed nucleosomes (LPN) and tightly packed nucleosomes (TPN); (**B**): Detailed structure of an individual nucleosome, showing DNA wrapped around a histone octamer composed of histones H2A, H2B, H3 and H4; (**C**): Interaction of transcription factors (TF) with chromatin, demonstrating the accessibility of LPN regions to TF binding, in contrast to the TPN regions. Some elements in this figure have been adapted from BioRender templates (biorender.com).

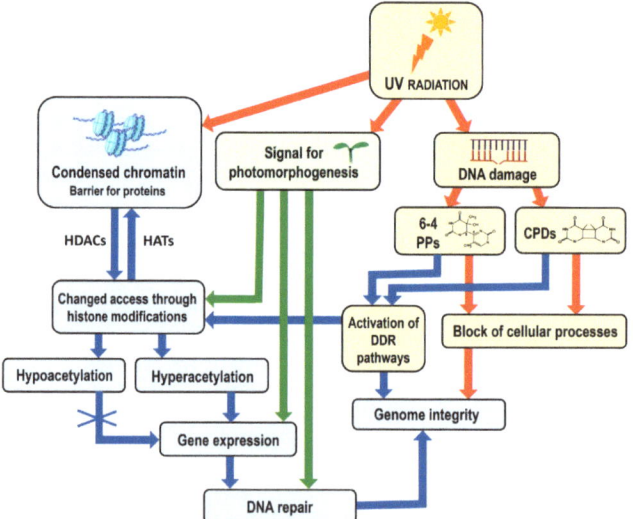

Figure 2. Diagram illustrating the impact of UV radiation on chromatin structure, gene expression and genome integrity, including the specific role of photomorphogenesis signals. UV radiation induces DNA damage, forming 6-4 PPs and CPDs, which block cellular processes and threaten genome integrity. Chromatin, structured into nucleosomes, acts as a barrier to the access of transcription factors and other regulatory proteins, which can be modified by histone modifications. Hyperacetylation allows gene expression necessary for DNA repair, whereas hypoacetylation condenses chromatin, restricting gene expression. UV radiation also signals photomorphogenesis, affecting gene expression related to developmental processes and enhancing repair mechanisms under light conditions. The DDR pathways are activated to recognize and initiate the repair of DNA damage and maintain genome integrity. The interplay between chromatin modifications, UV-induced DNA damage and cellular responses maintains genome integrity and regulates plant development. Red arrows indicate negative effects—blocking cellular processes and compromising genome integrity. Blue and green

arrows indicate positive effects—the activation of DDR pathways and chromatin remodeling processes, enhanced gene expression and DNA repair. Abbreviations: UV, Ultraviolet radiation; CPDs, cyclobutane pyrimidine dimers; 6-4 PPs, pyrimidine–pyrimidone (6-4) photoproducts; DDR, DNA damage response; HATs, histone acetyltransferases; HDACs, histone deacetylases. Some elements in this figure have been adapted from BioRender templates (biorender.com).

In the first mechanism, histone-modifying enzymes alter protein-binding affinities through covalent modifications. The second mechanism is coordinated by chromatin remodeling complexes that facilitate nucleosomes sliding to new positions. The third mechanism, methylation of DNA cytosine residues, interferes with some regulatory TFs affecting their binding to DNA [24,29]. Among these processes, covalent histone modifications are mechanisms that drive multistep cellular activities.

Additionally, recent studies have highlighted the importance of non-coding RNAs (ncRNAs) in chromatin dynamics. ncRNAs can guide chromatin-modifying complexes to specific genomic loci, influencing chromatin structure and gene expression [30], which adds another layer of regulation in chromatin accessibility and TF binding.

The role of environmental signals in modulating chromatin structure cannot be understated. Light, for example, not only triggers photomorphogenesis but also induces specific chromatin modifications that facilitate the binding of TFs involved in light-responsive gene expression (Figure 2) [22]. This interaction between environmental signals and chromatin dynamics underscores the complexity of gene regulation in plants.

2.2. Mechanisms of Chromatin Remodeling—"Open" vs. "Closed" States

The posttranslational modifications, such as acetylation, methylation, phosphorylation, ubiquitination, sumoylation and poly(ADP) ribosylation, play a key role in the regulation of gene expression [31,32]. Histone acetylation, a fundamental regulatory mechanism affecting chromatin organization, is controlled by the reversible actions of HATs, which add acetyl groups, and histone deacetylases (HDACs), which remove them. HATs transfer negatively charged acetyl (CH_3COO^-) groups to positively charged amino (NH^{3+}) groups of lysine residues, reducing the overall positive charge of histone tails. This modification loosens the bonds between positively charged histones and negatively charged DNA, facilitating the binding of various TFs, including those involved in DNA repair. Consequently, these processes impact chromatin organization and various aspects of plant growth and development [31,33]. Hyperacetylation of histones is generally associated with transcriptional activation, whereas hypoacetylation is linked to a condensed chromatin structure and the repression of gene transcription [34].

Other posttranslational modifications, like methylation and phosphorylation, can further modulate the chromatin state. For instance, histone methylation can either activate or repress transcription depending on the specific residues modified and the extent of methylation (mono-, di- or trimethylation) [35]. Phosphorylation events are often associated with chromatin condensation during mitosis but can also signal the initiation of transcription in interphase cells [36]. The interplay between these modifications constitutes the "histone code", a complex regulatory network that determines the chromatin state and, consequently, gene expression patterns [37]. This code is interpreted by various "reader" proteins that recognize specific histone modifications and recruit additional factors necessary for chromatin remodeling and transcriptional regulation.

Moreover, environmental factors such as light and stress conditions can influence the activity of HATs and HDACs, thereby modulating chromatin structure and gene expression. For example, light-induced activation of specific HATs can lead to the hyperacetylation of histones at promoters of light-responsive genes, facilitating their transcription and contributing to plant photomorphogenesis [21,38]. Similarly, stress conditions can alter HAT and HDAC activity, affecting the expression of stress-responsive genes and enabling plants to adapt to changing environments.

Understanding the mechanisms governing the "open" and "closed" states of chromatin is crucial for elucidating how plants integrate external and internal signals to fine-tune gene expression for optimal growth and survival. This knowledge can inform strategies to enhance plant resilience and productivity through targeted manipulation of chromatin-modifying enzymes.

3. HAT Families in Plants

In Arabidopsis, the four major HAT families have been classified based on sequence homology and their mode of action: the GNAT family (from GCN5-related N-acetyltransferase or HAG family, represented by HAG1, HAG2 and HAG3), the MYST family (from MOZ, Ybt2, Sas2 and Tip60-like or HAM family, represented by HAM1 and HAM2), the p300/CBP family (from the p300/CREB binding protein or HAC family, represented by HAC1, HAC2, HAC4, HAC5 and HAC12) and the TAFII250 family (from the TATA-binding protein (TBP)-associated factor or HAF family, represented by HAF1 and HAF2) (Figure 3).

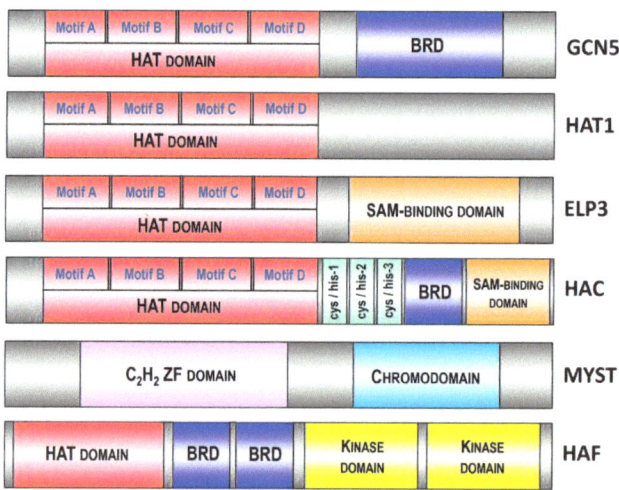

Figure 3. Domain architecture of various histone acetyltransferases (HATs) highlighting conserved motifs and domains. The diagram depicts the domain organization of GCN5, HAC, ELP3, HAT1, MYST and HAF, illustrating the presence of the HAT domain responsible for acetyltransferase activity across different enzymes. Additional domains such as the bromodomain (BRD), SAM-binding domain, C_2H_2 zinc finger (ZF) domain, chromodomain and kinase domain are shown, emphasizing the multifunctionality and regulatory mechanisms of these HATs in chromatin modification and gene expression. Conserved motifs (A, B, C, D) in the HAT domain are indicated. The size of different enzymes and domains is schematically presented and does not reflect the actual size of the structural elements of the proteins. Abbreviations: HAT, histone acetyltransferase; BRD, bromodomain; SAM, S-adenosylmethionine; ZF, zinc finger.

The GNAT family is subdivided into three subfamilies: the GCN5 subfamily (from General Control Non-derepressible protein 5 or HAG1), the ELP3 subfamily (from Elongator complex Protein 3 or HAG3) and the HAT1 subfamily (or HAG2) [39]. The structure of all three Arabidopsis GNAT subfamilies includes a HAT domain, containing four motifs—A, B, C and D [34]. These motifs are highly conserved across plant species, highlighting their essential roles in histone acetylation functions. For instance, motif A, which includes a critical aspartate residue for acetyl-CoA binding, shows over 90% conservation in a comparative study of monocots and dicots. Additionally, motifs B, C and D, involved in substrate recognition and catalytic activity, display more than 85% conservation across various plant species [40]. Additionally, GCN5 (HAG1) and ELP3 (HAG3) possess extra domains: a bromodomain (BRD) and a radical S-adenosylmethionine (SAM)-binding domain, respectively [41] (Figure 3). These structural differences underlie their diversified functions. The enzymes GCN5 (HAG1), HAT1 (HAG2) and ELP3 (HAG3) acetylate histones at different lysine residues: GCN5 acetylates H3K14 and HAT1 acetylates H4K12 [42]. Arabidopsis GCN5 is involved in plant development and the regulation of gene expression in response to light and cold [43]. HAT1 is associated with cell cycle progression and DNA replication [44], whereas ELP3 is linked to ABA sensitivity, resistance to oxidative stress, disease susceptibility and cell cycle progression [45,46].

Further exploration of the p300/CBP and TAFII250 families reveals their important roles in chromatin remodeling and gene regulation. Members of the p300/CBP family, such as HAC1, HAC2, HAC4, HAC5 and HAC12, integrate various signaling pathways and act as transcriptional co-activators, mediating histone acetylation to facilitate transcriptional activation of target genes involved in developmental processes and stress responses [47,48]. The TAFII250 family members, HAF1 and HAF2, are integral components of the transcription factor IID (TFIID) complex, which initiates transcription by RNA polymerase II, regulating genes involved in plant growth, development and environmental adjustment [49,50]. The TAFII250 homologs share conserved TBP-binding motifs, with a preservation degree of approximately 85% across analyzed plant species, which is essential for their function in the transcription initiation complex [39].

Investigating the diverse roles and mechanisms of HAT family members in plants reveals the complex regulation of chromatin dynamics and gene expression, essential for understanding photomorphogenesis and developing strategies to enhance growth and stress tolerance.

4. Light as a Dual Agent: Developmental Stimulus and Source of DNA Damage

Light is the most important environmental factor that regulates plant growth and development, serving as an energy source required for photosynthesis. Light signals also stimulate photomorphogenesis, the transition from scotomorphogenic (dark) to photomorphogenic (light) development [51].

Ultraviolet (UV) radiation, a natural component of sunlight with shorter wavelengths than the visible spectrum, is divided into three groups: UV-A (315–400 nm), UV-B (280–315 nm) and UV-C (<280 nm). UV light serves as a key growth modulator, which induces a wide range of physiological responses in plants [52]. UV-A radiation influences photomorphogenesis, promoting processes such as stem elongation and leaf expansion. UV-B radiation regulates the synthesis of secondary metabolites, which are important for plant defense mechanisms. Low doses of UV-B can enhance photosynthetic efficiency and stimulate the production of protective compounds like flavonoids and phenolics, which absorb UV light and mitigate its harmful effects. UV-C is mostly filtered out by the Earth's atmosphere, but it can still induce stress responses that activate repair mechanisms, thereby enhancing plant resilience to environmental stresses. On the other hand, UV-B light is the main genotoxic agent to which plants are continuously exposed. UV rays are generally categorized as non-ionizing radiation; however, UV photons possess sufficient energy to disrupt chemical bonds and induce cellular damage [6,53]. High doses of UV-B can damage DNA, RNA, lipids and proteins [5,54]. UV-B radiation primarily induces the formation of dimers between adjacent pyrimidines in the DNA strand, such as cyclobutane pyrimidine dimers (CPDs) and pyrimidine (6-4) pyrimidone photoproducts (6-4 PPs) (Figure 2), but can also generate oxidative DNA damage [55–58]. These lesions block DNA metabolism and disrupt genomic integrity, triggering DNA repair mechanisms to either remove or tolerate the damage [59,60].

UV-B induces numerous changes in the expression of genes involved in histone acetylation and DNA repair. Exposure of Arabidopsis and maize plants to UV-B increases CPD formation, leading to accumulation of DNA lesions. Campi et al. [61] have demonstrated that chromatin remodeling and histone acetylation significantly enhance DNA repair capacity. Arabidopsis MYST proteins HAM1 and HAM2, and the GNAT protein HAG3, are involved in the UV-B-induced DNA damage repair and signaling [41]. However, members of the p300/CBP family (HAC) and the TAFII250 family (HAF) do not contribute to DNA repair following UV-B exposure, although HAM1, HAM2 and HAG3 play a role in UV-B signaling [62]. Furthermore, modifications of histone–DNA interactions affect UV-B responses and DNA repair [6,61]. Treatment of Arabidopsis and maize plants with curcumin, an inhibitor of histone acetyltransferases, prior to UV-B exposure results in reduced DNA repair and increased DNA damage [61]. This demonstrates a clear link between UV-B response, chromatin state and DNA repair mechanisms.

Unlike UV-C and X-ray radiation, UV-B does not produce double-strand DNA breaks but causes oxidative DNA damage [54]. Consequently, UV-B exposure also triggers the expression of antioxidant defense genes, which mitigate the oxidative stress caused by UV-B radiation [13].

Thus, numerous lines of evidence indicate a broader role of acetyltransferases in plant UV response and the dual function of light as a developmental stimulus and a damaging factor, which is crucial for maintaining genome stability and overall plant health.

5. Key Transcription Factors in Photomorphogenesis and Their Interaction with HATs

As mentioned above, photomorphogenesis is the transition process from scotomorphogenic (dark) to photomorphogenic (light) development. During scotomorphogenesis, typical phenotypic features such as long hypocotyls, curved apical hooks and closed cotyledons ensure proper seedling development in dark conditions, providing protection against mechanical damage while emerging from the soil. Upon seedling emergence and exposure to light, numerous cellular changes occur, including inhibition of hypocotyl elongation, unfolding of the apical hook and cotyledon opening. These changes are triggered by a group of TFs that regulate gene expression [63]. The modulation of over 2000 nuclear genes and observed changes in chromatin structure contribute to the successful implementation of this transition [64–66].

Light signals of different wavelengths activate various families of photoreceptors like cryptochromes (CRY) and phytochromes (PHY), which mediate plant perception and response to light. Cryptochromes primarily perceive blue light, while phytochromes respond to the red/far-red light spectrum [67,68]. In the nucleus, phytochromes interact with multiple partners to modulate the transcription of downstream target genes linked to light responses [69,70], including the bZIP protein HY5 (ELONGATED HYPOCOTYL5) [71,72]. PHYTOCHROME-INTERACTING FACTORs (PIFs) are major partners of phytochromes and serve as key regulators of the transition from scotomorphogenesis to photomorphogenesis [73–75]. Light triggers the degradation of PIF proteins, thereby inhibiting COP1/SPA activity [76]. PIF1 protein is a substrate of the COP1/SPA E3 ligase in light-grown seedlings [77]. Both classes of photomorphogenic repressors (the COP1/SPA complex and the PIF family) synergistically suppress plant photomorphogenesis in the dark. PIF proteins regulate HY5 function via the COP1/SPA complex. COP1 activity is further regulated by two COP1-interacting proteins, CSU1 (COP1 Suppressor1) and CSU2 (COP1 Suppressor2). CSU1, a RING-finger E3 ligase, targets COP1 for degradation, whereas CSU2, a coiled-coil protein, interacts with the same domain of COP1. Inhibition of COP1/SPA activity is achieved through CSU2 blocking COP1 homodimerization or CSU1 blocking COP1/SPA heterodimerization [78]. Extensive studies have demonstrated that COP1 is a well-known regulator of light-mediated plant development [79–81]. This photomorphogenic repressor interacts directly and specifically with the photomorphogenic activator HY5, negatively modulating its activity through direct protein–protein interactions [82]. These antagonistic interactions likely function as a molecular switch, allowing plants to adapt to changing light conditions and implement the most appropriate and optimal developmental program. Additionally, a recent report indicates that light-regulated ubiquitination and degradation of PIFs and HY5 by COP1 are crucial for fine-tuning plant responses to fluctuating light environments [81].

Thus, histone acetylation, mediated by HATs, regulates these TFs by facilitating a more open chromatin structure, promoting the binding of TFs such as HY5 to their target genes and ensuring that light-responsive genes are properly expressed during photomorphogenesis [83].

5.1. COP1 as a Negative Regulator of Photomorphogenesis

The E3 ubiquitin ligase Constitutive Photomorphogenic 1 (COP1) is a negative regulator of photomorphogenesis in plant and animal cells. Initially identified as a single-copy gene in *Arabidopsis thaliana*, *COP1* is regulated by various light conditions including farred, red, blue and UV-B light [79]. COP1 plays an important role in many developmental processes [84,85], environmental stress responses [86] and dynamic interactions between signaling pathways [87,88]. Its function is intricately linked to light signaling pathways, affecting processes such as flowering [89,90], circadian rhythms [91], UV-B signaling [92], stomatal opening and development [93], plant defense [94], cold acclimation [86], light-induced root elongation [84] and the juvenile–adult phase change in rice [95], which underscores the central role of COP1 in photomorphogenic development [96]. Homologs of Arabidopsis COP1 have been identified in the genomes of pea [97], tomato [98], rice [99] and mammals [100]. The COP1 proteins from rice and Arabidopsis share a high level of amino acid sequence identity (73%) and similarity (83%) [99].

To understand how light affects *COP1* expression in different plant species, researchers have examined tissue-specific expression patterns of *COP1* in Arabidopsis and pea. In Arabidopsis, *COP1* transcript levels remain constant under light and dark conditions [101], indicating no light-dependent regulation of *COP1* expression. Similarly, pea COP1 protein levels are unaffected by light [97].

COP1 is a multifunctional 76 kDa enzyme consisting of three protein domains: an N-terminal RING-finger domain, a coiled-coil domain and seven C-terminal WD40 repeats [80,102]. Each domain is essential for COP1 functions, and the loss of any domain results in a non-functional protein [103]. The C-terminal WD40 repeat domain is responsible for substrate recognition and binding to DDB1 (DNA Damage-Binding Protein 1). In vitro studies have shown interaction between the human TRIB1 peptide and Arabidopsis COP1. The WD40 repeat domain forms a seven-bladed β-propeller structure with an inserted loop on the bottom face of the first blade, and connects to the conserved Val-Pro motif of the TRIB1 peptide, identified as a COP1-interacting site. This domain mediates the interaction of COP1 with substrates and regulatory proteins [104]. The N-terminal RING-finger domain of COP1 binds to ubiquitin-conjugating enzymes (E2s) that "attach" ubiquitin units to substrates targeted for degradation. The coiled-coil domain interacts with the coiled-coil domain of the transcription factor SPA1 (Suppressor of PhyA-105 1) [105]. SPA proteins, a small family of four members (SPA1, SPA2, SPA3 and SPA4), repress photomorphogenesis and elongation in dark-grown Arabidopsis. These proteins contain an N-terminal kinase-like domain, a central coiled-coil domain and a C-terminal WD repeats domain. Unlike COP1, which is conserved across higher plants and mammals, SPA proteins are plant-specific [106].

The COP1-SPA complex is a tetrameric assembly (440 kDa) comprising two COP1 and two SPA proteins with all possible combinations of the four SPA proteins [107]. Genetic and biochemical evidence indicates that SPA1 modulates E3 ubiquitin ligase activity on HY5 in vitro [108]. Several TFs serve as substrates for the COP1-SPA complex: HY5 induces seedling de-etiolation [109]; HFR1 (Long Hypocotyl in Far Red) contributes to shade avoidance [110,111]; PAP1 and PAP2 activate anthocyanin biosynthesis [112]; and CONSTANS is a key activator in photoperiodic flowering [89].

In the dark, COP1 forms a tetrameric complex with SPA proteins, associated with the CUL4 (Cullin4)-DDB1-RBX1 (Ring-Box Protein 1) core in the multimeric CUL4-DDB1-RBX1 COP1/SPA1 E3 ligase [113]. CUL4 acts as a scaffold for DDB1 and RBX1; DDB1 links the COP1–SPA complex, while RBX1 recruits E2s. The activated E2 enzyme attaches individual ubiquitin units in a poly-ubiquitin chain to the substrate, signaling for 26S proteasome activation and subsequent degradation. COP1 mediates the 26S proteasome-dependent degradation of TFs promoting photomorphogenesis, such as HY5, HYH (HY5 Homolog), LAF1 (Long After Far-Red Light1), HFR1 and UVR8 (UV RESISTANCE LOCUS 8), which repress photomorphogenesis [80] (Figure 4A).

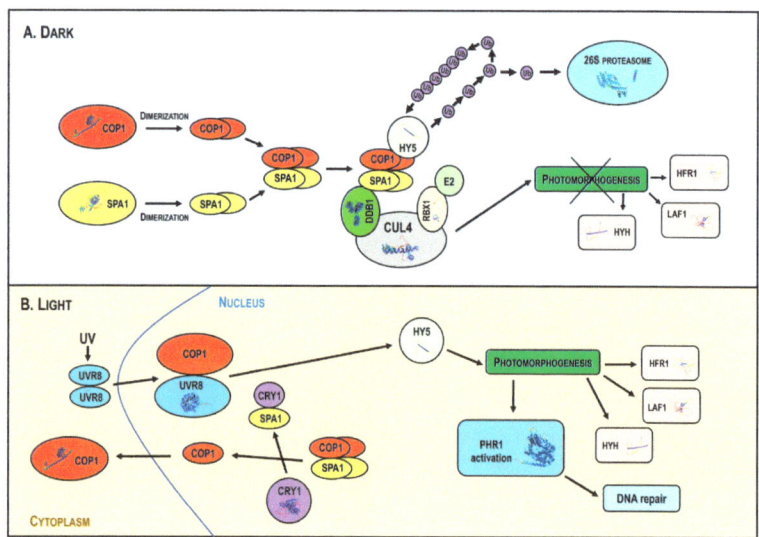

Figure 4. Mechanism of action of the multimeric CUL4-DDB1-RBX1-COP1-SPA1 E3 ligase under dark and light conditions. In the dark (**Panel A**), COP1 forms a complex with SPA proteins and the CUL4-DDB1-RBX1 core, targeting the transcription factors HY5, HYH, LAF1 and HFR1 for ubiquitin-mediated degradation, inhibiting photomorphogenesis. In light (**Panel B**), photoreceptors inhibit COP1, disassembling the COP1-SPA complex and promoting the nuclear export of COP1, allowing the accumulation of photomorphogenic regulators and activating DNA repair mechanisms. Abbreviations: CUL4, Cullin4; DDB1, DNA Damage-Binding Protein 1; RBX1, Ring-Box Protein 1; COP1, Constitutive Photomorphogenic 1; SPA, Suppressor of PhyA-105; HY5, Elongated Hypocotyl 5; Ub, ubiquitin; E2, Ub-conjugating enzyme; HYH, HY5 Homolog; LAF1, Long After Far-Red Light1; HFR1, Long Hypocotyl in Far Red; CRY1, cryptochrome; UVR8, UV RESISTANCE LOCUS 8; PHR1, Photolyase1; UV, Ultraviolet radiation.

In light, activated photoreceptors inhibit COP1 activity, leading to the disassembly of the COP1-SPA complex and promoting the nuclear export of COP1. This downregulates COP1 activity, allowing the accumulation of positive photomorphogenic regulators that promote plant photomorphogenesis. Light also stimulates *PHR1* expression and DNA repair (Figure 4B).

Plants employ different strategies to control COP1 activity. Previous studies have shown that COP1 transition from the nucleus to the cytoplasm requires at least 24 h of light exposure. However, recent findings demonstrate that this nucleocytoplasmic shuttling occurs within a few hours, potentially stabilizing HY5 protein levels rapidly [106,114]. Light not only excludes COP1 from the nucleus but also induces the degradation of SPA1 and SPA2 [68]. This degradation may be mediated by COP1 itself, interacting directly with SPA proteins via coiled-coil domains [106]. Another potential mechanism of light-induced COP1/SPA inactivation is the sumoylation of COP1 in the coiled-coil domain, which enhances COP1 activity. The Arabidopsis SUMO E3 ligase modifies the SUMO consensus motif (K193 residue) in the coiled-coil domain of COP1. Loss of sumoylation may inactivate COP1 in response to light [115]. These multifaceted regulatory mechanisms highlight the central role of COP1 in photomorphogenesis and its complex interplay with light signaling pathways.

5.2. External and Hormonal Factors Affecting COP1 Activity

Variable environmental conditions considerably influence the stability and functional activity of COP1, thus affecting the degradation or activation of its target proteins. There is a strong connection between light and temperature signaling that determines the subcellular localization of COP1 [116]. For instance, at relatively low temperatures (17 °C), COP1 is stabilized, leading to the degradation of the floral inducer GIGANTEA and delayed flowering [117]. Exposure to 4 °C reduces the nuclear abundance of COP1, preventing the degradation of the photomorphogenic activator HY5 in the dark. HY5 induces the expression of many cold-responsive genes, and its stabilization under cold conditions is linked to cold acclimation and enhanced freezing tolerance in plants [86]. High ambient temperatures (37 °C) also reduce nuclear COP1 levels, resulting in increased HY5 protein levels and subsequent photomorphogenic responses.

Hormones also modulate COP1 activity by either promoting or inhibiting the plant photomorphogenesis. The nucleocytoplasmic localization of COP1 is primarily regulated by strigolactones and ethylene. Strigolactones positively regulate photomorphogenesis under light conditions, leading to light-dependent inhibition of hypocotyl elongation and increased HY5 protein levels [118]. In contrast, under dark conditions, ethylene increases COP1 protein levels in the nucleus, mediates HY5 degradation and contributes to hypocotyl elongation [87]. When plants are exposed to light, ethylene enhances COP1 movement from the cytoplasm to the nucleus, regulating hypocotyl elongation by reducing HY5 protein levels. These findings underscore the intricate interplay between environmental cues and hormonal signals in regulating COP1 activity, thereby orchestrating plant development and stress responses.

COP1 regulation appears to be more complex than originally suggested, especially under light containing a short-wave UV component. In Arabidopsis, grown under low levels of UV-B, *COP1* acts as a positive regulator of UV-B response and photomorphogenesis by stimulating HY5 transcription. At the protein level, COP1 also mediates UV-B signaling through interaction with UVR8 [92,119,120]. Recent data reveal that dark-grown barley seedlings exhibit low *COP1* transcription levels, which increase significantly upon initial light exposure and remain consistently high under UV light [121]. This aligns with the positive light activation of *COP1* transcription in rice plants, indicating phytochrome involvement in the regulation of rice *COP1* expression [99]. Thus, both cereals show a positive light-dependent regulation of *COP1* gene expression in contrast to the results found in Arabidopsis and pea. These observations reveal intricate *COP1* regulation and expand our understanding of the complex mechanisms different plant species use to control photomorphogenesis and adapt to light-induced stress.

5.3. Regulatory Role of UVR8 and PHR1 in Photomorphogenesis

The UV-B photoreceptor is a key photomorphogenic regulator involved in two protective processes: UV-B acclimation and UV-B tolerance [92,122,123]. UV-B acclimation includes protective measures such as increased levels of DNA repair enzymes, enhanced antioxidant activity and the accumulation of UV-B absorbing metabolites [124]. These alterations provide plants with additional means to counteract and mitigate the negative effects of environmental stressors [125]. Beyond UV-B acclimation, UVR8 plays a broader role in plant growth and development, including responses to osmotic stress [126], induction of the circadian clock [127], inhibition of hypocotyl growth [92], stomatal closure [128], regulation of leaf morphogenesis [129] and phototropic bending [130]. These diverse physiological responses are related to UVR8 activity and contribute to the establishment of UV-B tolerance. The physiological role of UVR8 in UV-B tolerance has been demonstrated by comparing uvr8 mutants with wild-type controls under light conditions [92].

UVR8 is composed of two monomer units that form a stable homodimer through electrostatic interactions between oppositely charged amino acids [131]. Mutations in these amino acids can disrupt dimer integrity, weakening dimerization affinity or causing constitutive monomerization [132]. UVR8 is a seven-bladed β-propeller protein that does not use a bound chromophore to absorb light [131, but instead employs 14 specific tryptophans for UV-B photoreception [133]. The positions of these tryptophans are highly conserved through evolution with six located in the β-propeller blade, one in the carboxy-terminal domain of unknown function and seven on the surface interacting with the dimer [133–135]. The β-propeller core domain and the carboxy-terminal C27 domain of UVR8 mediate interaction with COP1. The β-propeller core domain facilitates UV-B-dependent interaction with COP1, whereas the C27 domain regulates COP1 activity [136,137]. UV-B radiation causes UVR8 homodimer disassembly into monomers, initiating a signaling cascade that leads to transcriptional regulation of target genes [138,139].

The inactive UVR8 exists as a homodimer localized in the cytoplasm. Upon UV-B absorption, UVR8 monomerizes and the monomers are translocated to the nucleus, where they bind directly to COP1. This interaction changes gene expression by dissociating the COP1/SPA complex from CUL4-DDB1 [140,141]. The UVR8-COP1 interaction stabilizes the HY5 transcription factor and stimulates the transcription of numerous UVR8-regulated genes associated with UV-B protection and DNA repair [142–144]. Among the main UV-B responsive targets controlled by UVR8 is the plant photolyase gene *PHR1* (or *UVR2*). Photolyases are major DNA repair proteins that directly split pyrimidine dimers, leading to error-free damage elimination [59,139,145]. *PHR1*-encoded photolyase specifically binds and repairs CPDs, whereas the *UVR3*-encoded protein repairs 6-4 PPs [146]. Both enzymes contribute to restoring the native DNA form and maintaining plant genome integrity under UV stress. Their inactivation results in a loss of photorepair activity and hypersensitivity to UV-B [147,148]. Thus, UV-B is a daily stress factor for plants in their natural habitats, necessitating a complex and tightly regulated interplay between multiple mechanisms to control plant genome integrity, light-induced stress tolerance and acclimation.

6. HATs and DNA Repair Capacity

Histone acetylation facilitates the accessibility of chromatin to the DNA repair machinery by loosening the chromatin structure, which is critical for the rapid response to DNA damage and the efficient repair of UV-induced lesions. HATs manage this chromatin remodeling process by acetylating histones, thus ensuring that repair proteins can access and correct the damaged DNA (Figure 5A,B). The consequences of DNA damage in mutant forms exhibit an inadequate response due to defective HAT function, resulting in ineffective DNA repair (Figure 5C,D). The restricted access to DNA in chromatin with insufficient histone acetylation leads to compacted chromatin and obstructed access for transcription factors.

Proteins involved in DNA damage response are closely linked to chromatin modifications and remodeling [149]. Histone acetylation is one of the major posttranslational modifications involved in the control of DNA repair [61]. In-depth analyses of different HAT members have revealed a complex yet essential role for different acetyltransferases in UV-B tolerance in plants. An important question has been whether the GNAT protein HAG3 could contribute to UV-B-induced DNA damage repair through the regulation of the expression of DNA repair genes. Experiments with *hag3* RNA interference (RNAi) transgenic plants have shown high expression levels of *PHR1* (*UVR2*) under control conditions (without UV-B exposure) and lower accumulation of CPDs, which could be linked to the higher basal levels of DNA repair enzymes. Similar observations have been made with *UVR7*, encoding the protein ERCC1, a subunit of the NER (nucleotide excision repair) complex, which performs excision of damaged DNA. Downregulation of *HAG3* gene leads to a specific phenotype under UV-B radiation, manifested by lower inhibition of Arabidopsis leaf and root growth, higher levels of UV-B-absorbing compounds and fewer DNA lesions compared to wild-type plants. Another important player in the UV-B-mediated regulation of various genes, including plant photolyases, is the bZIP transcription factor HY5. Under favorable conditions without UV-B radiation, higher expression levels of HY5 have been observed in *hag3* RNAi transgenic plants compared to wild-type plants. The *hag3* transgenic plants show improved adaptation to increased levels of UV-B radiation [41].

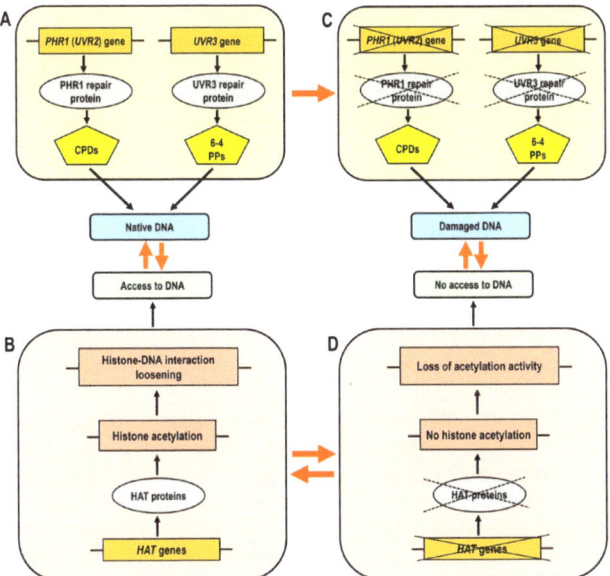

Figure 5. Simplified diagram illustrating the functionality of histone acetyltransferases (HATs) and DNA repair genes, which are essential for effective DNA damage responses. (**Panel A**): Normal chromatin structure where histone acetylation facilitates the loosening of DNA-histone bonds, allowing access of transcription factors to DNA. (**Panel B**): The accessibility of DNA in its native state, supported by proper gene function. (**Panel C**): The effects of DNA damage where mutant forms show a lack of correct response due to impaired HAT function, leading to improper DNA repair. (**Panel D**): Loss or decrease of histone acetylation leads to compacted chromatin and obstructed access of transcription factors to DNA. Abbreviations: HAT, histone acetyltransferase; CPDs, cyclobutane pyrimidine dimers; 6-4 PPs, pyrimidine–pyrimidone (6-4) photoproducts.

HAM1, HAM2 and HAG3 have been identified as participants in UV-B-induced DNA damage repair and signaling. However, *haf1* mutants display sensitivity to different genotoxic agents but not to UV-B radiation [62,150]. Specifically, light-dependent expression of CPD photolyase, which reverses pyrimidine dimerization, is not affected by the inactivation of HAF1 histone acetyltransferase from the TAFII250 family. Plants deficient in *HAF1* and wild-type plants exhibit similar *PHR1* transcript levels and both are able to upregulate the *PHR1* gene in response to CPD accumulation upon UV-B exposure. These findings imply that the photorepair system remains functional in HAF1-deficient lines (Figure 5D). Nevertheless, HAC1 and HAF1, although not critical for the removal of UV-B-induced lesions, have been implicated in other aspects of the UV-B response [62].

In summary, HATs are actively involved in UV-B-triggered DNA damage repair and signaling by regulating the expression of DNA repair genes and modifying the chromatin structure to provide access to damaged DNA, thereby maintaining genome integrity and enhancing plant tolerance to UV-B radiation (Figure 5).

7. Future Perspectives

Histone acetylation is a conserved mechanism that profoundly influences chromatin structure, regulates the cell cycle, maintains genome stability and ensures chromatin plasticity. Successful adaptation to various environmental constraints relies on genes that support plant repair potential and facilitate the transition from scotomorphogenic to photomorphogenic development. This transition involves the modulation of multiple nuclear genes, enhancing the acclimation efficiency of plants.

Future research will focus on developing systematic and innovative models that incorporate various epigenetic layers, including other histone modifications, such as methylation, phosphorylation, ubiquitination, sumoylation, ADP-ribosylation, citrullination and glycosylation, and different activators and inhibitors. New insights into the interplay between chromatin dynamics and DNA repair mechanisms will further elucidate UV tolerance mechanisms in plants. Understanding these mechanisms will support the development of cultivars with enhanced tolerance to UV radiation, thereby improving crop performance and yield under field conditions.

The intricate mechanisms by which higher plants acclimate and adapt to changing environmental conditions highlight the essential role of light in their development and stress responses. HATs modulate chromatin dynamics, which in turn regulates gene expression in response to light signals and other environmental factors. Understanding the interconnections between HATs and light signaling pathways has provided insights into the complex regulatory networks governing photomorphogenesis. However, several avenues remain for further exploration.

One promising direction is the detailed characterization of individual HAT family members and their specific roles in different plant species. The functions of Arabidopsis HATs such as HAG1, HAG2 and HAG3 have been extensively studied; however, similar research in other model plants and crop species could reveal conserved and unique regulatory mechanisms. This knowledge can be leveraged to enhance crop resilience and productivity. Another critical area of research is the interaction between HATs and other epigenetic factors. The crosstalk between histone acetylation, methylation and phosphorylation, as well as the involvement of non-coding RNAs in chromatin remodeling, represents a complex regulatory network that requires further elucidation. Advanced genomic and proteomic approaches, including chromatin immunoprecipitation sequencing (ChIP-seq) and mass spectrometry, can help map these interactions at high resolution, providing a comprehensive understanding of the epigenetic landscape in plants.

Investigating how HATs modulate the expression of DNA repair genes and other stress-responsive factors can uncover new strategies for enhancing plant tolerance to environmental stressors. Developing HAT inhibitors or activators as potential tools for modulating plant stress responses also holds great promise. Moreover, the application of CRISPR/Cas9 and other genome-editing technologies offers exciting opportunities to manipulate HAT genes and study their functions in planta. Creating loss-of-function and gain-of-function mutants can provide direct insights into the physiological roles of HATs in various developmental and stress-response pathways. In addition to these lines of inquiry, future action should consider the integration of multi-omics approaches, such as transcriptomics, proteomics and metabolomics, to build a holistic understanding of HAT function in plant biology. Collaboration with agricultural scientists and biotechnologists will be essential to translate basic research findings into practical applications that can enhance crop performance and resilience.

8. Conclusions

The study of HATs as key regulators of plant photomorphogenesis is a rapidly evolving field with significant implications for plant biology and agriculture. Further exploration of the diverse roles and mechanisms of HATs, particularly their influence on photomorphogenesis and UV-induced DNA repair, can uncover novel strategies to enhance plant growth and development, and improve stress resilience, contributing to sustainable agricultural practices in the face of global environmental challenges.

Understanding the precise mechanisms by which HATs regulate gene expression and chromatin dynamics in response to light and other environmental signals is essential for developing effective interventions. This knowledge can be applied to enhance crop performance, improve stress tolerance and ensure food security in an increasingly variable climate. Continued interdisciplinary research and collaboration will be crucial in unlocking the full potential of HATs for sustainable agriculture and plant biotechnology.

Author Contributions: Conceptualization, I.B., V.M. and V.V.; software, G.B.; resources, V.M.; writing—original draft preparation, I.B. and V.V.; writing—review and editing, I.B., G.B., V.M., L.S. and V.V.; visualization, I.B. and V.V.; project administration, V.V.; funding acquisition, G.B., V.M. and V.V. All authors have read and agreed to the published version of the manuscript.

Funding: This research was funded by the Ministry of Education and Science (MES) of Bulgaria, grant number 01-27/06.02.2024.

Acknowledgments: This work has been carried out in the framework of the National Science Program "Environmental Protection and Reduction of Risks of Adverse Events and Natural Disasters", approved by the Resolution of the Council of Ministers NO 577/17.08.2018 and supported by the Ministry of Education and Science (MES) of Bulgaria (Agreement No. 01-27/06.02.2024).

Conflicts of Interest: The authors declare no conflicts of interest. The funder had no role in the design of the study, in the writing of the manuscript, or in the decision to publish the results.

References

1. Sultan, S.E. Plant developmental responses to the environment: Eco-devo insights. *Curr. Opin. Plant Biol.* **2010**, *13*, 96–101. [CrossRef] [PubMed]
2. Von Wettberg, E.J.; Stinchcombe, J.R.; Schmitt, J. Early developmental responses to seedling environment modulate later plasticity to light spectral quality. *PLoS ONE* **2012**, *7*, e34121. [CrossRef] [PubMed]
3. Sharma, A.; Kumar, V.; Shahzad, B.; Ramakrishnan, M.; Singh Sidhu, G.P.; Bali, A.S.; Handa, N.; Kapoor, D.; Yadav, P.; Khanna, K.; et al. Photosynthetic response of plants under different abiotic stresses: A review. *J. Plant Growth Regul.* **2020**, *39*, 509–531. [CrossRef]
4. Muhammad, I.; Shalmani, A.; Ali, M.; Yang, Q.H.; Ahmad, H.; Li, F.B. Mechanisms regulating the dynamics of photosynthesis under abiotic stresses. *Front. Plant Sci.* **2021**, *11*, 615942. [CrossRef] [PubMed]
5. Casati, P.; Walbot, V. Rapid transcriptome responses of maize (*Zea mays*) to UV-B in irradiated and shielded tissues. *Genome Biol.* **2004**, *5*, R16. [CrossRef] [PubMed]
6. Casati, P.; Campi, M.; Chu, F.; Suzuki, N.; Maltby, D.; Guan, S.; Burlingame, A.L.; Walbot, V. Histone acetylation and chromatin remodeling are required for UV-B–dependent transcriptional activation of regulated genes in maize. *Plant Cell* **2008**, *20*, 827–842. [CrossRef]
7. Piccini, C.; Cai, G.; Dias, M.C.; Romi, M.; Longo, R.; Cantini, C. UV-B radiation affects photosynthesis-related processes of two Italian *Olea europaea* (L.) varieties differently. *Plants* **2020**, *9*, 1712. [CrossRef] [PubMed]
8. Liaqat, W.; Altaf, M.T.; Barutçular, C.; Nawaz, H.; Ullah, I.; Basit, A.; Mohamed, H.I. Ultraviolet-B radiation in relation to agriculture in the context of climate change: A review. *Cereal Res. Commun.* **2023**, *13*, 1–24. [CrossRef] [PubMed]
9. Georgieva, M.; Vassileva, V. Stress management in plants: Examining provisional and unique dose-dependent responses. *Int. J. Mol. Sci.* **2023**, *24*, 5105. [CrossRef]
10. Waterworth, W.M.; Jiang, Q.; West, C.E.; Nikaido, M.; Bray, C.M. Characterization of Arabidopsis photolyase enzymes and analysis of their role in protection from ultraviolet-B radiation. *J. Exp. Bot.* **2002**, *53*, 1005–1015. [CrossRef]
11. Bergo, E.; Segalla, A.; Giacometti, G.M.; Tarantino, D.; Soave, C.; Andreucci, F.; Barbato, R. Role of visible light in the recovery of photosystem II structure and function from ultraviolet-B stress in higher plants. *J. Exp. Bot.* **2003**, *54*, 1665–1673. [CrossRef]
12. Manova, V.; Georgieva, M.; Borisov, B.; Stoilova, B.; Gecheff, K.; Stoilov, L. Genomic and gene-specific induction and repair of DNA damage in barley. In *Induced Plant Mutations in the Genomics Era*; Shu, Q.Y., Ed.; Food and Agriculture Organization of the United Nations: Rome, Italy, 2009; pp. 133–136.
13. Shi, C.; Liu, H. How plants protect themselves from ultraviolet-B radiation stress. *Plant Physiol.* **2021**, *187*, 1096–1103. [CrossRef]
14. Selvam, K.; Wyrick, J.J.; Parra, M.A. DNA repair in nucleosomes: Insights from histone modifications and mutants. *Int. J. Mol. Sci.* **2024**, *25*, 4393. [CrossRef]
15. Novo, N.; Romero-Tamayo, S.; Marcuello, C.; Boneta, S.; Blasco-Machin, I.; Velázquez-Campoy, A.; Villanueva, R.; Moreno-Loshuertos, R.; Lostao, A.; Medina, M.; et al. Beyond a platform protein for the degradosome assembly: The Apoptosis-Inducing Factor as an efficient nuclease involved in chromatinolysis. *PNAS Nexus* **2023**, *2*, pgac312. [CrossRef]
16. Chua, Y.L.; Brown, A.P.C.; Gray, J.C. Targeted histone acetylation and altered nuclease accessibility over short regions of the pea plastocyanin gene. *Plant Cell* **2001**, *13*, 599–612. [CrossRef]
17. Chory, J.; Peto, C.; Feinbaum, R.; Pratt, L.; Ausubel, F. *Arabidopsis thaliana* mutant that develops as a light-grown plant in the absence of light. *Cell* **1989**, *58*, 991–999. [CrossRef] [PubMed]
18. Pepper, A.; Delaney, T.; Washburn, T.; Poole, D.; Chory, J. *DET1*, a negative regulator of light-mediated development and gene expression in arabidopsis, encodes a novel nuclear-localized protein. *Cell* **1994**, *78*, 109–116. [CrossRef]
19. Benvenuto, G.; Formiggini, F.; Laflamme, P.; Malakhov, M.; Bowler, C. The photomorphogenesis regulator DET1 binds the amino-terminal tail of histone H2B in a nucleosome context. *Curr. Biol.* **2002**, *12*, 1529–1534. [CrossRef] [PubMed]
20. Kim, J.H. Multifaceted chromatin structure and transcription changes in plant stress response. *Int. J. Mol. Sci.* **2021**, *22*, 2013. [CrossRef] [PubMed]

21. Martínez-García, J.F.; Moreno-Romero, J. Shedding light on the chromatin changes that modulate shade responses. *Physiol. Plant.* **2020**, *169*, 407–417. [CrossRef]
22. Perrella, G.; Kaiserli, E. Light behind the curtain: Photoregulation of nuclear architecture and chromatin dynamics in plants. *New Phytol.* **2016**, *212*, 908–919. [CrossRef] [PubMed]
23. Olins, A.L.; Olins, D.E. Spheroid chromatin units (ν bodies). *Science* **1974**, *183*, 330–332. [CrossRef] [PubMed]
24. Pfluger, J.; Wagner, D. Histone modifications and dynamic regulation of genome accessibility in plants. *Curr. Opin. Plant Biol.* **2007**, *10*, 645–652. [CrossRef] [PubMed]
25. Vaillant, I.; Paszkowski, J. Role of histone and DNA methylation in gene regulation. *Curr. Opin. Plant Biol.* **2007**, *10*, 528–533. [CrossRef] [PubMed]
26. Minnoye, L.; Marinov, G.K.; Krausgruber, T.; Pan, L.; Marand, A.P.; Secchia, S.; Greenleaf, W.J.; Furlong, E.E.M.; Zhao, K.; Schmitz, R.J.; et al. Chromatin accessibility profiling methods. *Nat. Rev. Methods Primers* **2021**, *1*, 10. [CrossRef] [PubMed]
27. Mansisidor, A.R.; Risca, V.I. Chromatin accessibility: Methods, mechanisms, and biological insights. *Nucleus* **2022**, *13*, 236–276. [CrossRef] [PubMed]
28. Nisa, M.-U.; Huang, Y.; Benhamed, M.; Raynaud, C. The plant DNA damage response: Signaling pathways leading to growth inhibition and putative role in response to stress conditions. *Front. Plant Sci.* **2019**, *10*, 653. [CrossRef] [PubMed]
29. Klemm, S.L.; Shipony, Z.; Greenleaf, W.J. Chromatin accessibility and the regulatory epigenome. *Nat. Rev. Genet.* **2019**, *20*, 207–220. [CrossRef] [PubMed]
30. Numan, M.; Sun, Y.; Li, G. Exploring the emerging role of long non-coding RNAs (lncRNAs) in plant biology: Functions, mechanisms of action, and future directions. *Plant Physiol. Biochem.* **2024**, *4*, 108797. [CrossRef]
31. Kouzarides, T. Chromatin modifications and their function. *Cell* **2007**, *128*, 693–705. [CrossRef]
32. Millán-Zambrano, G.; Burton, A.; Bannister, A.J.; Schneider, R. Histone post-translational modifications—Cause and consequence of genome function. *Nat. Rev. Genet.* **2022**, *23*, 563–580. [CrossRef] [PubMed]
33. Ramazi, S.; Allahverdi, A.; Zahiri, J. Evaluation of post-translational modifications in histone proteins: A review on histone modification defects in developmental and neurological disorders. *J. Biosci.* **2020**, *45*, 135. [CrossRef]
34. Sterner, D.E.; Berger, S.L. Acetylation of histones and transcription related factors. *Microbiol. Mol. Biol. Rev.* **2000**, *64*, 435–459. [CrossRef] [PubMed]
35. Zhao, T.; Zhan, Z.; Jiang, D. Histone modifications and their regulatory roles in plant development and environmental memory. *J. Genet. Genom.* **2019**, *46*, 467–476. [CrossRef] [PubMed]
36. Pecinka, A.; Chevalier, C.; Colas, I.; Kalantidis, K.; Varotto, S.; Krugman, T.; Michailidis, C.; Vallés, M.P.; Muñoz, A.; Pradillo, M. Chromatin dynamics during interphase and cell division: Similarities and differences between model and crop plants. *J. Exp. Bot.* **2020**, *71*, 5205–5222. [CrossRef] [PubMed]
37. Bhan, A.; Deb, P.; Mandal, S.S. Epigenetic code: Histone modification, gene regulation, and chromatin dynamics. In *Gene Regulation, Epigenetics and Hormone Signaling*; Mandal, S.S., Ed.; Wiley-VCH Verlag GmbH & Co. KGaA: Weinheim, Germany, 2017; Volume 12, pp. 29–58.
38. Patitaki, E.; Schivre, G.; Zioutopoulou, A.; Perrella, G.; Bourbousse, C.; Barneche, F.; Kaiserli, E. Light, chromatin, action: Nuclear events regulating light signaling in Arabidopsis. *New Phytol.* **2022**, *236*, 333–349. [CrossRef] [PubMed]
39. Pandey, R.; Muller, A.; Napoli, C.A.; Selinger, D.A.; Pikaard, C.S.; Richards, E.J.; Bender, J.; Mount, D.W.; Jorgensen, R.A. Analysis of histone acetyltransferase and histone deacetylase families of *Arabidopsis thaliana* suggests functional diversification of chromatin modification among multicellular eukaryotes. *Nucleic Acids Res.* **2002**, *30*, 5036–5055. [CrossRef] [PubMed]
40. Cserhati, M. Motif content comparison between monocot and dicot species. *Genom. Data* **2015**, *3*, 128–136. [CrossRef]
41. Fina, J.P.; Casati, P. HAG3, a histone acetyltransferase, affects UV-B responses by negatively regulating the expression of DNA repair enzymes and sunscreen content in *Arabidopsis thaliana*. *Plant Cell Physiol.* **2015**, *56*, 1388–1400. [CrossRef]
42. Earley, K.W.; Shook, M.S.; Brower-Toland, B.; Hicks, L.; Pikaard, C.S. In vitro specificities of Arabidopsis co-activator histone acetyltransferases: Implications for histone hyperacetylation in gene activation. *Plant J.* **2007**, *52*, 615–626. [CrossRef]
43. Servet, C.; Conde e Silva, N.; Zhou, D. Histone acetyltransferases AtGCN5/HAG1 is a versatile regulator of developmental and inducible gene expression in Arabidopsis. *Mol. Plant* **2010**, *3*, 670–677. [CrossRef] [PubMed]
44. Vandepoele, K.; Vlieghe, K.; Florquin, K.; Hennig, L.; Beemster, G.T.S.; Gruissem, W.; Van de Peer, Y.; Inzé, D.; De Veylder, L. Genome-wide identification of potential plant E2F target genes. *Plant Physiol.* **2005**, *139*, 316–328. [CrossRef] [PubMed]
45. Defraia, C.T.; Zhang, X.; Mou, Z. Elongator subunit 2 is an accelerator of immune responses in *Arabidopsis thaliana*. *Plant J.* **2010**, *64*, 511–523. [CrossRef] [PubMed]
46. Xu, D.; Huang, W.; Li, Y.; Wang, H.; Huang, H.; Cui, X. Elongator complex is critical for cell cycle progression and leaf patterning in Arabidopsis. *Plant J.* **2012**, *69*, 792–808. [CrossRef] [PubMed]
47. Chen, Y.; Guo, P.; Dong, Z. The role of histone acetylation in transcriptional regulation and seed development. *Plant Physiol.* **2024**, *194*, 1962–1979. [CrossRef] [PubMed]
48. Longo, C.; Lepri, A.; Paciolla, A.; Messore, A.; De Vita, D.; Bonaccorsi di Patti, M.C.; Amadei, M.; Madia, V.N.; Ialongo, D.; Di Santo, R.; et al. New inhibitors of the human p300/CBP acetyltransferase are selectively active against the Arabidopsis HAC proteins. *Int. J. Mol. Sci.* **2022**, *23*, 10446. [CrossRef] [PubMed]
49. Boycheva, I.; Vassileva, V.; Iantcheva, A. Histone acetyltransferases in plant development and plasticity. *Curr. Genom.* **2014**, *15*, 28. [CrossRef] [PubMed]

50. Chua, Y.L.; Gray, J.C. Histone modifications and transcription in plants. *Annu. Plant Rev. Online* **2018**, *15*, 79–111.
51. Wang, P.; Abid, M.A.; Qanmber, G.; Askari, M.; Zhou, L.; Song, Y.; Liang, C.; Meng, Z.; Malik, W.; Wie, Y.; et al. Photomorphogenesis in plants: The central role of phytochrome interacting factors (PIFs). *Environ. Exp. Bot.* **2022**, *194*, 104704. [CrossRef]
52. Brestic, M.; Zivcak, M.; Vysoka, D.M.; Barboricova, M.; Gasparovic, K.; Yang, X.; Kataria, S. Acclimation of photosynthetic apparatus to UV-B radiation. In *UV-B Radiation and Crop Growth*; Springer Nature: Singapore, 2023; pp. 223–260.
53. Manova, V.; Georgieva, R.; Borisov, B.; Stoilov, L. Efficient removal of cyclobutane pyrimidine dimers in barley: Differential contribution of light-dependent and dark DNA repair pathways. *Physiol. Plant.* **2016**, *158*, 236–253. [CrossRef]
54. Britt, A.B. DNA damage and repair in plants. *Annu. Rev. Plant Physiol. Plant Mol. Biol.* **1996**, *47*, 75–100. [CrossRef] [PubMed]
55. Banaś, A.K.; Zgłobicki, P.; Kowalska, E.; Bażant, A.; Dziga, D.; Strzałka, W. All you need is light. Photorepair of UV-induced pyrimidine dimers. *Genes* **2020**, *11*, 1304. [CrossRef] [PubMed]
56. Friedberg, E.C.; Walker, G.C.; Seide, W. *DNA Repair and Mutagenesis*; American Society for Microbiology: Washington, DC, USA, 1995.
57. Premi, S.; Han, L.; Mehta, S.; Knight, J.; Zhao, D.; Palmatier, M.A.; Kornacker, K.; Brash, D.E. Genomic sites hypersensitive to ultraviolet radiation. *Proc. Natl. Acad. Sci. USA* **2019**, *116*, 24196–24205. [CrossRef] [PubMed]
58. Bohm, K.A.; Morledge-Hampton, B.; Stevison, S.; Mao, P.; Roberts, S.A.; Wyrick, J.J. Genome-wide maps of rare and atypical UV photoproducts reveal distinct patterns of damage formation and mutagenesis in yeast chromatin. *Proc. Natl. Acad. Sci. USA* **2023**, *120*, e2216907120. [CrossRef] [PubMed]
59. Manova, V.; Gruszka, D. DNA damage and repair in plants–from models to crops. *Front. Plant Sci.* **2015**, *6*, 885. [CrossRef] [PubMed]
60. Szurman-Zubrzycka, M.; Jędrzejek, P.; Szarejko, I. How do plants cope with DNA damage? A concise review on the DDR pathway in plants. *Int. J. Mol. Sci.* **2023**, *24*, 2404. [CrossRef] [PubMed]
61. Campi, M.; D'Andrea, L.; Emiliani, J.; Casati, P. Participation of chromatin-remodeling proteins in the repair of ultraviolet-B-damaged DNA. *Plant Physiol.* **2012**, *158*, 981–995. [CrossRef]
62. Fina, J.P.; Masotti, F.; Rius, S.P.; Crevacuore, F.; Casatti, P. HAC1 and HAF1 histone acetyltransferases have different roles in UV-B responses in Arabidopsis. *Front. Plant Sci.* **2017**, *10*, 1179. [CrossRef] [PubMed]
63. Pan, Y.; Shi, H. Stabilizing the transcription Factors by E3 Ligase COP1. *Trends Plant Sci.* **2017**, *22*, 999–1001. [CrossRef]
64. Castells, E.; Molinier, J.; Drevensek, S.; Genschik, P.; Barneche, F.; Bowler, C. *det1-1*-induced UV-C hyposensitivity through *UVR3* and *PHR1* photolyase gene over-expression. *Plant J.* **2010**, *63*, 392–404. [CrossRef]
65. Guo, L.; Zhou, J.; Elling, A.A.; Charron, J.B.F.; Deng, X.W. Histone modifications and expression of light-regulated genes in Arabidopsis are cooperatively influenced by changing light conditions. *Plant Physiol.* **2008**, *147*, 2070–2083. [CrossRef]
66. Benhamed, M.; Bertrand, C.; Servet, C.; Zhou, D.X. *Arabidopsis GCN5, HD1*, and *TAF1/HAF2* interact to regulate histone acetylation required for light-responsive gene expression. *Plant Cell* **2006**, *18*, 2893–2903. [CrossRef]
67. Bae, G.; Choi, G. Decoding of light signals by plant phytochromes and their interacting proteins. *Annu. Rev. Plant Biol.* **2008**, *59*, 281–311. [CrossRef]
68. Balcerowicz, M.; Fittinghoff, K.; Wirthmueller, L.; Maier, A.; Fackendahl, P.; Fiene, G.; Koncz, C.; Hoecker, U. Light exposure of Arabidopsis seedlings causes rapid de-stabilization as well as selective post-translational inactivation of the repressor of photomorphogenesis SPA2. *Plant J.* **2011**, *65*, 712–723. [CrossRef] [PubMed]
69. Huq, E.; Quail, P.H. PIF4, a phytochrome-interacting bHLH factor, functions as a negative regulator of phytochrome B signaling in *Arabidopsis*. *EMBO J.* **2002**, *21*, 2441–2450. [CrossRef]
70. Su, J.; Liu, B.; Liao, J.; Yang, Z.; Lin, C.; Oka, Y. Coordination of cryptochrome and phytochrome signals in the regulation of plant light responses. *Agronomy* **2017**, *7*, 25. [CrossRef]
71. Jiao, Y.; Lau, O.S.; Deng, X.W. Light-regulated transcriptional networks in higher plants. *Nat. Rev. Genet.* **2007**, *8*, 217–230. [CrossRef] [PubMed]
72. Xu, X.; Paik, I.; Zhu, L.; Bu, Q.; Huang, X.; Deng, X.W.; Huq, E. PHYTOCHROME INTERACTING FACTOR1 enhances the E3 ligase activity of CONSTITUTIVE PHOTOMORPHOGENIC1 to synergistically repress photomorphogenesis in *Arabidopsis*. *Plant Cell* **2014**, *26*, 1992–2006. [CrossRef]
73. Castillon, A.; Shen, H.; Huq, E. Phytochrome Interacting Factors: Central players in phytochrome-mediated light signaling networks. *Trends Plant Sci.* **2007**, *12*, 514–521. [CrossRef] [PubMed]
74. Leivar, P.; Quail, P. PIFs: Pivotal components in a cellular signaling hub. *Trends Plant Sci.* **2011**, *16*, 19–28. [CrossRef]
75. Legris, M.; Ince, Y.Ç.; Fankhauser, C. Molecular mechanisms underlying phytochrome-controlled morphogenesis in plants. *Nat. Commun.* **2019**, *10*, 5219. [CrossRef]
76. Pham, V.N.; Kathare, P.K.; Huq, E. Phytochromes and phytochrome interacting factors. *Plant Physiol.* **2018**, *176*, 1025–1038. [CrossRef]
77. Zhu, L.; Bu, Q.; Xu, X.; Paik, I.; Huang, X.; Hoecker, U.; Deng, X.W.; Huq, E. CUL4 forms an E3 ligase with COP1 and SPA to promote light-induced degradation of PIF1. *Nat. Commun.* **2015**, *6*, 7245. [CrossRef]
78. Xu, D.; Lin, F.; Jiang, Y.; Ling, J.; Hettiarachchi, C.; Tellgren-Roth, C.; Holm, M.; Wei, N.; Deng, X.W. *Arabidopsis* COP1 SUPPRESSOR 2 represses COP1 E3 ubiquitin ligase activity through their coiled-coil domains association. *PLoS Genet.* **2015**, *11*, e1005747. [CrossRef]

79. Huang, X.; Ouyang, X.; Deng, X.W. Beyond repression of photomorphogenesis: Role switching of COP/DET/FUS in light signaling. *Curr. Opin. Plant Biol.* **2014**, *21*, 96–103. [CrossRef]
80. Lau, O.-S.; Deng, X.-W. The photomorphogenic repressors COP1 and DET1: 20 years later. *Trends Plant Sci.* **2012**, *17*, 10. [CrossRef]
81. Ponnu, J.; Hoecker, U. Illuminating the COP1/SPA ubiquitin ligase: Fresh insights into its structure and functions during plant photomorphogenesis. *Front. Plant Sci.* **2021**, *12*, 662793. [CrossRef]
82. Ang, L.H.; Chattopadhyay, S.; Wei, N.; Oyama, T.; Okada, K.; Batschauer, A.; Deng, X.W. Molecular interaction between COP1 and HY5 defines a regulatory switch for light control of *Arabidopsis* development. *Mol. Cell* **1998**, *1*, 213–222. [CrossRef]
83. Jing, Y.; Guo, Q.; Lin, R. The SNL-HDA19 histone deacetylase complex antagonizes HY5 activity to repress photomorphogenesis in Arabidopsis. *New Phytol.* **2021**, *229*, 3221–3236. [CrossRef]
84. Dyachok, J.; Zhu, L.; Liao, F.; He, J.; Huq, E.; Blancaflor, E.B. SCAR mediates light-induced root elongation in *Arabidopsis* through photoreceptors and proteasomes. *Plant Cell* **2011**, *23*, 3610–3626. [CrossRef]
85. Wang, F.F.; Lian, H.L.; Kang, C.Y.; Yang, H.Q. Phytochrome B is involved in mediating red light-induced stomatal opening in *Arabidopsis thaliana*. *Mol. Plant* **2010**, *3*, 246–259. [CrossRef]
86. Catala, R.; Medina, J.; Salinas, J. Integration of low temperature and light signaling during cold acclimation response in *Arabidopsis*. *Proc. Natl. Acad. Sci. USA* **2011**, *108*, 16475–16480. [CrossRef]
87. Yu, Y.; Wang, J.; Zhang, Z.; Quan, R.; Zhang, H.; Deng, X.W.; Ma, L.; Huang, R. Ethylene promotes hypocotyl growth and HY5 degradation by enhancing the movement of COP1 to the nucleus in the light. *PLoS Genet.* **2013**, *9*, e1004025. [CrossRef]
88. Bhatnagar, A.; Singh, S.; Khurana, J.P.; Burman, N. HY5-COP1: The central module of light signaling pathway. *J. Plant Biochem. Biotechnol.* **2020**, *29*, 590–610. [CrossRef]
89. Liu, L.J.; Zhang, Y.C.; Li, Q.H.; Sang, Y.; Mao, J.; Lian, H.L.; Wang, L.; Yang, H.Q. COP1-mediated ubiquitination of CONSTANS is implicated in cryptochrome regulation of flowering in *Arabidopsis*. *Plant Cell* **2008**, *20*, 292–306. [CrossRef]
90. Jang, S.; Marchal, V.; Panigrahi, K.C.S.; Wenkel, S.; Soppe, W.; Deng, X.D.; Valverde, F.; Coupland, G. *Arabidopsis* COP1 shapes the temporal pattern of CO accumulation conferring a photoperiodic flowering response. *EMBO J.* **2008**, *27*, 1277–1288. [CrossRef]
91. Yu, J.W.; Rubio, V.; Lee, N.Y.; Bai, S.; Lee, S.Y.; Kim, S.S.; Liu, L.; Zhang, Y.; Irigoyen, M.L.; Sullivan, J.A.; et al. COP1 and ELF3 control circadian function and photoperiodic flowering by regulating GI stability. *Mol. Cell* **2008**, *32*, 617–630. [CrossRef]
92. Favory, J.J.; Stec, A.; Gruber, H.; Rizzini, L.; Oravecz, A.; Funk, M.; Albert, A.; Cloix, C.; Jenkins, G.I.; Oakeley, E.J.; et al. Interaction of COP1 and UVR8 regulates UVB-induced photomorphogenesis and stress acclimation in *Arabidopsis*. *EMBO J.* **2009**, *28*, 591–601. [CrossRef]
93. Kang, C.Y.; Lian, H.L.; Wang, F.F.; Huang, J.R.; Yang, H.Q. Cryptochromes, phytochromes, and COP1 regulate light-controlled stomatal development in *Arabidopsis*. *Plant Cell* **2009**, *21*, 2624–2641. [CrossRef]
94. Jeong, R.D.; Chandra-Shekara, A.C.; Barman, S.R.; Navarre, D.; Klessig, D.F.; Kachroo, A.; Kachroo, P. Cryptochrome 2 and phototropin 2 regulate resistance protein-mediated viral defense by negatively regulating an E3 ubiquitin ligase. *Proc. Natl. Acad. Sci. USA* **2010**, *107*, 13538–13543. [CrossRef]
95. Tanaka, N.; Itoh, H.; Sentoku, N.; Kojima, M.; Sakakibara, H.; Izawa, T.; Itoh, J.; Nagato, Y. The *COP1* ortholog PPS regulates the juvenile-adult and vegetative-reproductive phase changes in rice. *Plant Cell* **2011**, *23*, 2143–2154. [CrossRef]
96. Wang, W.; Chen, Q.; Botella, J.R.; Guo, S. Beyond light: Insights into the role of constitutively photomorphogenic1 in plant hormonal signaling. *Front. Plant Sci.* **2019**, *10*, 557. [CrossRef]
97. Zhao, L.; Wang, C.; Zhu, Y.; Zhao, J.; Wu, X. Molecular cloning and sequencing of the cDNA of cop1 gene from *Pisum sativum*. *Biochim. Biophys. Acta* **1998**, *1395*, 326–328. [CrossRef]
98. Liu, Y.; Roof, S.; Ye, Z.; Barry, C.; van Tuinen, A.; Vrebalov, J.; Bowler, C.; Giovannoni, J. Manipulation of light signal transduction as a means of modifying fruit nutritional quality in tomato. *Proc. Natl. Acad. Sci. USA* **2004**, *101*, 9897–9902. [CrossRef]
99. Tsuge, T.; Inagaki, N.; Yoshizumi, T.; Shimada, H.; Kawamoto, T.; Matsuki, R.; Yamamoto, N.; Matsui, M. Phytochrome-mediated control of *COP1* gene expression in rice plants. *Mol. Genet. Genom.* **2001**, *265*, 43–50. [CrossRef]
100. Wang, H.; Kang, D.; Deng, X.-W.; Wei, N. Evidence for functional conservation of a mammalian homologue of light-responsive plant protein COP1. *Curr. Biol.* **1999**, *9*, 711–714. [CrossRef]
101. Deng, X.W.; Matsui, M.; Wei, N.; Wagner, D.; Chu, A.M.; Feldmann, K.A.; Quail, P.H. *COP1*, an Arabidopsis regulatory gene, encodes a protein with both a zinc-binding motif and a G_β homologous domain. *Cell* **1992**, *71*, 791–801. [CrossRef]
102. Yi, C.; Deng, X.W. COP1—From plant photomorphogenesis to mammalian tumorigenesis. *Trends Cell Biol.* **2005**, *15*, 618–625. [CrossRef]
103. Holtkotte, X.; Dieterle, S.; Kokkelink, L.; Artz, O.; Leson, L.; Fittinghoff, K.; Hayama, R.; Ahmad, M.; Hoecker, U. Mutations in the N-terminal kinase-like domain of the repressor of photomorphogenesis SPA1 severely impair SPA1 function but not light responsiveness in Arabidopsis. *Plant J.* **2016**, *88*, 205–218. [CrossRef]
104. Holm, M.; Hardtke, C.S.; Gaudet, R.; Deng, X.W. Identification of a structural motif that confers specific interaction with the WD40 repeat domain of *Arabidopsis* COP1. *EMBO J.* **2001**, *20*, 118–127. [CrossRef]
105. Hoecker, U.; Quail, P.H. The phytochrome A-specific signaling intermediate SPA1 interacts directly with COP1, a constitutive repressor of light signaling in *Arabidopsis*. *J. Biol. Chem.* **2001**, *276*, 38173–38178. [CrossRef]
106. Hoecker, U. The activities of the E3 ubiquitin ligase COP1/SPA, a key repressor in light signaling. *Curr. Opin. Plant Biol.* **2017**, *37*, 63–69. [CrossRef]

107. Zhu, D.; Maier, A.; Lee, J.H.; Laubinger, S.; Saijo, Y.; Wang, H.; Qu, L.J.; Hoecker, U.; Deng, X.W. Biochemical characterization of *Arabidopsis* complexes containing CONSTITUTIVELY PHOTOMORPHOGENIC1 and SUPPRESSOR OF PHYA proteins in light control of plant development. *Plant Cell* **2008**, *20*, 2307–2323. [CrossRef]
108. Saijo, Y.; Sullivan, J.A.; Wang, H.; Yang, J.; Shen, Y.; Rubio, V.; Ma, L.; Hoecker, U.; Deng, X.W. The COP1–SPA1 interaction defines a critical step in phytochrome A-mediated regulation of HY5 activity. *Genes Dev.* **2003**, *17*, 2642–2647. [CrossRef]
109. Osterlund, M.T.; Hardtke, C.S.; Wei, N.; Deng, X.W. Targeted destabilization of HY5 during light-regulated development of *Arabidopsis*. *Nature* **2000**, *405*, 462–466. [CrossRef]
110. Yang, J.; Lin, R.; Hoecker, U.; Liu, B.; Xu, L.; Wang, H. Repression of light signaling by Arabidopsis SPA1 involves post-translational regulation of HFR1 protein accumulation. *Plant J.* **2005**, *43*, 131–141. [CrossRef]
111. Rolauffs, S.; Fackendahl, P.; Sahm, J.; Fiene, G.; Hoecker, U. Arabidopsis *COP1* and *SPA* genes are essential for plant elongation but not for acceleration of flowering time in response to a low red light to far-red light ratio. *Plant Physiol.* **2012**, *160*, 2015–2027. [CrossRef]
112. Maier, A.; Schrader, A.; Kokkelink, L.; Falke, C.; Welter, B.; Iniesto, E.; Rubio, V.; Uhrig, J.F.; Hulskamp, M.; Hoecker, U. Light and the E3 ubiquitin ligase COP1/SPA control the protein stability of the MYB transcription factors PAP1 and PAP2 involved in anthocyanin accumulation in Arabidopsis. *Plant J.* **2013**, *74*, 638–651. [CrossRef]
113. Han, X.; Huang, X.; Deng, X.W. The photomorphogenic central repressor COP1: Conservation and functional diversification during evolution. *Plant Commun.* **2020**, *1*, 100044. [CrossRef]
114. Pacin, M.; Legris, M.; Casal, J.J. Rapid decline in nuclear COSTITUTIVE PHOTOMORPHOGENESIS1 abundance anticipates the stabilization of its target ELONGATED HYPOCOTYL5 in the light. *Plant Physiol.* **2014**, *164*, 1134–1138. [CrossRef]
115. Lin, X.L.; Niu, D.; Hu, Z.L.; Kim, D.H.; Jin, Y.H.; Cai, B.; Liu, P.; Miura, K.; Yun, D.J.; Kim, W.Y.; et al. An Arabidopsis SUMO E3 Ligase, SIZ1, negatively regulates photomorphogenesis by promoting COP1 activity. *PLoS Genet.* **2016**, *12*, e1006016. [CrossRef]
116. Delker, C.; Sonntag, L.; James, G.V.; Janitza, P.; Ibanez, C.; Ziermann, H.; Peterson, T.; Denk, K.; Mull, S.; Ziegler, J.; et al. The DET1–COP1–HY5 pathway constitutes a multipurpose signaling module regulating plant photomorphogenesis and thermomorphogenesis. *Cell Rep.* **2014**, *9*, 1983–1989. [CrossRef] [PubMed]
117. Jang, K.; Lee, H.G.; Jung, S.J.; Paek, N.C.; Seo, P.J. The E3 ubiquitin ligase COP1 regulates thermosensory flowering by triggering GI degradation in *Arabidopsis*. *Sci. Rep.* **2015**, *5*, 12071. [CrossRef] [PubMed]
118. Tsuchiya, Y.; Vidaurre, D.; Toh, S.; Hanada, A.; Nambara, E.; Kamiya, Y.; Yamaguchi, S.; McCourt, P. A small-molecule screen identifies new functions for the plant hormone strigolactone. *Nat. Chem. Biol.* **2010**, *6*, 741–749. [CrossRef]
119. Oravecz, A.; Baumann, A.; Máté, Z.; Brzezinska, A.; Molinier, J.; Oakeley, E.J.; Adam, E.; Schafer, E.; Nagy, F.; Ulm, R. CONSTITUTIVELY PHOTOMORPHOGENIC1 is required for the UV-B response in *Arabidopsis*. *Plant Cell* **2006**, *18*, 1975–1990. [CrossRef]
120. Yin, R.; Skvortsova, M.Y.; Loubéry, S.; Ulm, R. COP1 is required for UV-B–induced nuclear accumulation of the UVR8 photoreceptor. *Proc. Natl. Acad. Sci. USA* **2016**, *113*, E4415–E4422. [CrossRef]
121. Boycheva, I.; Georgieva, R.; Stoilov, L.; Manova, V. Effects of light and UV-C radiation on the transcriptional activity of *COP1* and *HY5* gene homologues in barley. In *Mutation Breeding, Genetic Diversity and Crop Adaptation to Climate Change*; CABI: Wallingford, UK, 2021; pp. 478–486.
122. Kliebenstein, D.J.; Lim, J.E.; Landry, L.G.; Last, R.L. Arabidopsis *UVR8* regulates ultraviolet-B signal transduction and tolerance and contains sequence similarity to human *Regulator of Chromatin Condensation 1*. *Plant Physiol.* **2002**, *130*, 234–243. [CrossRef] [PubMed]
123. Podolec, R.; Demarsy, E.; Ulm, R. Perception and signaling of ultraviolet-B radiation in plants. *Annu. Rev. Plant Biol.* **2021**, *72*, 793–822. [CrossRef] [PubMed]
124. Ulm, R.; Jenkins, G.I. Q&A: How do plants sense and respond to UV-B radiation? *BMC Biol.* **2015**, *13*, 45.
125. Hideg, E.; Jansen, M.A.; Strid, A. UV-B exposure, ROS, and stress: Inseparable companions or loosely linked associates? *Trends Plant Sci.* **2013**, *18*, 107–115. [CrossRef]
126. Fasano, R.; Gonzalez, N.; Tosco, A.; Dal Piaz, F.; Docimo, T.; Serrano, R.; Grillo, S.; Leone, A.; Inze, D. Role of Arabidopsis *UV RESISTANCE LOCUS 8* in plant growth reduction under osmotic stress and low levels of UV-B. *Mol. Plant* **2014**, *7*, 773–791. [CrossRef] [PubMed]
127. Feher, B.; Kozma-Bognar, L.; Kevei, E.; Hajdu, A.; Binkert, M.; Davis, S.J.; Schafer, E.; Ulm, R.; Nagy, F. Functional interaction of the circadian clock and UV RESISTANCE LOCUS 8-controlled UV-B signaling pathways in *Arabidopsis thaliana*. *Plant J.* **2011**, *67*, 37–48. [CrossRef] [PubMed]
128. Tossi, V.; Lamattina, L.; Jenkins, G.I.; Cassia, R.O. Ultraviolet-B-induced stomatal closure in Arabidopsis is regulated by the UV RESISTANCE LOCUS8 photoreceptor in a nitric oxide-dependent mechanism. *Plant Physiol.* **2014**, *164*, 2220–2230. [CrossRef] [PubMed]
129. Wargent, J.J.; Gegas, V.C.; Jenkins, G.I.; Doonan, J.H.; Paul, N.D. UVR8 in *Arabidopsis thaliana* regulates multiple aspects of cellular differentiation during leaf development in response to ultraviolet B radiation. *New Phytol.* **2009**, *183*, 315–326. [CrossRef] [PubMed]
130. Vandenbussche, F.; Van Der Straeten, D. Differential accumulation of ELONGATED HYPOCOTYL5 correlates with hypocotyl bending to ultraviolet-B light. *Plant Physiol.* **2014**, *166*, 40–43. [CrossRef] [PubMed]

131. Wu, D.; Hu, Q.; Yan, Z.; Chen, W.; Yan, C.; Huang, X.; Zhang, J.; Yang, P.; Deng, H.; Wang, J.; et al. Structural basis of ultraviolet-B perception by UVR8. *Nature* **2012**, *484*, 214–219. [PubMed]
132. Christie, J.M.; Arvai, A.S.; Baxter, K.J.; Heilmann, M.; Pratt, A.J.; O'Hara, A.; Kelly, S.M.; Hothorn, M.; Smith, B.O.; Hitomi, K.; et al. Plant UVR8 photoreceptor senses UV-B by tryptophan-mediated disruption of cross-dimer salt bridges. *Science* **2012**, *335*, 1492–1496. [CrossRef] [PubMed]
133. Jenkins, G.I. Structure and function of the UV-B photoreceptor UVR8. *Curr. Opin. Struct. Biol.* **2014**, *29*, 52–57. [CrossRef] [PubMed]
134. O'Hara, A.; Jenkins, G.I. In vivo function of tryptophans in the *Arabidopsis* UV-B photoreceptor UVR8. *Plant Cell* **2012**, *24*, 3755–3766. [CrossRef]
135. Li, X.; Liu, Z.; Ren, H.; Kundu, M.; Zhong, F.W.; Wang, L.; Gao, J.; Zhong, D. Dynamics and mechanism of dimer dissociation of photoreceptor UVR8. *Nat. Commun.* **2022**, *13*, 93. [CrossRef]
136. Cloix, C.; Kaiserli, E.; Heilmann, M.; Baxter, K.J.; Brown, B.A.; O'Hara, A.; Smith, B.O.; Christie, J.M.; Jenkins, G.I. C-terminal region of the UV-B photoreceptor UVR8 initiates signaling through interaction with the COP1 protein. *Proc. Natl. Acad. Sci. USA* **2012**, *109*, 16366–16370. [CrossRef] [PubMed]
137. Yin, R.; Arongaus, A.B.; Binkert, M.; Ulm, R. Two distinct domains of the UVR8 photoreceptor interact with COP1 to initiate UV-B signaling in Arabidopsis. *Plant Cell* **2015**, *27*, 202–213. [CrossRef] [PubMed]
138. Rizzini, L.; Favory, J.J.; Cloix, C.; Faggionato, D.; O'Hara, A.; Kaiserli, E.; Baumeister, R.; Schafer, E.; Nagy, F.; Jenkins, G.I.; et al. Perception of UV-B by the *Arabidopsis* UVR8 protein. *Science* **2011**, *332*, 103–106. [CrossRef] [PubMed]
139. Brown, B.A.; Cloix, C.; Jiang, G.H.; Kaiserli, E.; Herzyk, P.; Kliebenstein, D.J.; Jenkins, G.I. A UV-B-specific signaling component orchestrates plant UV protection. *Proc. Natl. Acad. Sci. USA* **2005**, *102*, 18225–18230. [CrossRef] [PubMed]
140. Huang, X.; Ouyang, X.; Yang, P.; Lau, O.S.; Chen, L.; Wei, N.; Deng, X.W. Conversion from CUL4-based COP1-SPA E3 apparatus to UVR8-COP1-SPA complexes underlies a distinct biochemical function of COP1 under UV-B. *Proc. Natl. Acad. Sci. USA* **2013**, *110*, 16669–16674. [CrossRef] [PubMed]
141. Volná, A.; Červeň, J.; Nezval, J.; Pech, R.; Špunda, V. Complex role of photoreceptors in light and temperature sensing: From mechanism to the target genes regulation. A focus on the genes related to the biosynthesis of phenolic compounds. *Preprints* **2024**, *24*, 2024012145. [CrossRef]
142. Ulm, R.; Baumann, A.; Oravecz, A.; Mate, Z.; Adam, E.; Oakeley, E.J.; Schafer, E.; Nagy, F. Genome-wide analysis of gene expression reveals function of the bZIP transcription factor HY5 in the UV-B response of *Arabidopsis*. *Proc. Natl. Acad. Sci. USA* **2004**, *101*, 1397–1402. [CrossRef]
143. Huang, X.; Ouyang, X.; Yang, P.; Lau, O.S.; Li, G.; Li, J.; Chen, H.; Deng, X.W. *Arabidopsis* FHY3 and HY5 positively mediate induction of *COP1* transcription in response to photomorphogenic UV-B light. *Plant Cell* **2012**, *24*, 4590–4606. [CrossRef]
144. Liang, T.; Yang, Y.; Liu, H. Signal transduction mediated by the plant UV-B photoreceptor UVR8. *New Phytol.* **2019**, *221*, 1247–1252. [CrossRef]
145. Heijde, M.; Ulm, R. Reversion of the *Arabidopsis* UV-B photoreceptor UVR8 to the homodimeric ground state. *Proc. Natl. Acad. Sci. USA* **2013**, *110*, 1113–1118. [CrossRef]
146. Britt, A.B. Repair of DNA damage induced by solar UV. *Photosynth. Res.* **2004**, *81*, 105–112. [CrossRef]
147. Landry, L.G.; Stapleton, A.E.; Lim, J.; Hoffman, P.; Hays, J.B.; Walbot, V.; Last, R.L. An *Arabidopsis* photolyase mutant is hypersensitive to ultraviolet-B radiation. *Proc. Natl. Acad. Sci. USA* **1997**, *94*, 328–332. [CrossRef] [PubMed]
148. Jansen, M.A.K.; Gaba, V.; Greenberg, B.M. Higher plants and UV-B radiation: Balancing damage, repair and acclimation. *Trends Plant Sci.* **1998**, *3*, 131–135. [CrossRef]
149. Schmidt, C.K.; Jackson, S.P. On your MARK, get SET(D2), go! H3K36me3 primers DNA mis match repair. *Cell* **2013**, *153*, 513–515. [CrossRef]
150. Waterworth, W.M.; Drury, G.E.; Blundell-Hunter, G.; West, C.E. Arabidopsis TAF1 is an MRE11-interacting protein required for resistance to genotoxic stress and viability of the male gametophyte. *Plant J.* **2015**, *84*, 545–557. [CrossRef]

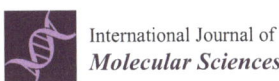

International Journal of
Molecular Sciences

MDPI

Article

Selenium Nanoparticle and Melatonin Treatments Improve Melon Seedling Growth by Regulating Carbohydrate and Polyamine

Lu Kang [1,2,3], Yujiao Jia [1], Yangliu Wu [4], Hejiang Liu [3], Duoyong Zhao [3], Yanjun Ju [3], Canping Pan [1,*] and Jiefei Mao [2,*]

1   Key Laboratory of National Forestry and Grassland Administration on Pest Chemical Control and Innovation Center of Pesticide Research, College of Science, China Agricultural University, Beijing 100193, China; 96208zx@163.com (L.K.)
2   State Key Laboratory of Desert and Oasis Ecology, Key Laboratory of Ecological Safety and Sustainable Development in Arid Lands, Xinjiang Institute of Ecology and Geography, Chinese Academy of Sciences, Urumqi 830011, China
3   Institute of Agricultural Quality Standards and Testing Technology, Xinjiang Academy of Agricultural Sciences, Urumqi 830091, China
4   School of Biological Science and Technology, University of Jinan, Jinan 250022, China
*   Correspondence: canpingp@cau.edu.cn (C.P.); mjf@ms.xjb.ac.cn (J.M.); Tel.: +86-10-6273197 (C.P.); +86-991-7827370 (J.M.); Fax: +86-10-62733620 (C.P.)

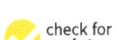

check for
updates

Citation: Kang, L.; Jia, Y.; Wu, Y.; Liu, H.; Zhao, D.; Ju, Y.; Pan, C.; Mao, J. Selenium Nanoparticle and Melatonin Treatments Improve Melon Seedling Growth by Regulating Carbohydrate and Polyamine. *Int. J. Mol. Sci.* **2024**, *25*, 7830. https://doi.org/10.3390/ijms25147830

Academic Editors: Philippe Jeandet and Mateusz Labudda

Received: 26 June 2024
Revised: 12 July 2024
Accepted: 15 July 2024
Published: 17 July 2024

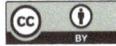

Abstract: Bio-stimulants, such as selenium nanoparticles and melatonin, regulate melon growth. However, the effects of individual and combined applications of selenium nanoparticles and melatonin on the growth of melon seedlings have not been reported. Here, two melon cultivars were sprayed with selenium nanoparticles, melatonin, and a combined treatment, and physiological and biochemical properties were analyzed. The independent applications of selenium nanoparticles, melatonin, and their combination had no significant effects on the plant heights and stem diameters of Jiashi and Huangmengcui melons. Compared with the controls, both selenium nanoparticle and melatonin treatments increased soluble sugars (6–63%) and sucrose (11–88%) levels, as well as the activity of sucrose phosphate synthase (171–237%) in melon leaves. The phenylalanine ammonia lyase (29–95%), trans cinnamate 4-hydroxylase (32–100%), and 4-coumaric acid CoA ligase (26–113%), as well as mRNA levels, also increased in the phenylpropanoid metabolism pathway. Combining the selenium nanoparticles and melatonin was more effective than either of the single treatments. In addition, the levels of superoxide dismutase (43–130%), catalase (14–43%), ascorbate peroxidase (44–79%), peroxidase (25–149%), and mRNA in melon leaves treated with combined selenium nanoparticles and melatonin were higher than in controls. The results contribute to our understanding of selenium nanoparticles and melatonin as bio-stimulants that improve the melon seedlings' growth by regulating carbohydrate, polyamine, and antioxidant capacities.

Keywords: bio-stimulants; melon; primary metabolism; secondary metabolism

1. Introduction

Melon (*Cucumis melo* L.) is a vital economic vegetable crop worldwide [1,2], with a global production of 27.3 million metric tons. For commercial cultivation, the cultivars Jiashi (JSG) and Huang mengcui (HMC) melon are the most important [3]. Selenium nanoparticles, melatonin, and other bio-stimulants have no negative effects on endophytic bacteria; therefore, they may be conducive to promoting plant health [4]. Plant primary metabolites are directly involved in growth, development, and reproduction [5]. Plant secondary metabolites are not only useful natural products, but they also play important roles in plant defense systems against pathogenic attacks and environmental stresses [6,7]. Plant secondary metabolites provide defense functions and regulate defense-signaling pathways that protect plants in response to herbivore invasion [8]. Plants produce three main types of secondary metabolites, phenols, terpenes, and nitrogen/sulfur compounds. The shikimic acid pathway leads to the formation of phenolic products involved in plant defenses. Terpenes, based on 5-C isoterpenoids, are toxins and deter herbivores, and nitrogen and sulfur compounds are synthesized mainly from amino acids [9].

Selenium nanoparticles are less toxic and more biocompatible than sodium selenate or sodium selenite [10]. Selenium nanoparticles increase the carboxylase activity of ribulose diphosphate and the chlorophyll content, especially through the activation of some key genes and proteins involved in the photosynthetic system. Treatments of 25–50 $\mu mol \cdot L^{-1}$ selenium nanoparticles reduce the large amount of reactive oxygen species (ROS) produced by nicotinamide adenine dinucleotide phosphate oxidase and enhance glutathione peroxidase (GSH-Px), thereby reducing protein carbonylation in rice seedlings [11]. Foliar applications of 25 $mg \cdot L^{-1}$ selenium nanoparticles increase cucumber height and leaf area [12]. The activities of antioxidant enzymes in plants are key factors in alleviating the effects of external stress [13,14]. The exogenous application of selenium nanoparticles improves the photosynthetic pigments of rape by increasing the activities of antioxidant enzymes, such as catalase (CAT), ascorbate peroxidase (APX), and superoxide dismutase (SOD). Additionally, the expression of stress-response genes enhances the drought and heat tolerances of rape [15,16].

Selenium nanoparticles enhance the antioxidant capacity mainly by improving the metabolic pathways of glutathione, carbon, and nitrogen, thereby improving various physiological indexes of maize that promote its growth [17]. Nanotechnology increases plant productivity, nutrient absorption, and agronomic soil properties, which result in improved plant growth and productivity [18–20]. Nanotechnology is widely considered to be on the cutting edge, with the potential to promote plant science research because nanoparticles have unique physicochemical properties compared with bulk particles [21,22].

Melatonin acts as a bio-stimulant of plant development, including germination, photosynthesis, and water utilization [23–25]. Melatonin is a key molecule in plant immune responses, along with nitric oxide, jasmonic acid, and salicylic acid [26,27]. Melatonin is involved in growth and photosynthetic processes. Melatonin causes multiple changes at the mRNA level and is a multi-regulatory molecule capable of coordinating many aspects of plant development [28]. Melatonin treatments significantly reduce hydrogen peroxide (H_2O_2) and malondialdehyde (MDA) contents, enhance the non-enzymatic antioxidant system's capacity, and increase CAT, peroxidase (POD), SOD, and APX activity levels [29]. Melatonin enhances the antioxidant capacity of cotton, improves photosynthetic efficiency, reduces chlorophyll degradation and ROS accumulation, inhibits ABA synthesis, and delays the drought-induced senescence of cotton leaves [30]. Strawberries soaked in melatonin maintain fresh weights and fruit firmness, and they have reduced *Botrytis cinerea* infection levels. Additionally, melatonin treatments increase 1,1-diphenyl-2-picrohydrazyl radical (DPPH) clearance, as well as CAT, SOD, POD, and APX activity levels [31]. The application of melatonin improves the internal nutrition and flavor quality of tomato fruit by regulating the accumulations of primary and secondary metabolites during the ripening process [32].

Foliar applications of selenium nanoparticles enhance the antioxidant ability and the cucurbitacin B level of melon [33]. However, there have been no systematic reports on the effects of melatonin or selenium nanoparticle + melatonin combination applications on melon. This study aimed to explore the effects of selenium nanoparticle + melatonin combination treatments on the physiological and biochemical characteristics of melon plants. We investigated the effects of single applications of selenium nanoparticles and melatonin on plants, and we hypothesized that the combined application of bio-stimulant selenium nanoparticles + melatonin would have a synergistic effect. The goals were to provide a theoretical basis and technical support for the rational use of the selenium nanoparticle + melatonin combination to regulate the amino acid, carbohydrate, polyamine, and antioxidant capacities of melon.

2. Results

2.1. Effects of Selenium Nanoparticles and Melatonin on Plant Biomass

The effects of selenium nanoparticles, melatonin, and their combination on fresh and dry weights, plant heights, and stem diameters are shown in Figure S1. The independent applications of selenium nanoparticles and melatonin did not have significant effects on melon plant height or stem diameter. Compared with the controls, independent foliar spraying of selenium nanoparticles, melatonin, and selenium nanoparticles + melatonin increased the stem fresh weights of JSG by 23%, 6%, and 6%, respectively, and those of HMC by 9%, 6%, and 10%, respectively. All three treatments increased stem dry weights of JSG by 13–25% and of HMC by 8–19% compared with controls.

2.2. Lipoxygenase and Plant Hormones after Selenium Nanoparticle and Melatonin Treatments

The effects of selenium nanoparticles, melatonin, and the selenium nanoparticle + melatonin combination on plant hormones in melon are shown in Figure 1. Compared with controls, melatonin and selenium nanoparticles + melatonin significantly increased the IAA in leaves of JSG and HMC by 291–236% and 41–83%, respectively (Figure 1A). The three treatments had no significant effects on JA and SA (Figure 1B,C) in leaves of JSG and HMC compared with controls. The effects of selenium nanoparticles, melatonin, and the selenium nanoparticle + melatonin combination on lipoxygenase and mRNA levels in melon are shown in Figure 1D–I. The selenium nanoparticles, melatonin, and selenium nanoparticle + melatonin foliar interventions had no significant effects on LOX activity or the transcription levels in JSG and HMC leaves, except for *LOX2* and *LOX9* mRNA levels.

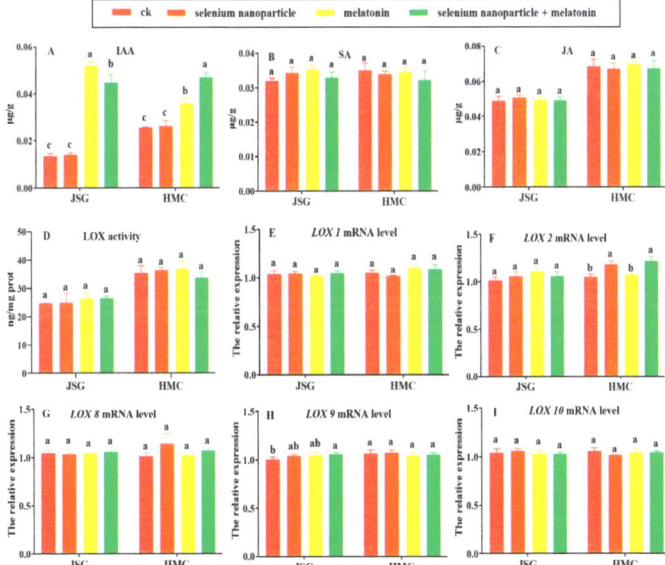

Figure 1. Effects of selenium nanoparticles and melatonin on plant hormone content and lipoxygenase in two melon cultivars. JSG and HMC refer to melon cultivars. Different letters indicate a significant difference ($p < 0.05$) between treatments. (**A**): IAA content, (**B**): SA content, (**C**): JA content, (**D**): LOX activity, (**E**): *LOX1* mRNA level, (**F**): *LOX2* mRNA level, (**G**): *LOX8* mRNA level, (**H**): *LOX9* mRNA level, (**I**): *LOX10* mRNA level.

2.3. Effects of Selenium Nanoparticle and Melatonin Treatments on Amino Acid and Carbohydrate Metabolism

The effects of selenium nanoparticles, melatonin, and the selenium nanoparticle + melatonin combination on amino acid and carbohydrate metabolism in melon leaves are shown in Figure 2. Compared with controls, melatonin and selenium nanoparticles + melatonin significantly increased the total amino acids of JSG, by 20% and 6%, respectively, and in HMC leaves by 26% and 16%, respectively (Figure 2A). The selenium nanoparticles and selenium nanoparticle + melatonin combination increased glutamate in leaves of JSG by 37% and 42%, respectively, and in HMC by 21% and 26%, respectively, compared with the controls (Figure 2B). The effects of the three treatments on the GS activity of JSG leaves were not significant. Compared with controls, the selenium nanoparticles and selenium nanoparticle + melatonin combination significantly increased the GS activity of HMC leaves, by 19% and 18%, respectively (Figure 2C). The three treatments significantly increased the GABA of JSG and HMC leaves by 279–386% and 16–57%, respectively, compared with controls (Figure 2D). Compared with controls, the three treatments significantly increased soluble sugars in the two cultivars by 6–63% (Figure 2E). The three treatments significantly increased the sucrose contents of the two cultivars by 11–88% compared with controls (Figure 2F). Compared with controls, the selenium nanoparticles and selenium nanoparticle + melatonin combination significantly increased the reducing sugars in JSG leaves by 12–14% and in HMC leaves by 30–36% (Figure 2G). The selenium nanoparticle, melatonin, and selenium nanoparticle + melatonin combination groups significantly increased SS activities in JSG leaves by 19–46% and in HMC leaves by 16–20% compared with controls (Figure 2H). The three treatments significantly increased the SPS activities in JSG leaves by 171–237% and in HMC leaves by 46–88% compared with controls (Figure 2I).

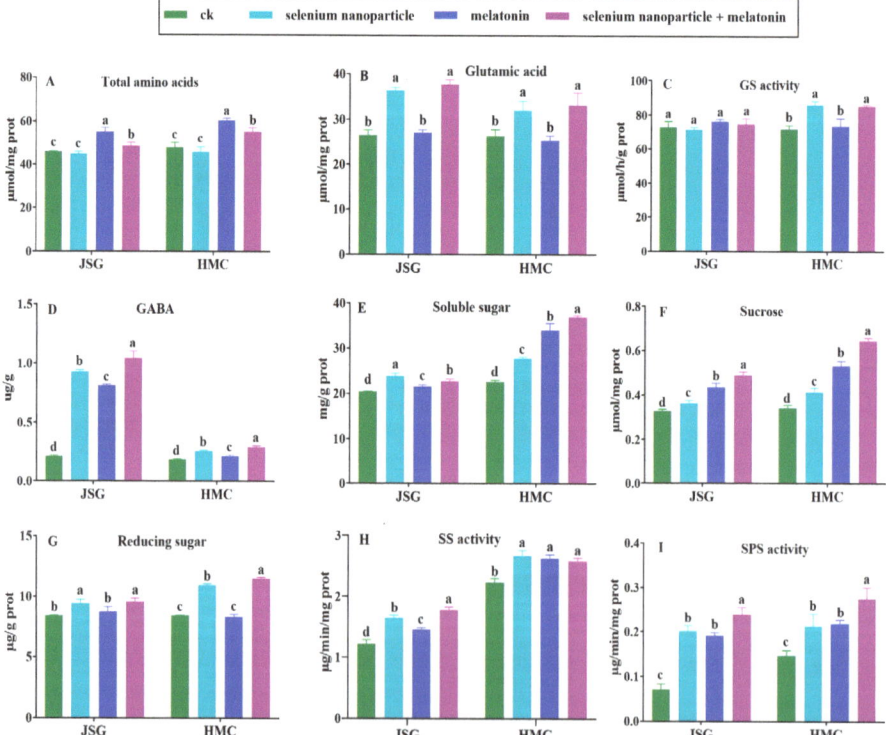

Figure 2. Effects of selenium nanoparticles and melatonin on amino acid content, carbohydrate metabolism in two melon cultivars. JSG and HMC refer to melon cultivars. Different letters indicate a significant difference ($p < 0.05$) between treatments. (**A**): Total amino acids content, (**B**): Glutamic acid content, (**C**): GS activity, (**D**): GABA content, (**E**): Soluble sugar content, (**F**): Sucrose content, (**G**): Reducing sugar content, (**H**): SS activity, (**I**): SPS activity.

2.4. Effects of Selenium Nanoparticle and Melatonin Treatments on Secondary Metabolism

2.4.1. Selenium Nanoparticle and Melatonin Effects on Lignin Synthesis

The effects of selenium nanoparticles, melatonin, and selenium nanoparticle + melatonin combination on lignin synthesis in melon are shown in Figure 3. Compared with controls, the selenium nanoparticles and selenium nanoparticles + melatonin significantly increased the lignin level in JSG leaves by 22% and 8%, respectively, and in HMC leaves by 18% and 8%, respectively (Figure 3A). The three treatments significantly increased the hydroxyproline level by 25–44% in JSG leaves and by 23–30% in HMC leaves compared with controls (Figure 3B). Compared with controls, selenium nanoparticles, melatonin, and the selenium nanoparticle + melatonin combination significantly increased CAD activities in JSG leaves by 50%, 24%, and 33%, respectively, and in HMC leaves by 40%, 54%, and 30%, respectively (Figure 3C). The three treatments significantly increased the *CAD* mRNA level in JSG leaves by 53–77% compared with controls (Figure 3D). The selenium nanoparticle, melatonin, and selenium nanoparticle + melatonin combination groups had no significant effects on *CCR* expression in either cultivar's leaves compared with controls (Figure 3E).

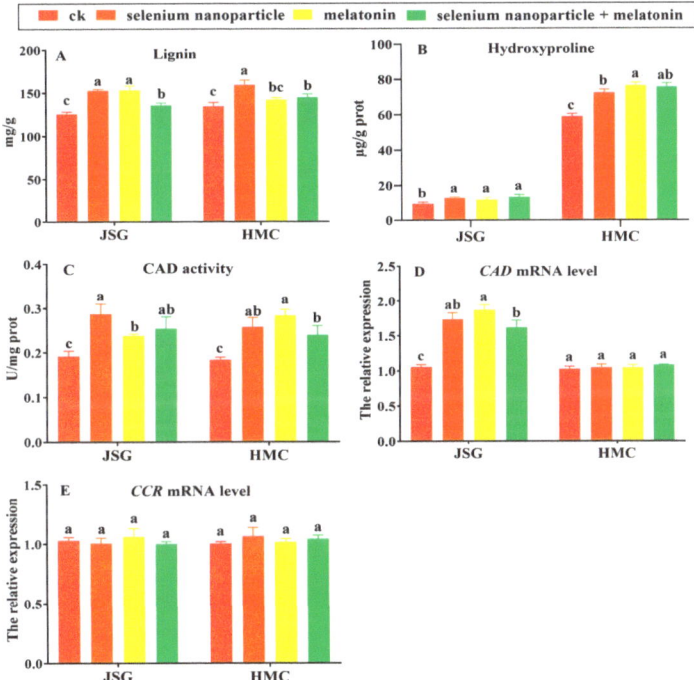

Figure 3. Effects of selenium nanoparticles and melatonin on lignin synthesis in two melon cultivars. JSG and HMC refer to melon cultivars. Different letters indicate a significant difference ($p < 0.05$) between treatments. (**A**): Lignin content, (**B**): Hydroxyproline content, (**C**): CAD activity, (**D**): *CAD* mRNA level, (**E**): *CCR* mRNA level.

2.4.2. Polyamine Metabolism after Selenium Nanoparticle and Melatonin Treatments

The effects of selenium nanoparticles, melatonin, and selenium nanoparticles + melatonin on polyamine metabolism in melon plants are shown in Figure 4. Compared with controls, the selenium nanoparticles and melatonin significantly increased PAO activity in JSG leaves by 26% and 23%, respectively, and in HMC leaves by 46% and 51%, respectively. The melatonin and selenium nanoparticle + melatonin combination treatments significantly increased the *PAO* mRNA level in JSG leaves by 22–29% and in HMC leaves by 24–23% compared with controls. The three treatments significantly increased the SPD level in JSG leaves by 202–288% and in HMC leaves by 39–80% compared with controls. Compared with controls, the selenium nanoparticle, melatonin, and selenium nanoparticle + melatonin combination treatments had no significant effects on the expression level of *SPD* in JSG and HMC leaves. The three treatments significantly increased SPM by 334–538% in JSG leaves and by 39–83% in HMC leaves compared with controls. Compared with controls, the selenium nanoparticle and selenium nanoparticle + melatonin combination treatments significantly up-regulated the *SPM* mRNA level in HMC leaves by 41% and 46%, respectively. The three treatments significantly increased PUT by 35–96% in JSG leaves and by 16–53% in HMC leaves compared with controls. The selenium nanoparticle, melatonin, and selenium nanoparticle + melatonin combination groups significantly increased the *SAMDC* mRNA level in JSG leaves by 38–180% and in HMC leaves by 64–229% compared with controls. Compared with controls, the three treatments significantly increased the expression level of *ADC* in HMC by 45–136%. Compared with controls, the selenium nanoparticles and selenium nanoparticle + melatonin combination significantly increased the *ODC* transcription level in HMC leaves by 71% and 73%, respectively. The three treatments significantly up-regulated the *CPA* expression in both cultivars by 31–78% compared with controls.

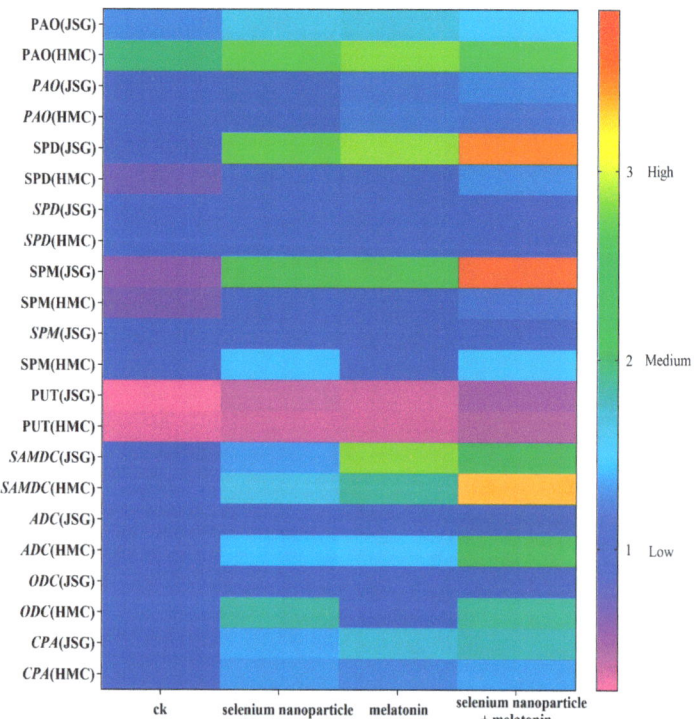

Figure 4. Effects of selenium nanoparticles and melatonin on polyamine metabolites in two melon cultivars. JSG and HMC refer to melon cultivars.

2.4.3. Effects of Selenium Nanoparticles and Melatonin on Phenylpropane Metabolism

The effects of selenium nanoparticles, melatonin, and the selenium nanoparticle + melatonin combination on phenylpropane metabolism in melon are shown in Figure 5. Compared with controls, the three treatments significantly increased total phenols in JSG leaves by 24–51% and in HMC leaves by 10–24% (Figure 5A). The selenium nanoparticle, melatonin, and selenium nanoparticle + melatonin combination groups significantly increased the flavonoid level in both cultivars by 19–64% compared with controls (Figure 5B). The three treatments significantly increased the PAL activity in JSG leaves by 31–95% and in HMC leaves by 29–43% compared with controls (Figure 5C). Compared with controls, the selenium nanoparticle and selenium nanoparticle + melatonin combination treatments significantly increased the *PAL* mRNA level in JSG leaves by 205% and 235%, respectively, and in HMC leaves by 226% and 222%, respectively (Figure 5D). The three treatments significantly increased the C4H activity in both cultivars by 32–100% compared with controls (Figure 5E). The selenium nanoparticle, melatonin, and selenium nanoparticle + melatonin combination groups significantly up-regulated the *C4H* expression in HMC leaves by 111–123% compared with controls (Figure 5F). Compared with controls, the melatonin and selenium nanoparticle + melatonin combination significantly increased 4CL activity by 26% and 26%, respectively, in JSG leaves and by 83% and 113%, respectively, in HMC leaves (Figure 5G). The three treatments significantly increased *4CL* expression in HMC leaves by 41–102% compared with controls (Figure 5H). The selenium nanoparticles, melatonin, and selenium nanoparticle + melatonin combination had no significant effects on the *CHS* expression in either cultivar (Figure 5I), but the three treatments significantly increased the *FLS* transcription level by 107–135% in HMC compared with controls (Figure 5J). Compared with controls, the selenium nanoparticle and selenium nanoparticle + melatonin combination groups significantly up-regulated the *LDOX* expression in HMC leaves by 44% and 75%, respectively (Figure 5K).

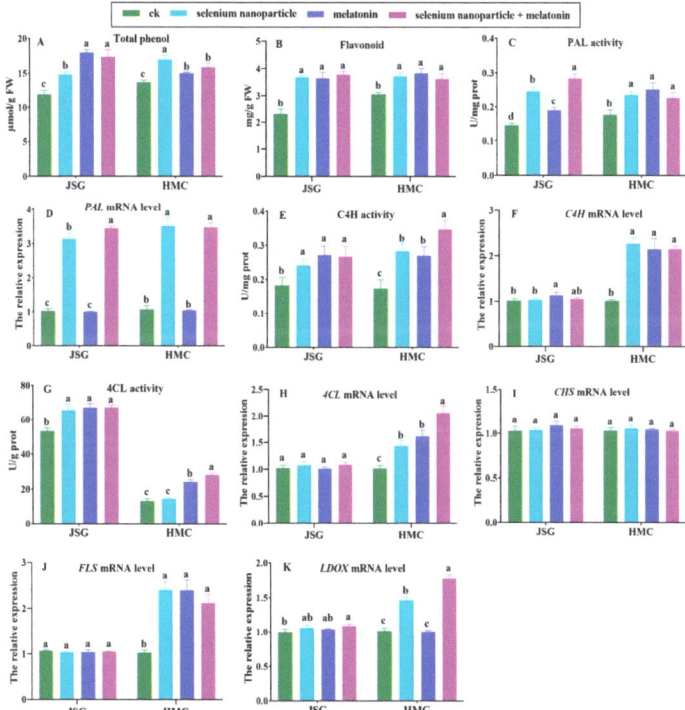

Figure 5. Effects of selenium nanoparticles and melatonin on phenylpropane metabolites in two melon cultivars. JSG and HMC refer to melon cultivars. Different letters indicate a significant difference ($p < 0.05$) between treatments. (**A**): Total phenol content, (**B**): Flavonoid content, (**C**): PAL activity, (**D**): *PAL* mRNA level, (**E**): C4H activity, (**F**): *C4H* mRNA level, (**G**): 4CL activity, (**H**): *4CL* mRNA level, (**I**): *CHS* mRNA level, (**J**): *FLS* mRNA level, (**K**): *LDOX* mRNA level.

2.5. Effects of Selenium Nanoparticle and Melatonin Treatment on Antioxidant Capacities

The effects of selenium nanoparticle, melatonin, and selenium nanoparticle + melatonin combination groups on the antioxidant capacities of melon are shown in Figure 6.

Compared with controls, the SOD activity after the three treatments significantly increased by 43–130% in the two cultivars (Figure 6A). The selenium nanoparticle and selenium nanoparticle + melatonin combination groups significantly increased the *SOD* mRNA level in JSG leaves by 93–96% and in HMC leaves by 54–71% compared with controls (Figure 6B). The three treatments significantly increased the CAT activity in both cultivars by 14–43% compared with controls (Figure 6C). Compared with controls, the selenium nanoparticle and selenium nanoparticle + melatonin combination treatments significantly up-regulated the *CAT* expression in JSG leaves by 148–128% and in HMC leaves by 51–56% (Figure 6D). The three treatments significantly increased the APX activity in both cultivars by 44–79% compared with controls (Figure 6E). The selenium nanoparticle + melatonin combination group significantly enhanced the *APX* transcription level in the two cultivars by 14–46% compared with controls (Figure 6F). The POD activity after the three treatments increased significantly by 25–149% in the two cultivars compared with controls (Figure 6G). Compared with controls, the selenium nanoparticle and selenium nanoparticle + melatonin combination treatments significantly increased the *POD* mRNA level in JSG leaves by 46–50% and in HMC leaves by 64–69% (Figure 6H).

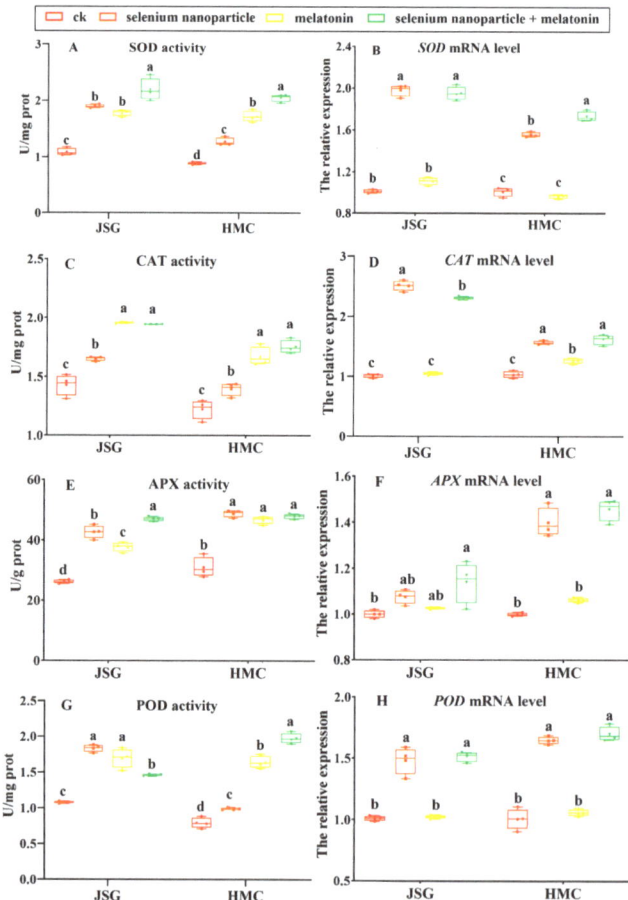

Figure 6. Effects of selenium nanoparticles and melatonin on the antioxidant capacities in two melon cultivars. JSG and HMC refer to melon cultivars. Different letters indicate a significant difference ($p < 0.05$) between treatments. (**A**): SOD activity, (**B**): *SOD* mRNA level, (**C**): CAT activity, (**D**): *CAT* mRNA level, (**E**): APX activity, (**F**): *APX* mRNA level, (**G**): POD activity, (**H**): *POD* mRNA level.

The effects of selenium nanoparticles, melatonin, and the selenium nanoparticle + melatonin combination on ROS and lipid peroxidation in melon are shown in Figure S2. Compared with controls, the three treatments had no significant effects on the H_2O_2 (Figure S2A) and MDA (Figure S2B) contents in JSG and HMC leaves. The selenium nanoparticles, melatonin, and selenium nanoparticle + melatonin combination significantly increased GSH by 12–47% in both cultivars compared with controls (Figure S2C). The proline level in both cultivars after the three treatments were significantly increased by 18–141% compared with controls (Figure S2D). Compared with controls, the scavenging ability of DPPH after the selenium nanoparticle, melatonin, and selenium nanoparticle + melatonin combination treatments significantly increased by 19–38% in the two cultivars (Figure S2E). These results indicated that selenium nanoparticles and melatonin increased the GSH level, proline level, and DPPH scavenging ability, whereas the treatments decreased the ROS level in melon leaves.

3. Discussion

Bio-stimulants are used to enhance the growth of plants, whose demand increases 12% per year on the global market [34]. In this study, bio-stimulants had certain promotional effects on the biomasses of melon seedlings, which were related to the increased production of IAA after selenium nanoparticle and melatonin treatments. Exogenous melatonin enhances immunity to the bacterial pathogen *Pseudomonas syringae* through SA [35]. It also promotes the production of sugar, resulting in an increasing SA content [36]. Melatonin plays roles in plant innate immunity against pathogens through SA/JA pathways, and the resulting up-regulation of the gene encoding SA biosynthetic heteromeric acid synthetase (*ICS1*) leads to an increased SA content [37]. The resistance of plants to biological stresses, including crop resistance to fungi, is induced by melatonin through endogenous hormones [38]. After selenium-containing treatments, the level of the defense hormone JA, which induces sulfur assimilation and GSH biosynthesis gene expression, and those of the defense genes related to SA synthesis increase [39]. The selenium nanoparticles and melatonin had no effect on the SA and JA contents in melon seedlings, which was related to the experimental conditions in which melon seedlings were under abiotic stress.

The mechanisms by which selenium nanoparticles and melatonin regulate carbohydrate and polyamine in melon are illustrated in Figure 7. The external stress increases LOX activity, accelerates the oxidation of unsaturated fatty acids catalyzed by LOX, and increases the MDA content [40]. Melatonin inhibits LOX activity and decreases *PbLOX1* and *PbLOX2* mRNA levels [41]. Proline, sugars, and free amino acids are bio-soluble solutes that protect plants from stress through osmotic regulation, ROS clearance, and plasma membrane integrity, and exogenous melatonin increases the selenium-induced contents of proline, free amino acids, and soluble sugars [42]. This was consistent with the selenium nanoparticle, melatonin, and selenium nanoparticle + melatonin combination treatments, which increased levels of primary metabolites, such as melon sugars and amino acids, in the present study. Melatonin improves the activities of sucrose-metabolism-related enzymes, hydrolyzing a large amount of sucrose into glucose and fructose. The increased soluble sugar and antioxidant enzyme activities lead to a greater stress resistance in grape seedlings and increase adaptability to environmental changes [43]. These findings are consistent with the results of the present study. The selenium nanoparticles and melatonin, as bio-stimulants, promoted the primary metabolic abilities of soluble sugar and amino acids in melon seedlings, providing a basis for the utilization of selenium nanoparticles and melatonin in melon cultivation.

Melatonin increases the lignification degree of tea by altering the expression levels of enzymes involved in the lignin synthesis pathway [44]. The hydroxyproline in plant cell walls plays important roles in plant growth, development, and defense [45]. This same trend was shown in the current study, with selenium nanoparticles, melatonin, and selenium nanoparticles + melatonin increasing levels of secondary metabolites, such as lignin and phenylpropane, in melon. Melatonin is involved in signaling in plants through its receptors and downstream signal transduction pathways [46]. The applications of 50 and 100 μmol·L^{-1} melatonin on leaves have greater effects on fruit quality than on leaf quality, and this significantly increases the phenolic content (including total phenols and flavonoids) [47]. Melatonin mitigates heat stress by increasing levels of soy phenols, flavonoids, prolines, and endogenous melatonin and polyamine [48]. In our study, selenium nanoparticles, melatonin, and selenium nanoparticles + melatonin increased SPM, SPD, PUT, and mRNA levels. Selenite up-regulates the expression of genes related to the biosynthesis of phenylpropane compounds and the activities of related enzymes, such as PAL, C4H, chalcone synthase, chalcone isomerase, and CAD [49]. Melatonin enhances the postharvest disease resistance of blueberry fruit by regulating phenylpropane metabolism (PAL, C4H, 4CL, and CAD activities) and mRNA levels [50]. This is consistent with the results of selenium nanoparticle, melatonin, and selenium nanoparticle + melatonin treatments used in this study.

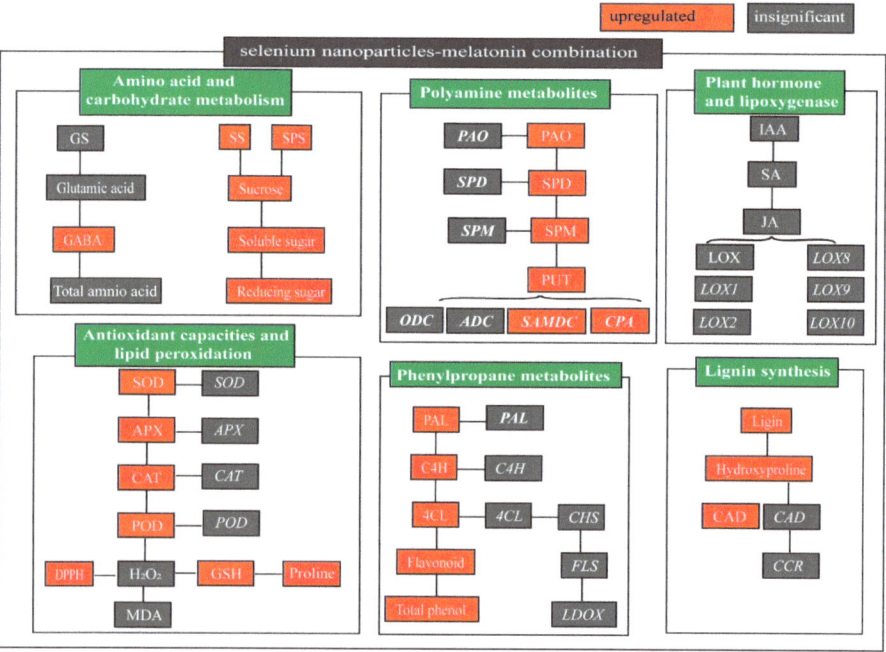

Figure 7. The mechanism of selenium nanoparticles and melatonin regulated carbohydrate, polyamines, and antioxidant capacity of melon plant. Red indicates upregulation, while gray indicates insignificance.

Melatonin plays different roles in plants, enhancing the activities of a variety of antioxidant enzymes, including SOD, CAT, and POD, and controlling ROS, as well as other free radicals, present in plant cells [51]. The combination treatment of melatonin and Na$_2$SeO$_3$ enhances the resistance of fruit to gray mold by increasing the activities of SOD, POD, and CAT, as well as the expression levels of disease-related genes [52]. Melatonin–selenium nanoparticles increase the activity levels of antioxidant enzymes, such as SOD, POD, CAT, APX, and GSH, and decrease the contents of MDA and H$_2$O$_2$ [53]. The application of selenium nanoparticles significantly increased the antioxidant capacity and decreased the MDA content. Compared with soil selenium applications, foliar selenium applications are efficient and safe, resulting in the delayed development of plaques on sunflower leaves. The application method leads to the absorption of selenite and efficient conversion to selenomethionine (80%) and selenium-containing proteins, which not only have enzymatic functions but also act as antioxidants through the direct scavenging of free radicals [54]. In future research, the effects of selenium nanoparticles and melatonin on the fruit quality of melon should be determined using carotenoids or other quality indicators. Additionally, the effects of bio-stimulants on the incidence of melon disease under biotic stress should be explored to provide evidence for the safe cultivation of melon.

4. Materials and Methods

4.1. Experimental Design

JSG and HMC melons were used as the study materials. The seeds of JSG and HMC were provided by the Hami Melon Research Center of the Xinjiang Academy of Agricultural Sciences (Urumqi, China). Full seeds were soaked, germinated, and planted in plastic pots (30 cm × 30 cm), with two plants per pot. The preparation and characterization of selenium nanoparticles has been reported previously [55]. The concentrations of selenium nanoparticles [33] and melatonin [56] used in this study were based on previous studies by our research group. When the seedlings grew to the 3–4 leaf stage, the leaves were spray-treated. Three treatments were established. There was a control (CK), as well as 5 mg·L^{-1} selenium nanoparticles, 5 mg·L^{-1} melatonin and 5 mg·L^{-1} selenium nanoparticles + melatonin combination groups, and each treatment was repeated three times. The water (control), selenium nanoparticles (5.0 mg·L^{-1}), melatonin (5.0 mg·L^{-1}), and selenium nanoparticle + melatonin combination (5.0 mg·L^{-1}) were sprayed on the seedling leaves. All the melon seedlings were placed outdoors, at 20 °C to 30 °C. The foliar spraying was carried out from 9:00 to 10:00 AM on windless and sunny days, and the spraying was based on no dripping from the foliar surface. After 7 days, melon leaves were collected, frozen in liquid nitrogen, and stored at −80 °C. The plant heights and stem diameters of melon seedlings were measured using a ruler and a vernier caliper, respectively. The fresh weights of the stems were measured after the leaves were collected, and the dry weights of the stems were measured after drying.

4.2. Determination of Lipid Peroxidation Products

The leaves were ground after being frozen in liquid nitrogen. Then, 0.1 g of each powdered sample was placed independently in a tube containing 1 mL extraction solution in accordance with the instructions of the appropriate test kit. Samples were homogenized and centrifuged at $12,000 \times g$ at 4 °C for 10 min for H_2O_2 and DPPH determinations, or at $4000 \times g$ at 4 °C for 10 min for MDA, proline, and reducing glutathione determinations. The obtained supernatants were treated using kits for H_2O_2 (Kit number: A064-1-1), MDA (Kit number: MDA, A003-1-1), proline (Kit number: A107-1-1), and DPPH (Kit number: A153-1-1) from Nanjing Jiancheng Bioengineering Institute (Nanjing, China). Reducing glutathione (GSH) was determined using a kit (Kit number: E-BC-K030-M, Elabscience Biotechnology Co., Ltd., Wuhan, China). The H_2O_2, MDA, proline, and DPPH levels were determined using a UV–visible spectrophotometer (Shanghai Shunyu Hengping Instrument Co., Ltd., Shanghai, China). GSH was determined using a multi-scan spectroscopic microporous plate spectrophotometer (Bio Tek Instruments Inc., Winooski, VT, USA). Obtained liquid samples were used to measure absorbance at 405 nm for H_2O_2, at 517 nm for DPPH, at 532 nm for MDA, at 520 nm for proline, and at 405 nm for GSH. The standard curve values for GSH, proline, and DPPH are shown in Table S1.

4.3. Determinations of Plant Primary and Secondary Metabolites

The SOD (Kit number: A001-3), CAT (Kit number: A007-1-1), APX (Kit number: A123-1-1), peroxidase (POD, Kit number: A084-3), phenylalanine ammonia lyase (PAL, Kit number: A137-1-1), glutamine synthetase (GS, Kit number: A047-1-1), total phenols (Kit number: A143-1-1), flavonoids (Kit number: A142-1-1), proteins (Kit number: A045-4), total amino acids (Kit number: A026-1-1), glutamic acid (Kit number: A074-1-1), lipoxygenase (LOX, H550-1), soluble sugar (Kit number: A145-1-1), sucrose (Kit number: A099-1-1), sucrose synthetase (SS, Kit number: A097-1-1), and sucrose phosphate synthetase (SPS, Kit number: A098-1-1) kits were procured from Nanjing Jiancheng Bioengineering Institute. The reducing sugar (Kit number: BC0235), trans-cinnamate 4-hydroxylase (C4H, Kit number: BC4080), co-A ligase (4CL, Kit number: BC4220), cinnamyl alcohol dehydrogenase (CAD, Kit number: BC4170), lignin (Kit number: BC4200), and hydroxyproline (Kit number: BC0255) kits were purchased from Solarbio Science and Technology Company Ltd. (Beijing, China). The polyamine oxidase (PAO) kit was procured from Shanghai Enzyme Linked Biotechnology Co., Ltd. (Shanghai, China).

The main steps for determining plant primary and secondary metabolite levels were as follows: melon leaves were ground with a pestle and a mortar containing liquid nitrogen. In total, 0.1 g of each powdered sample was placed in a tube containing 1 mL of the appropriate extraction solution in accordance with the instructions of an appropriate kit. Then, samples were homogenized and centrifuged at $800 \times g$ at 4 °C for 10 min for SOD, CAT, and POD; at $10,000 \times g$ at 4 °C for 10 min for APX and flavonoids, at $12,000 \times g$ at 4 °C for 10 min for PAL, at $4000 \times g$ at 4 °C for 10 min for GS and total phenols, at $2500 \times g$ at 4 °C for 10 min for proteins, at $3500 \times g$ at 4 °C for 10 min for total amino acids, at $2500 \times g$ at 4 °C for 10 min for glutamic acid, at $2000 \times g$ at 4 °C for 20 min for LOX, at $4000 \times g$ at 4 °C for 10 min for soluble sugar, at $8000 \times g$ at 4 °C for 10 min for SS and SPS, at $8000 \times g$ at 4 °C for 10 min for reducing sugar, at $8000 \times g$ for 10 min for lignin, at $16,000 \times g$ for 5 min for hydroxyproline, at $12,000 \times g$ at 4 °C for 10 min for C4H, at $8000 \times g$ at 4 °C for 10 min for 4CL, at $10,000 \times g$ at 4 °C for 10 min for CAD, and at $10,000 \times g$ at 4 °C for 10 min for PAO. The SOD, CAT, POD, LOX, reducing sugar, and PAO levels were determined from obtained supernatants using the appropriate kit and a multi-scan spectrum microplate spectrophotometer, and APX, PAL, SS, SPS, flavonoids, GS, total phenols, proteins, total amino acids, glutamic acid, soluble sugar, reducing sugar, lignin, hydroxyproline, C4H, 4CL, and CAD levels were obtained using appropriate kits and a UV–vis spectrophotometer (Shanghai Shunyu Hengping Instruments Co., Ltd., Shanghai, China) following the manufacturer's instructions. Obtained liquid samples were used to measure absorbance at 450 nm for SOD, at 405 nm for CAT, at 420 nm for POD, at 290 nm for APX and PAL, at 540 nm for GS, at 760 nm for total phenols, at 502 nm for flavonoids, at 562 nm for proteins, at 650 nm for total amino acids, at 340 nm for glutamic acid, at 450 nm for LOX, at 620 nm for soluble sugar, at 480 nm for SS and SPS, at 540 nm for reducing sugar, at 280 nm for lignin, at 560 nm for hydroxyproline, at 340 nm for C4H, at 333 nm for 4CL, at 340 nm for CAD, and at 450 nm for PAO. The standard curve values for POD, total phenols, flavonoids, total amino acids, glutamic acid, LOX, soluble sugar, SS, SPS, reducing sugar, and PAO are shown in Table S1.

4.4. Ultra Performance Liquid Chromatography Tandem Mass Spectrometry (UPLC–MS/MS) Analyses of Polyamines, γ-Aminobutyric Acid (GABA), and Plant Hormones

The samples were homogenized in 3.0 mL acetonitrile solution (8:2, v/v) and centrifuged at $4500 \times g$ at 4 °C for 10 min. The detection conditions for polyamines were as follows: HILIC column (100 mm × 2.1 mm, 1.7 μm), mobile phase: (A) 5 mmol/L ammonium acetate acetonitrile solution and (B) 0.1% formic acid solution; gradient elution: 0–1.0 min, 80% A; 1.0–1.5 min, 80–40% A; 1.5–6.0 min, 40% A; 6.0–6.5 min, 40–80% A; 6.5–9.5 min, 80% A; injection volume: 2 μL; flow rate: 0.3 mL/min; column temperature: 30 °C. In positive ion mode, the ion source temperature was 150 °C, and the solvent temperature was 350 °C. The N_2 flow rate of the cone hole was 650 L/h, and the N_2 flow rate was 250 L/h. The mass spectrum conditions of putrescine (PUT), spermine (SPM), spermidine (SPD), GABA, jasmonic acid (JA), salicylic acid (SA), and indoleacetic acid (IAA) are shown in Table S2. The samples were homogenized in 1.0 mL methanol/water/formic acid (15:4:1, $v/v/v$) and centrifuged at 4 °C for 5 min at $16,000 \times g$. The chromatographic conditions of the three plant hormones have been published previously [33]. The chromatographic conditions for melatonin were as follows: chromatographic column: ACQUITY UPLC BEH C18 (1.7 μm, 2.1 mm × 100 mm); mobile phase A: 0.1% (v/v) formic acid aqueous solution; mobile phase B: acetonitrile; injection volume 1 μL; flow rate of 0.2 mL/min. The mass spectrometry conditions were as follows: electrospray ionization (ESI$^+$); multiple reaction monitoring mode detection; detected ion pair: m/z 233→174. The other mass spectrometry tuning parameters were the same as those for plant hormones. The standard curve of melatonin was y = 318917x + 914976, R^2 = 0.9967. The mass spectra of the standard for melatonin is shown in Figure S3.

4.5. RT-qPCR Analysis

Total RNA was extracted using kits and reverse-transcribed into cDNA (Transgen Biotech Company Ltd., Beijing, China). The cDNA synthesis system is shown in Table S3. Primer sequences for target and actin control genes are shown in Table S4. Relative mRNA levels were calculated using $2^{-\Delta\Delta Ct}$.

4.6. Statistical Analyses

SPSS (version 26 SPSS Inc., Chicago, IL, USA) was used for the one-way analysis of variance (ANOVA). Tukey's tests were used for multiple comparisons to determine significant differences ($p < 0.05$). Graph Pad Prism software (version 8.02; San Diego, CA, USA) was used to calculate data statistics.

5. Conclusions

Selenium nanoparticle and melatonin foliar treatments facilitated melon seedling growth by regulating primary, secondary, and oxidative-stress metabolism. Independent applications of 5 mg·L^{-1} selenium nanoparticles, melatonin, and the selenium nanoparticle + melatonin combination increased stem dry weights of the JSG and HMC melon cultivars. Compared with control, selenium nanoparticles, melatonin, and the selenium nanoparticle + melatonin combination increased soluble sugar, sucrose, and SPS contents. Additionally, selenium nanoparticles, melatonin, and selenium nanoparticles + melatonin enhanced GABA, hydroxyproline, SPM, SPD, PUT, total phenols, flavonoids, GSH, and proline contents, as well as PAL, C4H, SOD, CAT, APX, and POD activities.

Supplementary Materials: The following supporting information can be downloaded at: https://www.mdpi.com/article/10.3390/ijms25147830/s1.

Author Contributions: L.K.: writing—original draft, methodology, data curation, investigation. Y.J. (Yujiao Jia): conceptualization, resources, formal analysis. Y.W.: conceptualization, resources, formal analysis. H.L.: conceptualization, formal analysis, data curation. D.Z.: conceptualization, formal analysis, data curation. Y.J. (Yanjun Ju): conceptualization, formal analysis, data curation. C.P. and J.M.: conceptualization, methodology, writing—review and editing. All authors have read and agreed to the published version of the manuscript.

Funding: The work was supported by the Key Laboratory of Forest Plant Ecology, Ministry of Education (KLP2024B1), the Tianshan Talent Plan of Xinjiang Uygur Autonomous Region Phase III (2021–2023), the Key Cultivation Project of Scientific and Technological Innovation of Xinjiang Academy of Agricultural Sciences (xjkcpy-2022002), and the 2115 Talent Development Program of China Agricultural University.

Institutional Review Board Statement: Not applicable.

Informed Consent Statement: Not applicable.

Data Availability Statement: Data are available upon request from the corresponding author.

Conflicts of Interest: The authors declare no conflicts of interest.

References

1. López-Martín, M.; Pérez-de-Castro, A.; Picó, B.; Gómez-Guillamón, M.L. Advanced Genetic Studies on Powdery Mildew Resistance in TGR-1551. *Int. J. Mol. Sci.* **2022**, *23*, 2553. [CrossRef] [PubMed]
2. Zhang, H.; Zhang, X.; Li, M.; Yang, Y.; Li, Z.; Xu, Y.; Wang, H.; Wang, D.; Zhang, Y.; Wang, H.; et al. Molecular mapping for fruit-related traits, and joint identification of candidate genes and selective sweeps for seed size in melon. *Genomics* **2022**, *114*, 110306. [CrossRef] [PubMed]

3. Sharma, S.P.; Leskovar, D.I.; Crosby, K.M.; Volder, A.; Ibrahim, A.M.H. Root growth, yield, and fruit quality responses of reticulatus and inodorus melons (*Cucumis melo* L.) to deficit subsurface drip irrigation. *Agric. Water Manag.* **2014**, *136*, 75–85. [CrossRef]
4. Husen, A.; Siddiqi, K.S. Plants and microbes assisted selenium nanoparticles: Characterization and application. *J. Nanobiotechnol.* **2014**, *12*, 28. [CrossRef] [PubMed]
5. Matsuura, H.N.; Malik, S.; de Costa, F.; Yousefzadi, M.; Mirjalili, M.H.; Arroo, R.; Bhambra, A.S.; Strnad, M.; Bonfill, M.; Fett-Neto, A.G. Specialized Plant Metabolism Characteristics and Impact on Target Molecule Biotechnological Production. *Mol. Biotechnol.* **2018**, *60*, 169–183. [CrossRef]
6. Yang, L.; Wen, K.S.; Ruan, X.; Zhao, Y.X.; Wei, F.; Wang, Q. Response of Plant Secondary Metabolites to Environmental Factors. *Molecules* **2018**, *23*, 762. [CrossRef]
7. Bakhoum, G.S.; Sadak, M.S.; Thabet, M.S. Induction of Tolerance in Groundnut Plants Against Drought Stress and Cercospora Leaf Spot Disease with Exogenous Application of Arginine and Sodium Nitroprusside Under Field Conditions. *J. Soil. Sci. Plant Nutruition* **2023**, *23*, 6612–6631. [CrossRef]
8. Divekar, P.A.; Narayana, S.; Divekar, B.A.; Kumar, R.; Gadratagi, B.G.; Ray, A.; Singh, A.K.; Rani, V.; Singh, V.; Singh, A.K.; et al. Plant Secondary Metabolites as Defense Tools against Herbivores for Sustainable Crop Protection. *Int. J. Mol. Sci.* **2022**, *23*, 2690. [CrossRef]
9. Zaynab, M.; Fatima, M.; Abbas, S.; Sharif, Y.; Umair, M.; Zafar, M.H.; Bahadar, K. Role of secondary metabolites in plant defense against pathogens. *Microb. Pathog.* **2018**, *124*, 198–202. [CrossRef]
10. Karthik, K.K.; Cheriyan, B.V.; Rajeshkumar, S.; Gopalakrishnan, M. A review on selenium nanoparticles and their biomedical applications. *Biomed. Technol.* **2024**, *6*, 61–74. [CrossRef]
11. Wang, C.; Cheng, T.; Liu, H.; Zhou, F.; Zhang, J.; Zhang, M.; Liu, X.; Shi, W.; Cao, T. Nano-selenium controlled cadmium accumulation and improved photosynthesis in indica rice cultivated in lead and cadmium combined paddy soils. *J. Environ. Sci.* **2021**, *103*, 336–346. [CrossRef] [PubMed]
12. Shalaby, T.A.; Abd-Alkarim, E.; El-Aidy, F.; Hamed, E.-S.; Sharaf-Eldin, M.; Taha, N.; El-Ramady, H.; Bayoumi, Y.; dos Reis, A.R. Nano-selenium, silicon and H₂O₂ boost growth and productivity of cucumber under combined salinity and heat stress. *Ecotoxicol. Environ. Saf.* **2021**, *212*, 111962. [CrossRef] [PubMed]
13. Iwaniuk, P.; Kaczyński, P.; Pietkun, M.; Łozowicka, B. Evaluation of titanium and silicon role in mitigation of fungicides toxicity in wheat expressed at the level of biochemical and antioxidant profile. *Chemosphere* **2022**, *308*, 136284. [CrossRef] [PubMed]
14. Iwaniuk, P.; Łuniewski, S.; Kaczyński, P.; Łozowicka, B. The Influence of Humic Acids and Nitrophenols on Metabolic Compounds and Pesticide Behavior in Wheat under Biotic Stress. *Agronomy* **2023**, *13*, 1378. [CrossRef]
15. Omar, A.A.; Heikal, Y.M.; Zayed, E.M.; Shamseldin, S.A.M.; Salama, Y.E.; Amer, K.E.; Basuoni, M.M.; Abd Ellatif, S.; Mohamed, A.H. Conferring of Drought and Heat Stress Tolerance in Wheat (*Triticum aestivum* L.) Genotypes and Their Response to Selenium Nanoparticles Application. *Nanomaterials* **2023**, *13*, 998. [CrossRef] [PubMed]
16. Mu, M.; Wang, Z.; Chen, Z.; Wu, Y.; Nie, W.; Zhao, S.; Yin, X.; Teng, X. Physiological characteristics, rhizosphere soil properties, and root-related microbial communities of Trifolium repens L. in response to Pb toxicity. *Sci. Total Environ.* **2024**, *907*, 167871. [CrossRef] [PubMed]
17. Wang, M.; Wang, Y.; Ge, C.; Wu, H.; Jing, F.; Wu, S.; Li, H.; Zhou, D. Foliar Selenium Nanoparticles Application Promotes the Growth of Maize (*Zea mays* L.) Seedlings by Regulating Carbon, Nitrogen and Oxidative Stress Metabolism. *Sci. Hortic.* **2023**, *311*, 111816. [CrossRef]
18. Salama, D.M.; Abd El-Aziz, M.E.; Rizk, F.A.; Abd Elwahed, M.S.A. Applications of nanotechnology on vegetable crops. *Chemosphere* **2021**, *266*, 129026. [CrossRef] [PubMed]
19. Sadak, M.; Bakhoum, G.; Tawfic, M. Chitosan and chitosan nanoparticle effect on growth, productivity and some biochemical aspects of *Lupinus termis* L plant under drought conditions. *Egypt. J. Chem.* **2022**, *65*, 537–549. [CrossRef]
20. Sadak, M.S.; Bakry, B.A.; El-Karamany, M.F. Agrophysiological variation in flax affected by folic acid and Ag nanoparticles foliar applications. *Asian J. Plant Sci.* **2022**, *21*, 339–346. [CrossRef]
21. Siddiqui, M.H.; Kalaji, H.M.; Zhang, Z.; Ma, X. Nanoparticles in environment and plant system: A boon or bane. *Chemosphere* **2022**, *308*, 136320. [CrossRef] [PubMed]
22. El-Bassiouny, H.M.S.; Abdallah, M.M.-S.; El-Enany, M.A.M.; Sadak, M.S. Nano-Zinc Oxide and Arbuscular mycorrhiza Effects on Physiological and Biochemical Aspects of Wheat Cultivars under Saline Conditions. *Pak. J. Biol. Sci. PJBS* **2020**, *23*, 478–490. [CrossRef] [PubMed]
23. Arnao, M.B.; Hernandez-Ruiz, J. Melatonin as a plant biostimulant in crops and during post-harvest: A new approach is needed. *J. Sci. Food Agric.* **2021**, *101*, 5297–5304. [CrossRef] [PubMed]
24. Sadak, M.S.; Bakry, B.A. Alleviation of drought stress by melatonin foliar treatment on two flax varieties under sandy soil. *Physiol. Mol. Biol. Plants* **2020**, *26*, 907–919. [CrossRef] [PubMed]
25. Sadak, M. Mitigation of salinity adverse effects of on wheat by grain priming with melatonin. *Int. J. ChemTech Res.* **2016**, *9*, 85–97.
26. Arnao, M.B.; Hernández-Ruiz, J. Melatonin and its relationship to plant hormones. *Ann. Bot.* **2018**, *121*, 195–207. [CrossRef] [PubMed]

27. Sadak, M.S. Nitric oxide and hydrogen peroxide as signaling molecules for better growth and yield of wheat plant exposed to water deficiency. *Egypt. J. Chem.* **2022**, *65*, 209–223. [CrossRef]
28. Arnao, M.B.; Hernández-Ruiz, J. Functions of melatonin in plants: A review. *J. Pineal Res.* **2015**, *59*, 133–150. [CrossRef]
29. Wu, C.; Hao, W.; Yan, L.; Zhang, H.; Zhang, J.; Liu, C.; Zheng, L. Postharvest melatonin treatment enhanced antioxidant activity and promoted GABA biosynthesis in yellow-flesh peach. *Food Chem.* **2023**, *419*, 136088. [CrossRef]
30. Yang, K.; Sun, H.; Liu, M.; Zhu, L.; Zhang, K.; Zhang, Y.; Li, A.; Zhang, H.; Zhu, J.; Liu, X.; et al. Morphological and Physiological Mechanisms of Melatonin on Delaying Drought-Induced Leaf Senescence in Cotton. *Int. J. Mol. Sci.* **2023**, *24*, 7269. [CrossRef]
31. Promyou, S.; Raruang, Y.; Chen, Z.Y. Melatonin Treatment of Strawberry Fruit during Storage Extends Its Post-Harvest Quality and Reduces Infection Caused by Botrytis cinerea. *Foods* **2023**, *12*, 1445. [CrossRef] [PubMed]
32. Dou, J.; Wang, J.; Tang, Z.; Yu, J.; Wu, Y.; Liu, Z.; Wang, J.; Wang, G.; Tian, Q. Application of Exogenous Melatonin Improves Tomato Fruit Quality by Promoting the Accumulation of Primary and Secondary Metabolites. *Foods* **2022**, *11*, 4097. [CrossRef] [PubMed]
33. Kang, L.; Wu, Y.; Zhang, J.; An, Q.; Zhou, C.; Li, D.; Pan, C. Nano-selenium enhances the antioxidant capacity, organic acids and cucurbitacin B in melon (*Cucumis melo* L.) plants. *Ecotoxicol. Environ. Saf.* **2022**, *241*, 113777. [CrossRef] [PubMed]
34. Kang, L.; Wu, Y.; Jia, Y.; Chen, Z.; Kang, D.; Zhang, L.; Pan, C. Nano-selenium enhances melon resistance to Podosphaera xanthii by enhancing the antioxidant capacity and promoting alterations in the polyamine, phenylpropanoid and hormone signaling pathways. *J. Nanobiotechnol.* **2023**, *21*, 377. [CrossRef] [PubMed]
35. Zhou, C.; Luo, L.; Miao, P.; Dong, Q.; Cheng, H.; Wang, Y.; Li, D.; Pan, C. A novel perspective to investigate how nanoselenium and melatonin lengthen the cut carnation vase shelf. *Plant Physiol. Biochem.* **2023**, *196*, 982–992. [CrossRef] [PubMed]
36. Calvo, P.; Nelson, L.; Kloepper, J.W. Agricultural uses of plant biostimulants. *Plant Soil.* **2014**, *383*, 3–41. [CrossRef]
37. Lee, H.Y.; Back, K. Melatonin is required for $H_2 O_2$- and NO-mediated defense signaling through MAPKKK3 and OXI1 in Arabidopsis thaliana. *J. Pineal Res.* **2017**, *62*, 12379. [CrossRef]
38. He, H.; He, L.F. Crosstalk between melatonin and nitric oxide in plant development and stress responses. *Physiol. Plant* **2020**, *170*, 218–226. [CrossRef] [PubMed]
39. Sun, C.; Liu, L.; Wang, L.; Li, B.; Jin, C.; Lin, X. Melatonin: A master regulator of plant development and stress responses. *J. Integr. Plant Biol.* **2021**, *63*, 126–145. [CrossRef]
40. Sharif, R.; Xie, C.; Zhang, H.; Arnao, M.B.; Ali, M.; Ali, Q.; Muhammad, I.; Shalmani, A.; Nawaz, M.A.; Chen, P.; et al. Melatonin and Its Effects on Plant Systems. *Molecules* **2018**, *23*, 2352. [CrossRef]
41. Wang, J.; Cappa, J.J.; Harris, J.P.; Edger, P.P.; Zhou, W.; Pires, J.C.; Adair, M.; Unruh, S.A.; Simmons, M.P.; Schiavon, M.; et al. Transcriptome-wide comparison of selenium hyperaccumulator and nonaccumulator Stanleya species provides new insight into key processes mediating the hyperaccumulation syndrome. *Plant Biotechnol. J.* **2018**. [CrossRef]
42. Kang, Y.; Liu, W.; Guan, C.; Guan, M.; He, X. Evolution and functional diversity of lipoxygenase (LOX) genes in allotetraploid rapeseed (*Brassica napus* L.). *Int. J. Biol. Macromol.* **2021**, *188*, 844–854. [CrossRef]
43. Liu, J.; Liu, H.; Wu, T.; Zhai, R.; Yang, C.; Wang, Z.; Ma, F.; Xu, L. Effects of Melatonin Treatment of Postharvest Pear Fruit on Aromatic Volatile Biosynthesis. *Molecules* **2019**, *24*, 4233. [CrossRef]
44. Ulhassan, Z.; Huang, Q.; Gill, R.A.; Ali, S.; Mwamba, T.M.; Ali, B.; Hina, F.; Zhou, W. Protective mechanisms of melatonin against selenium toxicity in Brassica napus: Insights into physiological traits, thiol biosynthesis and antioxidant machinery. *BMC Plant Biol.* **2019**, *19*, 507. [CrossRef] [PubMed]
45. Zhong, L.; Lin, L.; Yang, L.; Liao, M.; Wang, X.; Wang, J.; Lv, X.; Deng, H.; Liang, D.; Xia, H.; et al. Exogenous melatonin promotes growth and sucrose metabolism of grape seedlings. *PLoS ONE* **2020**, *15*, e0232033. [CrossRef] [PubMed]
46. Han, M.H.; Yang, N.; Wan, Q.W.; Teng, R.M.; Duan, A.Q.; Wang, Y.H.; Zhuang, J. Exogenous melatonin positively regulates lignin biosynthesis in Camellia sinensis. *Int. J. Biol. Macromol.* **2021**, *179*, 485–499. [CrossRef] [PubMed]
47. Liu, X.; Wolfe, R.; Welch, L.R.; Domozych, D.S.; Popper, Z.A.; Showalter, A.M. Bioinformatic Identification and Analysis of Extensins in the Plant Kingdom. *PLoS ONE* **2016**, *11*, e0150177. [CrossRef]
48. Back, K. Melatonin metabolism, signaling and possible roles in plants. *Plant J.* **2021**, *105*, 376–391. [CrossRef]
49. Xia, H.; Shen, Y.; Shen, T.; Wang, X.; Zhang, X.; Hu, P.; Liang, D.; Lin, L.; Deng, H.; Wang, J.; et al. Melatonin Accumulation in Sweet Cherry and Its Influence on Fruit Quality and Antioxidant Properties. *Molecules* **2020**, *25*, 753. [CrossRef]
50. Imran, M.; Aaqil Khan, M.; Shahzad, R.; Bilal, S.; Khan, M.; Yun, B.W.; Khan, A.L.; Lee, I.J. Melatonin Ameliorates Thermotolerance in Soybean Seedling through Balancing Redox Homeostasis and Modulating Antioxidant Defense, Phytohormones and Polyamines Biosynthesis. *Molecules* **2021**, *26*, 5116. [CrossRef]
51. Wang, G.; Wu, L.; Zhang, H.; Wu, W.; Zhang, M.; Li, X.; Wu, H. Regulation of the Phenylpropanoid Pathway: A Mechanism of Selenium Tolerance in Peanut (*Arachis hypogaea* L.) Seedlings. *J. Agric. Food. Chem.* **2016**, *64*, 3626–3635. [CrossRef] [PubMed]
52. Qu, G.; Wu, W.; Ba, L.; Ma, C.; Ji, N.; Cao, S. Melatonin Enhances the Postharvest Disease Resistance of Blueberries Fruit by Modulating the Jasmonic Acid Signaling Pathway and Phenylpropanoid Metabolites. *Front. Chem.* **2022**, *10*, 957581. [CrossRef] [PubMed]
53. Arnao, M.B.; Hernandez-Ruiz, J. Melatonin: A New Plant Hormone and/or a Plant Master Regulator? *Trends Plant Sci.* **2019**, *24*, 38–48. [CrossRef] [PubMed]
54. Zang, H.; Ma, J.; Wu, Z.; Yuan, L.; Lin, Z.Q.; Zhu, R.; Banuelos, G.S.; Reiter, R.J.; Li, M.; Yin, X. Synergistic Effect of Melatonin and Selenium Improves Resistance to Postharvest Gray Mold Disease of Tomato Fruit. *Front. Plant Sci.* **2022**, *13*, 903936. [CrossRef]

55. Farooq, M.A.; Islam, F.; Ayyaz, A.; Chen, W.; Noor, Y.; Hu, W.; Hannan, F.; Zhou, W. Mitigation effects of exogenous melatonin-selenium nanoparticles on arsenic-induced stress in Brassica napus. *Environ. Pollut.* **2022**, *292 Pt B*, 118473. [CrossRef]
56. Chen, Z.; Sun, H.; Hu, T.; Wang, Z.; Wu, W.; Liang, Y.; Guo, Y. Sunflower resistance against Sclerotinia sclerotiorum is potentiated by selenium through regulation of redox homeostasis and hormones signaling pathways. *Environ. Sci. Pollut. Res. Int.* **2022**, *29*, 38097–38109. [CrossRef]

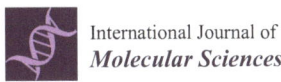

International Journal of
Molecular Sciences

MDPI

Review

Association between Reactive Oxygen Species, Transcription Factors, and Candidate Genes in Drought-Resistant Sorghum

Jiao Liu [1,2], Xin Wang [1,2], Hao Wu [1,2], Yiming Zhu [1,2], Irshad Ahmad [1,2] ⬭, Guichun Dong [2], Guisheng Zhou [1,2,*] and Yanqing Wu [1,2,*]

1   Joint International Laboratory of Agriculture and Agri-Product Safety, Yangzhou University, Yangzhou 225000, China; jiaoliu0407@163.com (J.L.); wangxin2203@163.com (X.W.); yzuwuhao@163.com (H.W.); mx120220721@stu.yzu.edu.cn (Y.Z.); irshadgadoon737@yahoo.com (I.A.)
2   Jiangsu Key Laboratory of Crop Cultivation and Physiology, Yangzhou University, Yangzhou 225000, China; gcdong@yzu.edu.cn
*   Correspondence: gszhou@yzu.edu.cn (G.Z.); yqwu@yzu.edu.cn (Y.W.); Tel.: +86-514-87973290 (G.Z.); Fax: +86-514-87973203 (G.Z.)

Abstract: Drought stress is one of the most severe natural disasters in terms of its frequency, length, impact intensity, and associated losses, making it a significant threat to agricultural productivity. Sorghum (*Sorghum bicolor*), a C4 plant, shows a wide range of morphological, physiological, and biochemical adaptations in response to drought stress, paving the way for it to endure harsh environments. In arid environments, sorghum exhibits enhanced water uptake and reduced dissipation through its morphological activity, allowing it to withstand drought stress. Sorghum exhibits physiological and biochemical resistance to drought, primarily by adjusting its osmotic potential, scavenging reactive oxygen species, and changing the activities of its antioxidant enzymes. In addition, certain sorghum genes exhibit downregulation capabilities in response to drought stress. Therefore, in the current review, we explore drought tolerance in sorghum, encompassing its morphological characteristics and physiological mechanisms and the identification and selection of its functional genes. The use of modern biotechnological and molecular biological approaches to improving sorghum resistance is critical for selecting and breeding drought-tolerant sorghum varieties.

Keywords: drought stress; sorghum; agronomic traits; reactive oxygen species; transcription factor; genes

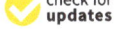

check for
updates

Citation: Liu, J.; Wang, X.; Wu, H.; Zhu, Y.; Ahmad, I.; Dong, G.; Zhou, G.; Wu, Y. Association between Reactive Oxygen Species, Transcription Factors, and Candidate Genes in Drought-Resistant Sorghum. *Int. J. Mol. Sci.* **2024**, *25*, 6464. https://doi.org/10.3390/ijms25126464

Academic Editors: Philippe Jeandet and Mateusz Labudda

Received: 8 May 2024
Revised: 4 June 2024
Accepted: 8 June 2024
Published: 12 June 2024

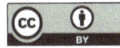

1. Introduction

Drought stress, one of the primary abiotic stresses, affects plant growth and development, potentially leading to disastrous outcomes. It hinders plant metabolic activities, such as gas exchange between leaves and cells, and it causes oxidative damage, which decreases yields [1,2]. Drought stress is a multidimensional abiotic stress that affects plants at molecular, morphological, physiological, and biochemical levels [3]. Drought stress may cause photosynthesis to stop and metabolic issues to occur, which can lead to plant death.

Sorghum (*Sorghum bicolor*) is a C4 "high-energy plant" known for its exceptional growth characteristics, as well as its high stress tolerance, rapid growth rate, and high biomass production [4]. It serves as a valuable source of cereals, fodder, and sugar. Sorghum is regarded as an exemplary example of excellent plant drought tolerance due to its inherent ability to withstand drought, diploid genome structure, and efficient photosynthetic system [5]. However, sorghum, a high-quality feed crop grown around the world, has been struggling in recent years due to climate change [6]. This has had a significant impact on its growth and crop quality, particularly during droughts. As a result, to ensure long-term sorghum production, it is critical to increase the crop's drought tolerance and investigate the processes underlying its drought resistance [7].

The main ways that sorghum can handle drought are through its agronomic traits, antioxidant defense mechanisms, ability to scavenge reactive oxygen species (ROS), and related transcription factors [8]. Drought tolerance is a polygenic trait that involves multiple genes in physio-morphological, molecular, and biochemical processes and pathways. Therefore, this review aimed to understand how drought-tolerant sorghum functions under drought stress. Section 1 emphasizes how drought affects the morphological characteristics of sorghum roots and how to mitigate those effects. Section 2 focuses on sorghum's physiological drought response mechanisms, focusing on its ROS scavenging and antioxidant systems for maintaining its normal cellular metabolism. Section 3 involves the identification of functional genes in drought-resistant sorghum and related transcription factors. This review's investigation will assist agronomists and breeders with developing and implementing drought-tolerant sorghum varieties capable of adjusting to changing production settings in arid locations. Integrating traditional and molecular breeding techniques with rapid generational advancement methods can reduce sorghum's breeding cycle and improve the effectiveness of introducing new types.

2. Agronomic Traits of Sorghum under Drought Stress

Under drought stress, sorghum exhibits a variety of agronomic traits, including reduced plant height, leaf wilting and crumpling, decreased numbers of spikes, and deficient grain filling [9]. These modifications eventually lead to changes in its growth and phenotype, and such morphological traits are clear signs of how well different types of sorghum can handle drought, and thus, they are useful tools for identifying drought-tolerant sorghum [4]. Numerous studies have indicated close correlations between sorghum's plant height morphology and its drought tolerance [5,10]. Under drought-tolerant conditions, sorghum biomass was significantly higher than that of drought-sensitive plants [11,12]. Emendack et al. [13] demonstrated that plant height, particularly in the early and late stages of growth, can serve as an indicator of drought tolerance in sorghum. In the early growth stages, drought-prone sorghum cultivars showed little-to-no germination, and in the later growth stages, they showed signs of male sterility, poor seed sets, and decreased yields. Bai et al. [14] showed that plant height and spike length were positively correlated with yield in sorghum under constant environmental conditions. Similarly, Zhou et al. [15] demonstrated that plant height and spike length diversity indices were greater than other agronomic characteristics in a study on sorghum germplasm resources, examining them as indicators of drought tolerance in sorghum under drought conditions. Under drought conditions, sorghum growth status not only determines the plant's photosynthetic area, production potential, and final yield but also exerts feedback regulation on its internal metabolism. Therefore, we can identify drought resistance in crops using indicators such as the seed germination rate, survival rate, plant height, dry matter accumulation rate, leaf area, number of yellow and withered leaves, leaf expansion rate, and interval between pollen shedding and silk emergence.

Under drought stress conditions, the root system's ability to absorb water directly affects sorghum's drought resistance [16]. Various factors, including drought tolerance and different sorghum varieties, influence the growth and development of the root system. For example, under drought stress conditions, the root systems of drought-resistant varieties are more developed than those of non-drought-resistant varieties [17]. Additionally, the same sorghum varieties have more developed root systems under moderate drought stress conditions compared to normal growth conditions. These research findings have been confirmed by Meyer et al. [16], who showed a strong positive correlation between drought tolerance and sorghum root lengths. Habyarimana et al. [17] also sought to address this association, observing that sorghum drought tolerance was dependent on its ability to acquire water from deeper soil regions in order to maintain an appropriate water content. Similar studies have also shown that sorghum roots can keep plants from drying out. This is accomplished by increasing root biomass, root length, and root volume expansion and improving root length density (RDL) [17]. Under limited water conditions, Blum et al., found that the length of the roots directly influenced the amount of water absorbed [18]. Additionally, Stone et al. [19] demonstrated that sorghum roots exhibited a consistent penetration rate of 3.4 cm per day, reaching a plateau approximately 10 days after flowering. These studies emphasized the importance of sorghum roots extending beyond the reach of accessible water during drought circumstances, with increased root lengths allowing the plants to acquire water from deeper soil layers and ameliorate the consequences of drought stress. There are significant genetic differences in root characteristics among varieties, with high heritability for traits such as root diameter, root dry weight, root length, and root density, while the heritability of root pulling force is relatively low. Dominant, additive, and cascading genetic effects control the expression of many genes related to drought resistance, influencing the phenotypic changes in sorghum roots under drought stress [20]. Notably, a drought-tolerant sorghum line possessed roots that extended at least 40 cm deeper than a drought-sensitive one, and deeper rooting of stay-green lines under drought conditions was reported [21]. In another study, under drought stress, drought-tolerant sorghum varieties exhibited larger root–shoot ratios, longer total root lengths, and greater root surface areas, emphasizing the critical function of increased root length in conferring drought tolerance [22].

QTL Mapping of Drought Tolerance in Sorghum Pre- and Post-Flowering under Drought Stress Conditions

Drought tolerance in sorghum is a complex quantitative trait influenced by a combination of major and minor genes, as well as genotypic and environmental factors [23]. Molecular marker technology has been extensively utilized to investigate the genetic basis of drought tolerance in sorghum, aiding in the identification and localization of QTLs associated with drought tolerance [24]. Sorghum has exhibited distinct response traits to drought stress, including pre-bloom and post-bloom drought tolerance, which may govern different genetic mechanisms. This explanation of genetic control and response traits has provided valuable insights into the molecular mechanisms of drought tolerance in sorghum [25–27].

Rosenow et al. [28] studied drought-tolerant sorghum hybrid cultivar selection and breeding for agricultural purposes, focusing on both the pre- and post-flowering stages. In particular, the location of the QTL for pre-flowering drought tolerance affected important yield-related traits in sorghum, such as the number of spike grains, the weight of one thousand kernels, and the overall seed yield. Tuinstra et al. [29] showed that a cross between pre-flowering drought-tolerant RTx7078 and pre-flowering drought-sensitive B35 developed a recombinant inbred line (RIL) population comprising 98 individuals. Their study identified six QTLs associated with pre-flowering drought resistance, with two QTLs in linkage group D, three in linkage group F, and one in linkage group M. Similarly, Kebede et al., used an RIL population of 125 individuals derived from a cross between pre-flowering drought-resistant SC56 and pre-flowering drought-sensitive RTx7000 [30]. Their research showed that four QTLs—Prf C, Prf E, Prf F, and Prf G—were linked to pre-flowering drought resistance. These QTLs explained 11.9% to 37.7% of the phenotypic variation. Notably, Prf E and Prf F originated from the drought-tolerant parental SC56, while Prf C and Prf G originated from the drought-sensitive parental RTx7000. These findings offer valuable insights into the genetic basis of pre-flowering drought tolerance in sorghum and provide essential information for breeding programs aimed at enhancing drought resilience in this important crop.

The localization of QTLs for drought tolerance after flowering in sorghum is critical due to the impact of post-flowering drought on plant physiology and yield. Post-flowering drought stress in sorghum leads to early leaf senescence, reduced chlorophyll content, diminished photosynthetic capacity, hindered grain filling, and, ultimately, reduced yield [31]. These effects can be primarily attributed to variations in flowering time, resulting in phenological differences. Sabadin et al., identified significant co-localization between flowering times and grain yields in sorghum, along with three QTLs, one of which was located on chromosome 9 and controlled both flowering time and plant height [32]. Their study provides valuable insights into the genetic basis of seed yields and QTLs in sorghum after flowering, with potential associations with plant height and seed yield. In another study, Sakhi et al., investigated 107 sorghum germplasm resources under drought treatments, starting at the spikelet stage [33]. Using ninety-eight pairs of SSR markers, they analyzed the association of twenty-three drought-tolerance traits and detected a total of nine QTLs associated with eight drought-tolerance traits, including stem thickness, leaf drying rate, flowering time, spikelet stipe protruding length, and flag leaf length. The identified QTLs and molecular markers can serve as a solid foundation for the precise localization of post-flowering drought-tolerance genes and the elucidation of their mechanisms of action in sorghum. These findings have contributed to a deeper understanding of the genetic basis of drought tolerance after flowering in sorghum, offering potential targets for molecular breeding strategies aimed at enhancing drought resilience in this important crop.

The integration of marker-assisted selection is pivotal in the screening and localization of QTLs for enhancing drought tolerance in sorghum lines [34]. A population was developed through pre-flowering and post-flowering backcrosses of sorghum with drought stress-sensitive lines, enabling the identification of QTLs on chromosomes controlling flowering time and plant height, thereby enhancing tolerance. The optimization of existing markers for the efficient detection of QTLs associated with drought tolerance in sorghum is crucial for advancing breeding efforts in this crop.

3. Mechanism of Physiological Response in Drought-Resistant Sorghum

3.1. Response of Photosynthetic System to Drought Stress

Under drought stress, the regulation of photosynthesis in leaves is an important phenomenon in controlling plant water loss [35]. During drought stress, plants reduce photosynthesis activity as a result of increased water loss, disturbed cellular functions, stomatal conductance, and gas exchange (Figure 1). Gas exchange is a key mechanism in plant tissues for maintaining cellular functions and energy production. Stomatal regulation plays an important role in preventing transpiration and water loss through the stomata, with stomatal opening often resulting in up to 90% water loss [36,37]. When transpiration rates increase, stomatal closure reduces water loss in sorghum. The negative correlation between sorghum's stomatal conductance and drought tolerance serves as a potential marker of drought tolerance [38]. Moreover, stomatal regulation is a key mechanism of an important cellular activity involving the maintenance of cellular water regulation [39]. Stomatal conductance (Gs) and transpiration rate (Tr) have been suggested as traits that can be used for marker-assisted selection in sorghum [40]. When soil moisture is insufficient, stomata tend to reduce transpiration rates through partial or total closure, which reduces water loss while reducing CO_2 entry, thus leading to decreases in the photosynthetic rates (Pn). It was found that the net photosynthetic rate (Pn), photochemical efficiency (Fv/Fm), photochemical burst (qP), and actual photosystem efficiency (ΦPSII) of sorghum decreased under drought stress.

These physiological and ecological characteristics reflect sorghum seedlings' physiological tolerance to drought stress. Is this physiological expression present in sorghum under drought stress at all reproductive stages? Can sorghum show similar physiological incentives to other crops after relieving stress? These questions require in depth study as they are important in guiding the development of appropriate field-management measures such as timely irrigation.

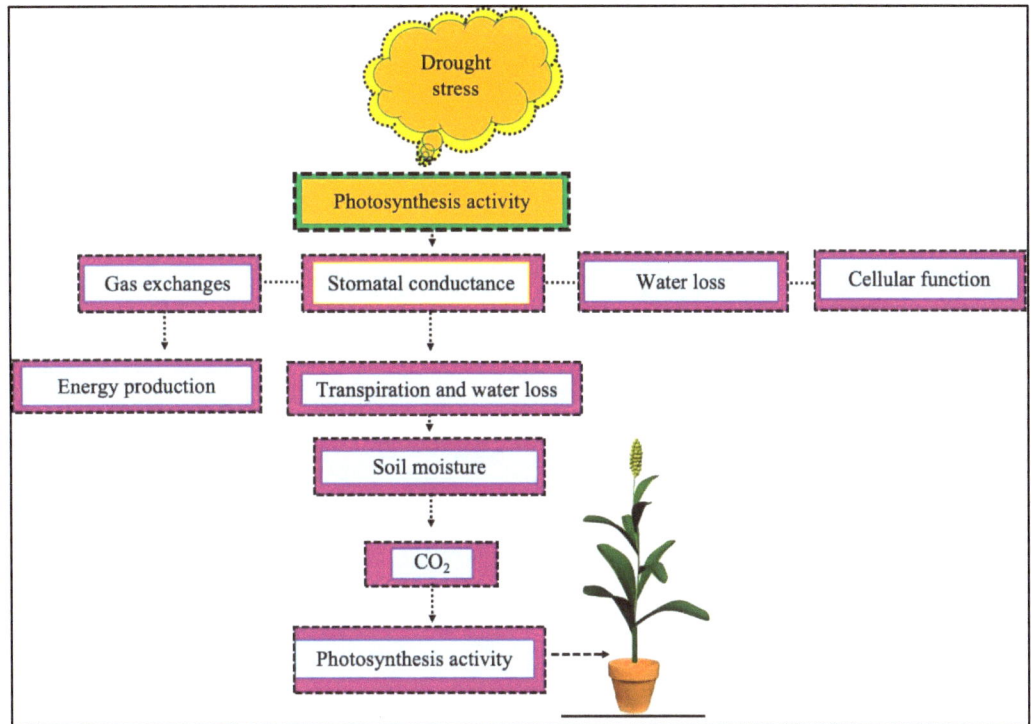

Figure 1. Drought stress adversely affects plant photosynthesis, and as a result, it affects gas exchange, stomatal conductance, water loss, and cellular functions. Gas exchange plays a key role in energy production. In addition, stomatal conductance regulates transpiration rates and water loss. When moisture content is limited during drought stress, it reduces the entry of CO_2 and, as a result, decreases photosynthesis activity in sorghum.

3.2. Response of Reactive Oxygen Metabolism System to Drought Stress

ROS are important signaling molecules in the cellular response to abiotic stress [41]. Drought stress induces the production of ROS such as superoxide radicals ($\cdot O_2^-$), hydroxyl radicals ($\cdot OH$), and H_2O_2. Previous research has shown that the $\cdot OH$ in ROS directly induces the peroxidative catabolism of unsaturated fatty acid chains in phospholipids, disrupting the overall membrane. This leads to metabolic dysregulation in vivo.

3.2.1. Participation in Signal Transduction

Previous research has demonstrated that ROS, as second messengers, are involved in various responses such as cell growth and development [42], programmed cell death (PCD) [43], hormone signaling [44], and different biotic and abiotic stresses by altering the redox states of cells [45].

In recent years, the investigation of plant adversity stress signal transduction (ROS) has become an essential component of cellular signal regulation and transmission [2]. NADPH oxidase at the plasma membrane is one of the major pathways for ROS production in plants. When plants are exposed to biotic or abiotic stress, NADPH oxidase rapidly catalyzes the production of large amounts of O_2- from O_2. The superoxide is then converted into other ROS, such as hydrogen peroxide (H_2O_2), by SOD hydroxyl (OH) radicals [46]. In sorghum, NADPH generates ROS which act as signaling molecules that activate stress response pathways and enzymes and lead gene expression changes under drought stress [47]. Moreover, NADPH-mediated ROS production maintains cellular homeostasis in these plants. ROS can modulate ion-channel activities in sorghum, trigger the synthesis of osmoprotectants, and regulate cell-wall strengthening, and as a result, cell structures and functions are maintained under drought stress conditions [48]. The Ca^{2+} concentrations in plasma membranes depend on the degree of plasma membrane Ca^{2+} channel activity or opening, the degree of activation of cytosolic Ca^{2+} pumps, etc. Among the aforementioned regulatory elements, ROS demonstrate a distinct regulatory influence (Figure 2).

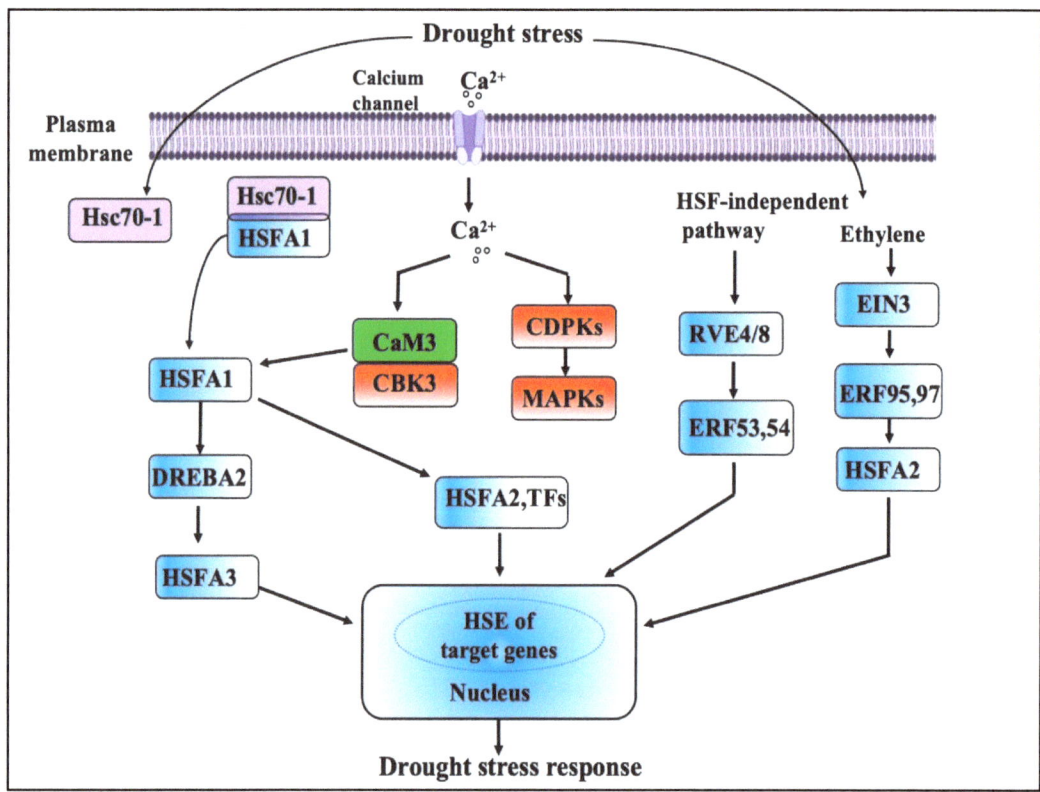

Figure 2. Plant ROS transcription-factor signaling network.

In turn, Ca^{2+} initiates NADPH oxidase, which induces ROS production and a greater cytoplasmic Ca^{2+} inward flow. Additionally, ROS act as second messengers in *Arabidopsis thaliana*, using HCN to break down seed dormancy [42]. ROS are also involved in signal transduction for the development of PCD in plants. Previous studies have shown that different ROS have specific functions in inducing signal transduction for PCD [43]. The mutant fluorescent (flu) produces monoclinic oxygen species in alternating light/dark environments, and the mutant stimulates a cell-death response immediately after the release of monoclinic oxygen species [49].

3.2.2. Involvement in ROS Metabolism

Stress primarily affects a plant's ROS-free-radical metabolism, the extent of lipid peroxidation in its cell membranes, and the activities of its antioxidant enzymes. There are two types of processes involved in ROS metabolism. The first are enzymatic antioxidants such as SOD, CAT, and APX, and the second are non-enzymatic antioxidants such as ASH, GSH, and alkaloids, which also remove intracellular ROS. CAT is a peroxisome signature enzyme that can convert H_2O_2 into O_2 and water and plays an indispensable role in the clearance of H_2O_2 from peroxisomes. Also, glutathione peroxidases (GPXs), GSTs, and peroxiredoxin (PRXs) [50] lower H_2O_2 and organic hydroperoxides through a thiol-mediated pathway that does not depend on ascorbate [50], and they do so using an ascorbate-independent thiol-mediated pathway to decrease H_2O_2 and organic hydroperoxides. These pathways work together to eliminate ROS. The antioxidant enzymes such as SOD, CAT, ascorbate peroxidase (APX), NADH-dependent dehydroascorbate reductase (NADH), glutathione reductase (GR), and glutathione peroxidase (GPX), and monodehydroascorbate reductase (MDAR), APX, GR, and NADH mitigate H_2O_2 through the Halliwell–Asada pathway [51,52]. The two primary approaches now used to represent major antioxidant enzyme activities (e.g., SOD, CAT, and APX) are as follows: first, comparing two control groups under two different drought and water situations [53], and second, summarizing the activities of the total extracted enzymes [54]. In order to examine the impacts of drought stress on the expression and activity of the major antioxidant enzymes such as SOD, CAT, and APX in a more comprehensive manner, it is common practice to utilize antioxidant enzyme expression and activity levels across a range of drought conditions [55]. In sorghum, ROS generated by NADPH oxidase activate antioxidant defense mechanisms. These mechanisms consist of the upregulation of antioxidant enzymes such as CAT, POD, and SOD, which alleviate the adverse effects of oxidative stress caused by the excessive accumulation of ROS under drought stress [48].

Harb et al., conducted transcriptomics research to investigate the effects of moderate drought stress on *Arabidopsis* [56]. To conduct a comprehensive analysis, they identified 406 *Arabidopsis* genes that encode fundamental components of antioxidant and redox homeostasis. Although this group of genes does not represent all proteins that may be involved in ROS-related metabolism or repair, it represents many known antioxidant and reductant regeneration enzymes. Finding redox-linked genes that are sensitive to drought shows how different antioxidative and redox homeostatic systems respond. However, the response within each class is complex and unique. Most notably, there is no general upregulation of ROS-producing enzymes or antioxidative and redox homeostatic pathways. In all categories, as many genes are repressed as are induced.

In 2022, Zheng et al., overexpressed *SbNAC9* in sorghum and discovered that the transgenic lines had better photosynthesis abilities, root structures, and ROS scavenging abilities, which made the sorghum more resistant to drought [57]. *SbNAC9* can also directly turn on the putative peroxidase gene *SbC5YQ75* and the putative enzyme gene *SbNCED3*, both of which are involved in making ABA [58]. Silencing *SbC5YQ75* and *SbNCED3* via VIGS resulted in reduced drought tolerance and decreased ABA content in the sorghum seedlings.

4. Transcription Factors Involved in the Drought Stress Response

During drought stress signal transduction, transcription factors (TFs) play crucial roles in plant growth and development under abiotic stress by initiating multiple pathways to regulate and reduce plant stress damage at multiple levels [59]. Over 1700 family genes encoding more than 50 transcription factors have been isolated from a model *Arabidopsis* plant. Among them, the main transcription factor gene families related to drought, salt, and heavy metal stress were AP2/ERF, HD-ZIP/bZIP, NAC, MYB, C2HC, and WRKY.

4.1. Response of HD-ZIP Transcription Factors to Drought Stress

HD-ZIP transcription factors are transcription factors that are only found in higher plants. They have a structure that includes a homodimeric domain (HD) that binds DNA and a zipper domain (ZIP) that interacts with proteins, with leucine at the C-terminus of the homodimeric domain [60,61]. Research has demonstrated that drought, excessive salt, ABA, and cold damage trigger genes belonging to subfamilies I and II of the HD-ZIP family of transcription factors. These two genes are involved in the hormone signaling pathway and regulate plant-cell expansion, division, and differentiation by interacting with hormone pathway genes and downstream genes, thus improving plant stress resistance [62–64].

Depending on the structures, conserved sequences, physiological functions, and other structural domains contained in the HD-ZIP protein genes, this family of proteins can be classified into four major classes (I–IV) [65,66], of which the first two are predominant in number (Figure 3).

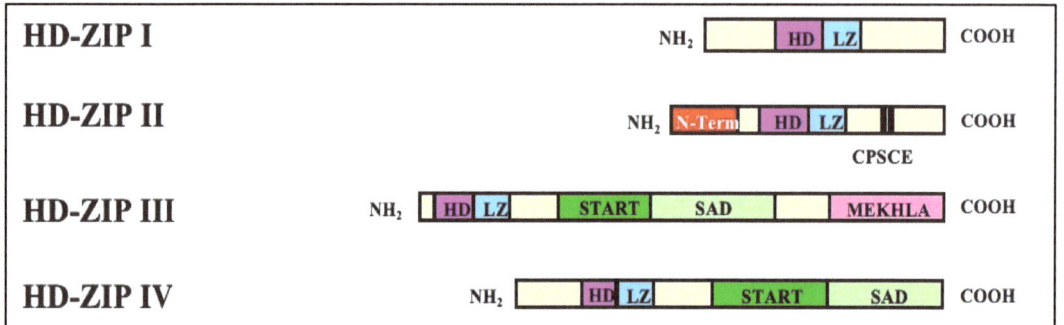

Figure 3. The classifications and structures of the HD-ZIP transcription factors.

The HD-ZIP transcription factors can improve the morphological characteristics of plants under abiotic stress. Sorghum is characterized by its small genome and short life cycle [67]. A relevant study indicated that, among the 1644 common differentially expressed genes (DEGs) in sorghum roots under severe drought stress and rehydration treatments, 2 HD-ZIP genes were upregulated under drought stress and downregulated under rehydration treatments while 4 HD-ZIP genes were downregulated under drought stress and upregulated under rehydration treatments. This suggested that HD-ZIP transcription factors have different expression patterns in sorghum roots [68].

Also, as a C4 crop, maize can lay the foundation for sorghum research. Using the pre-sequencing data for the maize transcriptome, a functional validation of the HD-ZIP transcription factors in maize plants found 42 genes that coded for HD-ZIP proteins [69]. The evolutionary tree analysis classified the 42 Zmhdz genes into 4 major categories, which aligned with the classification of the HD-ZIP genes in rice and *Arabidopsis*, demonstrating a high degree of sequence conservation in HD-ZIP genes. Researchers have found that overexpressing the HD-ZIP class genes *HaHB1* and *ATHB13* not only improved the drought tolerance of transgenic plants but also increased their biomass [70].

Transgenic rice that overexpressed the HD-ZIP class I gene *Zmhdz4* became more resistant to drought [71]. However, the overexpression of this gene in rice decreased its tolerance to salt stress [72], with a similar function to the *Arabidopsis thaliana* HD-ZIP class I transcription factor *ATHB6* [73,74]. In addition, it has been shown that members of the HD-ZIP class I family respond to stress through either the ABA-dependent pathway or the non-ABA-dependent pathway [75,76].

HD-ZIP II genes are mainly regulated by illumination conditions and auxin responses [77,78]. As a negative regulator, *ATHB2* can recognize its promoter region and participate in regulating the *Arabidopsis* shade-avoidance response [79]. *HAHB10*, an HD-ZIP II gene, shares a similar gene structure and expression pattern with *ATHB2*, which mainly regulates a plant's response to light quality and quantity as related to plant development [80]. Recent research has shown that the expression of two cotton HD-ZIP II genes, *GhHB2* and -4, can be upregulated in hypocotyls, cotyledons, and roots by external GA_3 treatments. These genes are crucial components of the phytohormone signaling system that controls early seedling development [81].

The HD-ZIP class III family of proteins contains the following five members: *ATHB88*, *CORONA (CNA)*, *PHABULOSA (PHB)*, *PHA VOLUTA (PHV)*, and *REV*. These genes are HD-ZIP class III family proteins, and increasing evidence has shown that they play major roles in embryonic development, cell differentiation, xylem formation, and lateral organ polarity transportation [82,83]. Previous studies on *Arabidopsis* have identified five HD-ZIP class III genes (*IFL1*, *ATHB8*, *ATHB9*, *ATHB14*, and *ATHB15*), and IFL1, *ATHB-9*, and *ATHB-14* were found to be connected to the development of the proximal axial regions of the apical meristematic tissues, the vascular bundles, and the lateral tissues, and they influenced the development of the root tips in the embryonic period [84]. Phytohormones and KANS transcriptionally regulate HD-ZIP III-mediated root development, while miR165/166 post-transcriptionally regulates it [85]. In addition, the overexpression of miR166G in *Arabidopsis* Jabba-1D (JBA-1D) mutant plants has been found to affect the transcription of HD-ZIP III homologous structural domain-leucine zip family genes [86]. HD-ZIP III genes all have ABRE and MBS action elements, but relevant analyses of their resistance abilities have yet to be reported, and further studies are needed to investigate their roles in response to drought stress. HD-ZIP IV genes are generally involved in determining outer cell fates [87,88]. The HD-ZIP class IV gene *AtHDG11* enhances drought tolerance in transgenic plants [89,90], and its homologous genes *Zmhdz14* and *Zmhdz13* also enhance drought tolerance in transgenic plants [69]. It has been hypothesized that genes in the same branch of the evolutionary tree have similar functions in sorghum resistance to abiotic stress [91]. Overexpression of the HD-ZIP class IV genes *Zmhdz14* and *Zmhdz13* not only enhanced the drought tolerance of transgenic plants but also their sensitivity to ABA [89]. Further, the leaf epidermis expressed OCL4, which encodes the maize HD-ZIP IV gene. *Arabidopsis* transgenic plants overexpressing OCL4 showed suppressed trichome development, while OCL4 RNAi transgenic plants showed ectopic trichome differentiation in their leaf margins [92].

Adverse hormone response elements have been detected in all 42 maize HD-ZIP genes. The ABA response elements appeared most frequently at 185, accounting for 47.07% of the total number of promoters in the study. Except for the HD-ZIP class I gene *Zmhdz41*, the HD-ZIP class II genes *Zmhdz37* and *Zmhdz14*, and the HD-ZIP class IV genes *Zmhdz35* and *Zmhdz30*, which did not contain ABA response elements, the remaining 37 (88.10% of the total number of genes) had 1 or more ABA response elements. Among the stress elements, the highest number of genes containing MBS elements was 23 (54.76% of the total number of genes), and these were shown to be positively induced by drought stress in the transcriptome data, with numbers of 10, 9, 0, and 4 in HD-ZIP I-IV, respectively. All 21 genes had MBS elements except for *Zmhdz14* (HD-ZIP II) and *Zmhdz35* (HD-ZIP IV), which did not contain ABRE elements.

As a C4 crop, sorghum's HD-ZIP transcription factors have received less attention, though maize, another C4 crop, has contributed to genetic, evolutionary, and other fundamental biological investigations. The availability of the sorghum genome sequences has provided an excellent opportunity for whole-genome annotation, classification, and comparative genomics research. Although HD-ZIP genes have been extensively characterized in *Arabidopsis* [93], rice [94], and other species [95], systemic analyses of the HD-ZIP gene family, especially for the potential stress-responsive members, have not been reported for many important species. The HD-ZIP genes in the maize genome have been found and are described at the beginning of this subsection. Furthermore, we investigated the transcript levels of HD-ZIP I genes in response to drought stress, which severely affects sorghum yields. The regulatory network of HD-ZIP proteins in the drought stress response is shown in Figure 4. The results provide a biological reference for future studies on the functions of the HD-ZIP genes and will be helpful for breeding drought-resistant sorghum.

Int. J. Mol. Sci. **2024**, *25*, 6464

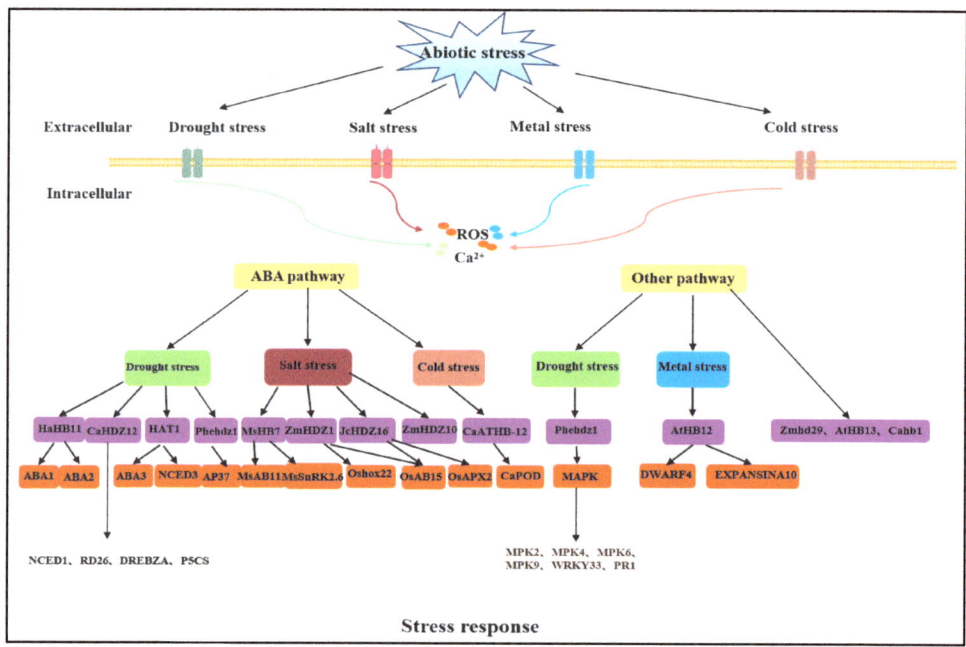

Figure 4. Molecular mechanisms of the HD-ZIP proteins under abiotic stress.

4.2. Roles of the MYB Transcription Factors in Sorghum under Drought Stress

MYB functions have been extensively investigated in different plant species. An extensive review by Ambawat et al., described the roles of MYB TFs in different plant processes, including abiotic and biotic stress responses [96]. There has been a lot of research on MYB TFs; therefore, it is important to explore how they may improve stress tolerance in agricultural crops. For example, Fang et al., demonstrated that MYB TFs are active factors in abiotic stress signaling, and MYBs have been found to regulate downstream genes in response to abiotic stresses and potentially act at both the transcriptional and post-transcriptional levels [97]. Last, but not least, Baldoni et al., reviewed the roles of MYB TFs in drought response mechanisms, providing specific examples of MYB functions and discussing potential applications of MYBs [98].

Under drought stress, MYB-like transcription factors regulate cell division and differentiation, biosynthesis, stomatal development, transpiration, photosynthesis, and root development. *AMYB60* and *AMYB44* in the model crop *Arabidopsis* are transcriptional repressors that regulate guard-cell development and stomatal movement. According to Scully et al., the overexpression of *SbMYB60* promoted monophenol production in drought-tolerant sorghum [99]. The MYB TF gene has also been an area of interest in other cereals. A new gene, *OsMYB48-1*, induced ABA, hydrogen peroxide, dehydration, and PEG under salt and drought stress treatments, according to a study [100] on the role of MYB TFs in drought tolerance in rice. RNA sequencing studies have shown that transgenic maize that overexpressed OsMYB55 was better able to handle drought and high temperatures. It also turned on a lot of genes that deal with stress [101]. More recently, Tang et al., found that *OsMYB6* overexpression in rice enhanced salt and drought stress tolerance compared to wild-type plants [102]. The overexpression of *MYB15* increased the sensitivity of plants to signals such as ABA and early drying, and it caused a greater number of stomata to close. Genes such as *ABA1/2*, *ABI3*, *AiADH1*, *RD22*, *RD29B*, and *AtEM6*, which are involved in ABA production, signal transduction, and response, had increased expression at the same time. Under drought stress, the overexpression lines showed significantly better water loss and survival than the control plants at both the nutrient and reproductive stages. The presence of *MYB15* homologous genes in plants such as tobacco, tomato, barley, and wheat is important for improving the drought tolerance of these plants. The overexpression of *OSMYB4* or its homologous genes significantly improved the tolerance to drought stress in *Arabidopsis* and tomato and apple plants.

MYB transcription factors, in addition to reacting to drought stress, play essential roles in plant responses to other environmental factors such as nutrient deficiencies, salt stress, and hypoxia stress. For example, the $R_1R_2R_3MYB$ transcription factor gene *OsMYB3R-2*, cloned from rice, was overexpressed in *Arabidopsis thaliana*, and the transgenic plants were significantly more tolerant to freezing, drought, and high-salt stress [103]. In sorghum plants under drought stress, MYB TFs were shown to regulate genes involved in water conversation, osmotic balance, and the antioxidant defense system [68]. This included the genes that encode enzymes for osmolyte biosynthesis (proline and glycine betain). Moreover, the MYB TFs helped to minimize water loss through transpiration, thereby conserving water in sorghum plants under drought stress [68].

Although several MYB genes have been functionally characterized in model and non-model species, the characterization of these TF genes in sorghum is limited. The genome-wide identification of MYB TFs in sorghum will be critical for understanding their stress-related functions and developing improved varieties.

4.3. NAC Improves Reactive Oxygen Species' Scavenging Capacities

NAC family transcription factors have numerous biological activities in different plants. So far, researchers have identified 117 NAC transcription factors in *Arabidopsis* and 151 in rice, 147 *ZmNAC* transcription factors in maize [104], and 131 NAC transcription factors in sorghum [105]. Many NAC TFs have been reported to be involved in plant responses to abiotic stress.

The *SNAC1* gene in rice was cloned in drought and high-salt conditions. The over-expression of this gene significantly improved drought and salt tolerance in rice, with a 22–34% increase in yield compared to wild-type rice [106]. Similarly, the overexpression of the *SNAC2* gene increased drought resistance in rice yields compared to wild-type rice yields [107,108]. Tran et al., cloned three *Arabidopsis* NAC family genes, *ANAC019*, *ANAC055*, and *ANAC072*, and they discovered that the overexpression of these genes dramatically increased drought tolerance compared to the wild type, with *ANAC072* being engaged in the ABA signaling system [109]. These results indicated that, as a transcription factor, *SNAC1* can actively regulate the expression of stress-related genes, and it may find application value in the improvement of drought resistance in crops.

It has been shown that the *GsNAC2* gene of the NAC family modulates sorghum's response to salt stress via various mechanisms. A total of 20 genes associated with the ABA signaling pathway were identified as being differentially expressed in the plant hormone signaling pathway. Among these, the negative regulator SbPP2C15 was downregulated following salt-stress-induced overexpression of the *GsNAC2* gene in sorghum. The positive regulator genes *SbSAPK9* and *SbABCI12* were found to be upregulated. The GA signaling pathway enriched 19 differentially expressed genes, and following the salt–alkali stress-induced overexpression of the *GsNAC2* gene in sorghum, the receptor genes *SbChitin1* and *SbChitin2* were elevated, while the negative regulators SbSHORT-ROOT1 and SbRGL1 were downregulated. The JA signaling pathway was enriched in 23 differentially expressed genes, with the receptor genes *SbTIFY9* and *SbTIFY11e*, the positive regulator *SbJAR1*, and the negative regulator *SbbHLH61* being significantly upregulated after the salt–alkali stress-induced overexpression of the *GsNAC2* gene in sorghum. Sorghum has shown the significant upregulation of key genes *GCL*, *GS*, *GSH-Px*, and *GR* following the salt–alkali stress-induced overexpression of the *GsNAC2* gene, and *GSH-Px* and GR enzyme activities were also significantly higher than those in the control group, with 18 differentially expressed genes enriched in the glutathione metabolism pathway.

In conclusion, the *GsNAC2* gene is important to sorghum's ability to deal with stress because it helps plants grow and develop, makes them better at getting rid of reactive oxygen species, controls glutathione metabolism pathways, and boosts the production of reduced glutathione. During drought stress conditions, sorghum accumulates proline, betainan, and soluble sugar to maintain cell turgor and protect cellular structures [8]. *GsNAC2* improves the expression of the genes involved in these osmolytes' biosynthesis, thereby contributing to better adjustment and enhanced drought tolerance in sorghum [110]. In sorghum, the GsNAC2 genes are involved in the regulation of the antioxidant defense mechanism by upregulating the genes that encode antioxidant enzymes such as SOD, CAT, and POD, which mitigate the excessive production of ROS and protect sorghum cells from oxidative damage [111]. All of these processes improve transgenic sorghum's stress tolerance.

To validate their RNA-Seq results, Zhang et al., utilized gene-specific primers and the qRT-PCR method to validate differentially expressed genes (DEGs) with NAC expression patterns [68]. In the leaves, five different regulatory factors in response to drought (mild and severe) and rehydration treatments were confirmed. The expression level ratios of drought and the corresponding control treatments determined by qRT-PCR were compared with the expression level ratios determined by RNA-Seq. There were significant correlations between the RNA-Seq and qRT-PCR data ($r^2 = 0.786$). The qRT-PCR results showed that the expression patterns of these genes were similar to those in the RNA-Seq analysis results.

5. Genes and Mechanisms Related to Drought Resistance in Sorghum

The completion of the sorghum genome sequence provides an effective guarantee for the cloning of genes related to drought and stress tolerance in sorghum, despite the fact that the primary QTL for drought resistance in sorghum has not yet been available in the form of corresponding candidate genes through the mapping and cloning technique. Abdel-Ghany et al., identified a set of genes (BTx623 [DR1] and SC56 [DR2]) that exhibited differential expression only in resistant genotypes in response to PEG-induced drought [20]. This group of genes encodes known transcription factors, other proteins (signaling and metabolic enzymes) associated with drought response, and many novel proteins with no known functions. A bioinformatics analysis revealed potential regulatory elements in these genes and cognate transcription factors that may modulate their expression. To further understand seedling-stage drought tolerance in sorghum and aid in the development of drought-resistant crops, future functional investigations using the uncharacterized genes expressed only in the drought-resistant genotypes are required.

Han et al. [112] isolated and cloned the sorghum *ERECTA* gene and analyzed its sequence structure as well as its expression pattern in response to drought stress during the seedling stage. The results showed that both the *Sb ER1* and *Sb ER2* genes were expressed in sorghum stems and leaves, and their expression levels gradually increased with the severity of drought stress, and so the two genes, *Sb ER1* and *Sb ER2*, may be prime candidates for genetic engineering. Liu et al. [110] cloned the *Sb SKIP* gene from sorghum and transferred it into tobacco for a drought function analysis. The findings provided the groundwork for further studies on the role of the *Sb SKIP* gene by demonstrating that its expression enhanced the tobacco plants' drought tolerance. In contrast, the cloning and functional analysis of the gene provided basic information for the creation of transgenic drought-resistant materials.

6. Conclusions

Abiotic stress severely reduces plant growth and yield. To mitigate the adverse effects of abiotic stress on sorghum, the plant uses a variety of responses, such as biochemical, physiological, and molecular responses.

Expanding China's food production is a great strategy to ensure food security and alleviate resource deficiencies under abiotic stress, including drought stress in sorghum. However, progress has yet to be made in selecting and improving drought-resistant plants.

It is still a challenge to reach the greatest yield potential due to issues with low planting efficiency and lower yields of drought-prone species in the promotion and use of their new varieties.

7. Future Recommendations

The current investigation provides a comprehensive review of the agronomic traits, reactive oxygen species metabolism mechanisms, and genetic basis of drought tolerance in sorghum. We presented the latest advances in sorghum morphology, physiology, and transcription factors, providing a broad understanding of these aspects. Additionally, we discussed the interactions between drought-induced ROS and the MAPK, NAC, and MYB signaling pathways. The various mechanisms that enable plant cells to withstand stress appear to be interconnected, and the degree of their interrelation is influenced by environmental factors. Due to the complexity of drought tolerance and the challenges in phenotypic aspects, the molecular genetic bases and foundations of these mechanisms have not been fully explored. Despite previous improvements, there is still tremendous potential for enhancing drought tolerance. Understanding the interplay between plant biology, cellular physiology, and plant–environment interactions requires the latest genetic information.

It has been confirmed that drought, salt, and heavy metals stresses can be alleviated via HD-ZIP transcription factor genes, such as AP2/ERF, HD-ZIP/bZIP, NAC, MYB, C2HC, and WRKY, which can be isolated from a model *Arabidopsis* plant and rice plants. However, the roles of these various genes in stressed sorghum have yet to be studied in order to alleviate the adverse effects of drought.

Author Contributions: J.L. participated in the writing (review and editing) of the original manuscript. G.Z. and Y.W. conceived the idea and acquired funding. X.W. contributed to the reviewing and editing of the manuscript. H.W. conceptualized the idea. Y.Z. assisted with the literature review. G.D. assisted with supervision. I.A. edited the manuscript and eliminated grammatical errors. All authors have read and agreed to the published version of the manuscript.

Funding: This work was supported by the China National Key R & D Program (2022YFE0113400), the Jiangsu Provincial Fund for Realizing Carbon Emission Peaking and Neutralization (BE2022305) and the National Natural Science Funds (32102411) (a project funded by the China Postdoctoral Science Foundation (2022M722698)), and the Postgraduate Research and Practice Innovation Program of Jiangsu Province (Yangzhou University) (KYCX23_3570).

Data Availability Statement: Data used in this article are present in the tables and figures.

Conflicts of Interest: The authors declare that they have no competing interests.

References

1. Zandalinas, S.I.; Fritschi, F.B.; Mittler, R. Global Warming, Climate Change, and Environmental Pollution: Recipe for a Multifactorial Stress Combination Disaster. *Trends Plant Sci.* **2021**, *26*, 588–599. [CrossRef]
2. Zhang, H.M.; Zhu, J.H.; Gong, Z.Z.; Zhu, J.K. Abiotic stress responses in plants. *Nat. Rev. Genet.* **2022**, *23*, 104–119. [CrossRef]
3. Abreha, K.B.; Enyew, M.; Carlsson, A.S.; Vetukuri, R.R.; Feyissa, T.; Motlhaodi, T.; Ng'uni, D.; Geleta, M. Sorghum in dryland: Morphological, physiological, and molecular responses of sorghum under drought stress. *Planta* **2022**, *255*, 20. [CrossRef]
4. Sarshad, A.; Talei, D.; Torabi, M.; Rafei, F.; Nejatkhah, P. Morphological and biochemical responses of *Sorghum bicolor* (L.) Moench under drought stress. *SN Appl. Sci.* **2021**, *3*, 81. [CrossRef]
5. Hossain, M.S.; Islam, M.N.; Rahman, M.M.; Mostofa, M.G.; Khan, M.A.R. Sorghum: A prospective crop for climatic vulnerability, food and nutritional security. *J. Agric. Food Res.* **2022**, *8*, 100300. [CrossRef]
6. Carr, T.W.; Mkuhlani, S.; Segnon, A.C.; Ali, Z.; Zougmoré, R.; Dangour, A.D.; Green, R.; Scheelbeek, P. Climate change impacts and adaptation strategies for crops in West Africa: A systematic review. *Environ. Res. Lett.* **2022**, *17*, 053001. [CrossRef]
7. Ahmad, R.; Alsahli, A.A.; Alansi, S.; Altaf, M.A. Exogenous melatonin confers drought stress by promoting plant growth, photosynthetic efficiency and antioxidant defense system of pea (*Pisum sativum* L.). *Sci. Hortic.* **2023**, *322*, 112431. [CrossRef]
8. Badigannavar, A.; Teme, N.; de Oliveira, A.C.; Li, G.Y.; Vaksmann, M.; Viana, V.E.; Ganapathi, T.R.; Sarsu, F. Physiological, genetic and molecular basis of drought resilience in sorghum [*Sorghum bicolor* (L.) Moench]. *Indian J. Plant Physiol.* **2018**, *23*, 670–688. [CrossRef]
9. Ndlovu, E.; van Staden, J.; Maphosa, M. Morpho-physiological effects of moisture, heat and combined stresses on *Sorghum bicolor* [Moench (L.)] and its acclimation mechanisms. *Plant Stress* **2021**, *2*, 100018. [CrossRef]

10. Rad, R.D.; Sharifabad, H.H.; Torabi, M.; Azizinejad, R.; Salemi, H.; Soltanabadi, M.H. Drought stress tolerance based on selection indices of resistant crops variety. *Glob. J. Environ. Sci. Manag.* **2023**, *9*, 287–298. [CrossRef]
11. Yahaya, M.A.; Shimelis, H. Drought stress in sorghum: Mitigation strategies, breeding methods and technologies—A review. *J. Agron. Crop Sci.* **2022**, *208*, 127–142. [CrossRef]
12. Dehnavi, A.R.; Zahedi, M.; Ludwiczak, A.; Cardenas Perez, S.; Piernik, A. Effect of salinity on seed germination and seedling development of sorghum (*Sorghum bicolor* (L.) Moench) genotypes. *Agronomy* **2020**, *10*, 859. [CrossRef]
13. Emendack, Y.; Herzog, H.; Götz, K.P.; Malinowski, D.P. Mid-Season water stress on yield and water use of millet (Panicum miliaceum) and sorghum (*Sorghum bicolour* L. Moench). *Aust. J. Crop Sci.* **2012**, *5*, 1486–1492.
14. Bai, X.Q.; Yu, P.P.; Li, Y.L.; Gao, J.M.; Pei, Z.Y.; Luo, F.; Sun, S.J. Genetic Analysis of Agronomic Characters in F2 Population of *Sorghum bicolor*. *Acta Agric.* **2019**, *34*, 107–114. (In Chinese) [CrossRef]
15. Zhou, Y.; Li, Z.B.; Huang, J.; Wu, Y.; Zhang, Y.Q.; Zhang, Z.L.; Zhang, X.C. Genetic Diversity of Sorghum Germplasms Based on Phenotypic Traits. *J. Plant Genet. Resour.* **2021**, *22*, 654–664. (In Chinese) [CrossRef]
16. Meyer, W.S. Resistance to water flow in the Sorghum plant. *Plant Physiol.* **1980**, *65*, 33–39. [CrossRef]
17. Habyarimana, E.; Laureti, D.; de Ninno, A.; Lorenzoni, C. Performance of biomass sorghum (*Sorghum bicolor* L. Moench) under different water regimes in Mediterranean region. *Ind. Crops Prod.* **2003**, *20*, 23–28. [CrossRef]
18. Blum, A. Drought resistance, water-use efficiency, and yield potential-are they compatible, dissonant, or mutually exclusive? *Aust. J. Agric. Res.* **2005**, *56*, 1159–1168. [CrossRef]
19. Stone, L.R.; Goodrum, D.E.; Schlegel, A.J.; Jaafar, M.N.; Khan, A.H. Water depletion depth of grain sorghum and sunflower in the central High Plains. *Agron.* **2002**, *94*, 936–943. [CrossRef]
20. Abdel-Ghany, S.E.; Ullah, F.; Ben-Hur, A.; Reddy, A.S.N. Transcriptome Analysis of Drought-Resistant and Drought-Sensitive Sorghum (*Sorghum bicolor*) Genotypes in Response to PEG-Induced Drought Stress. *Int. J. Mol. Sci.* **2020**, *21*, 772. [CrossRef]
21. Demissie, H.S.; Mindaye, T.T.; Teklu, D.N.; Kebede, F.G. Root system architecture analysis of sorghum genotypes and its effect on drought adaptation. *Rhizosphere* **2023**, *27*, 100772. [CrossRef]
22. Borrell, A.K.; Mullet, J.E.; George-Jaeggli, B.; van Oosterom, E.J.; Hammer, G.L.; Klein, P.E.; Jordan, D.R. Drought adaptation of stay-green sorghum is associated with canopy development, leaf anatomy, root growth, and water uptake. *J. Exp. Bot.* **2014**, *65*, 6251–6263. [CrossRef]
23. Mwamahonje, A.; Eleblu, J.S.Y.; Ofori, K.; Feyissa, T.; Deshpande, S.; Garcia-Oliveira, A.L.; Bohar, R.; Kigoni, M.; Tongoona, P. Introgression of QTLs for Drought Tolerance into Farmers' Preferred Sorghum Varieties. *Agriculture* **2021**, *11*, 883. [CrossRef]
24. Somegowda, V.K.; Prasad, K.V.S.V.; Naravula, J.; Vemula, A.; Selvanayagam, S.; Rathore, A.; Jones, C.S.; Gupta, R.; Deshpande, S.P. Genetic Dissection and Quantitative Trait Loci Mapping of Agronomic and Fodder Quality Traits in Sorghum Under Different Water Regimes. *Front. Plant Sci.* **2022**, *13*, 810632. [CrossRef]
25. Pereira, M.G.; Lee, M. Identification of genomic regions affecting plant height in sorghum and maize. *Theor. Appl. Genet.* **1995**, *90*, 380–388. [CrossRef]
26. Tuinstra, M.R.; Ejeta, G.; Goldsbrough, P. Evaluation of near isogenic sorghum lines contrasting for QTL markers associated with drought tolerance. *Crop Sci.* **1998**, *38*, 835–842. [CrossRef]
27. Haussmann, B.I.G.; Mahalakshmi, V.; Reddy, B.V.S.; Seetharama, N.; Hash, C.T.; Geiger, H.H. QTL mapping of stay-green in two sorghum recombinant inbred populations. *Theor. Appl. Genet.* **2002**, *106*, 133–142. [CrossRef]
28. Rosenow, D.T.; Clark, L.E.; Peterson, G.C.; Odvody, G.N.; Rooney, W.L. Registration of Tx3440 through Tx3482 sorghum germplasm. *J. Plant Regist.* **2021**, *15*, 379–387. [CrossRef]
29. Tuinstra, M.R.; Grote, E.M.; Goldsbrough, P.B.; Ejeta, G. Identification of quantitative trait loci associated with pre-flowering drought tolerance in sorghum. *Crop Sci.* **1996**, *36*, 1337–1344. [CrossRef]
30. Kebede, H.; Subudhi, P.K.; Rosenow, D.T.; Nguyen, H.T. Quantitative trait loci influencing drought tolerance in grain sorghum (*Sorghum bicolor* L. Moench). *Theor. Appl. Genet.* **2001**, *103*, 266–276. [CrossRef]
31. Hart, G.E.; Schertz, K.F.; Peng, Y.; Syed, N.H. Genetic mapping of *Sorghum bicolor* (L.) Moench QTLs that control variation in tillering and other morphological characters. *Theor. Appl. Genet.* **2001**, *103*, 1232–1242. [CrossRef]
32. Sabadin, P.K.; Malosetti, M.; Boer, M.P.; Tardin, F.D.; Santos, F.G.; Guimaraes, C.L.T.; Albuquerque, P.E.P.; Caniato, F.F.; Mollinari, M.; Margarido, G.R.A.; et al. Studying the genetic basis of drought tolerance in sorghum by managed stress trials and adjustments for phenological and plant height differences. *Theor. Appl. Genet.* **2012**, *124*, 1389–1402. [CrossRef]
33. Sakhi, S.; Shehzad, T.; Rehman, S.; Okuno, K. Mapping the QTLs underlying drought stress at developmental stage of sorghum [*Sorghum bicolor* (L.) Moench] by association analysis. *Euphytica* **2013**, *193*, 433–450. [CrossRef]
34. Rami, J.F.; Dufour, P.; Trouche, G.; Fliedel, G.; Mestres, C.; Davrieux, F.; Blanchard, P.; Hamon, P. Quantitative trait loci for grain quality, productivity, morphological and agronomical traits in sorghum (*Sorghum bicolor* L. Moench). *Theor. Appl. Genet.* **1998**, *97*, 605–616. [CrossRef]
35. Liu, J.; Wu, Y.Q.; Dong, G.C.; Zhu, G.L.; Zhou, G.S. Progress of Research on the Physiology and Molecular Regulation of Sorghum Growth under Salt Stress by Gibberellin. *Int. J. Mol. Sci.* **2023**, *24*, 6777. [CrossRef]
36. Gruss, S.M.; Souza, A.; Yang, Y.; Dahlberg, J.; Tuinstra, M.R. Expression of stay-green drought tolerance in dhurrin-free sorghum. *Crop Sci.* **2023**, *63*, 1270–1283. [CrossRef]
37. Ohashi, Y.; Nakayama, N.; Saneoka, H.; Fujita, K. Effects of drought stress on photosynthetic gas exchange, chlorophyll fluorescence and stem diameter of soybean plants. *Biol. Plant.* **2006**, *50*, 138–141. [CrossRef]

38. Borrell, A.K.; Christopher, J.T.; Kelly, A.; Collins, B.; Chenu, K. Balancing pre- and post-anthesis growth to maximise water-limited yield in cereals. *Field Crops Res.* **2023**, *296*, 108919. [CrossRef]
39. Khanthavong, P.; Yabuta, S.; Malik, A.; Hossain, M.A.; Akagi, I.; Sakagami, J.I. Combinational variation temperature and soil water response of stomata and biomass production in maize, millet, sorghum and rice. *Plants* **2022**, *11*, 1039. [CrossRef]
40. Ortiz, D.; Hu, J.Y.; Fernandez, M.G.S. Genetic architecture of photosynthesis in *Sorghum bicolor* under non-stress and cold stress conditions. *J. Exp. Bot.* **2017**, *68*, 4545–4557. [CrossRef]
41. del Río, L.A. ROS and RNS in plant physiology: An overview. *J. Exp. Bot.* **2015**, *66*, 2827–2837. [CrossRef]
42. Lee, S.; Park, C. Regulation of reactive oxygen species generation under drought conditions in arabidopsis. *Plant Signal. Behav.* **2012**, *7*, 599–601. [CrossRef]
43. Ye, C.J.; Zheng, S.Y.; Jiang, D.G.; Lu, J.Q.; Huang, Z.N.; Liu, Z.L.; Zhou, H.; Zhuang, C.X.; Li, J. Initiation and Execution of Programmed Cell Death and Regulation of Reactive Oxygen Species in Plants. *Int. J. Mol. Sci.* **2021**, *22*, 12942. [CrossRef]
44. Cui, S.Y.; Zhang, Z.F.; Fu, X.F.; Liu, J.Q.; Yang, H.S. Key Genes in Response to Drought Stress in Plant Hormone Signal Transduction Pathway of Oat. *J. Triticeae Crops* **2023**, *43*, 1384–1393. (In Chinese) [CrossRef]
45. Miller, G.; Suzuki, N.; Ciftci-Yilmaz, S.; Mittler, R. Reactive oxygen species homeostasis and signalling during drought and salinity stresses. *Plant. Cell Environ.* **2010**, *33*, 453–467. [CrossRef]
46. Choudhury, F.K.; Rivero, R.M.; Blumwald, E.; Mittler, R. Reactive oxygen species, abiotic stress and stress combination. *Plant J.* **2017**, *90*, 856–867. [CrossRef]
47. Rajarajan, K.; Ganesamurthy, K.; Raveendran, M.; Jeyakumar, P.; Yuvaraja, A.; Sampath, P.; Prathima, P.T.; Senthilraja, C. Differential responses of sorghum genotypes to drought stress revealed by physio-chemical and transcriptional analysis. *Mol. Biol. Rep.* **2021**, *48*, 2453–2462. [CrossRef]
48. Devnarain, N.; Crampton, B.G.; Olivier, N.; van der Westhuyzen, C.; Becher, J.V.M.; O'Kennedy, M.M. Transcriptomic analysis of a *Sorghum bicolor* landrace identifies a role for beta-alanine betaine biosynthesis in drought tolerance. *S. Afr. J. Bot.* **2019**, *127*, 244–255. [CrossRef]
49. op den Camp, R.G.L.; Przybyla, D.; Ochsenbein, C.; Laloi, C.; Kim, C.H.; Danon, A.; Wagner, D.; Hideg, É.; Göbel, C.; Feussner, I.; et al. Rapid induction of distinct stress responses after the release of singlet oxygen in arabidopsis. *Plant Cell* **2003**, *15*, 2320–2332. [CrossRef]
50. Dietz, K.J. Peroxiredoxins in plants and cyanobacteria. *Antioxid. Redox Sign.* **2011**, *15*, 1129–1159. [CrossRef]
51. Uzilday, B.; Turkan, I.; Sekmen, A.H.; Ozgur, R.; Karakaya, H.C. Comparison of ROS formation and antioxidant enzymes in Cleome gynandra (C4) and Cleome spinosa (C3) under drought stress. *Plant Sci.* **2012**, *182*, 59–70. [CrossRef] [PubMed]
52. Wu, S.W.; Hu, C.X.; Tan, Q.L.; Li, L.; Shi, K.L.; Zheng, Y.; Sun, X.C. Drought stress tolerance mediated by zinc-induced antioxidative defense and osmotic adjustment in cotton (Gossypium Hirsutum). *Acta Physiol. Plant.* **2015**, *37*, 167. [CrossRef]
53. Laxa, M.; Liebthal, M.; Telman, W.; Chibani, K.; Dietz, K.J. The Role of the Plant Antioxidant System in Drought Tolerance. *Antioxidants* **2019**, *8*, 94. [CrossRef] [PubMed]
54. Wang, Z.H.; Wei, Y.Q.; Zhao, Y.R.; Wang, Y.J.; Zou, F.; Huang, S.Q.; Yang, X.L.; Xu, Z.W.; Hu, H. Physiological and transcriptional evaluation of sweet sorghum seedlings in response to single and combined drought and salinity stress. *S. Afr. J. Bot.* **2022**, *146*, 459–471. [CrossRef]
55. Li, H.B.; Li, Y.L.; Ke, Q.B.; Kwak, S.S.; Zhang, S.Q.; Deng, X.P. Physiological and Differential Proteomic Analyses of Imitation Drought Stress Response in *Sorghum bicolor* Root at the Seedling Stage. *Int. J. Mol. Sci.* **2021**, *21*, 9174. [CrossRef] [PubMed]
56. Harb, A.; Krishnan, A.; Ambavaram, M.M.R.; Pereira, A. Molecular and Physiological Analysis of Drought Stress in Arabidopsis Reveals Early Responses Leading to Acclimation in Plant Growth. *Plant Physiol.* **2010**, *154*, 1254–1271. [CrossRef] [PubMed]
57. Zheng, Y.C.; Jin, X.Y.; Wang, J.Y.; Chen, W.; Yang, Z.; Chen, Y.X.; Yang, Y.H.; Lu, G.H.; Sun, B. SbNAC9 Improves Drought Tolerance by Enhancing Scavenging Ability of Reactive Oxygen Species and Activating Stress-Responsive Genes of Sorghum. *Int. J. Mol. Sci.* **2023**, *24*, 2401. [CrossRef]
58. Ngara, R.; Ramulifho, E.; Movahedi, M.; Shargie, N.G.; Brown, A.P.; Chivasa, S. Identifying differentially expressed proteins in sorghum cell cultures exposed to osmotic stress. *Sci. Rep.* **2018**, *8*, 8671. [CrossRef]
59. Hirayama, T.; Shinozaki, K. Research on plant abiotic stress responses in the post-genome era: Past, present and future. *Plant J.* **2010**, *61*, 1041–1052. [CrossRef]
60. Johannesson, H.; Wang, Y.; Engström, P. DNA-binding and dimerization preferences of Arabidopsis homeodomain-leucine zipper transcription factors in vitro. *Plant Mol. Biol.* **2001**, *45*, 63–73. [CrossRef]
61. Roodbarkelari, F.; Groot, E.P. Regulatory function of homeodomain-leucine zipper (HD-ZIP) family proteins during embryogenesis. *New Phytol.* **2017**, *213*, 95–104. [CrossRef] [PubMed]
62. Wang, Y.; Henriksson, E.; Soderman, E.; Henriksson, K.N.; Sundberg, E.; Engstrom, P. The Arabidopsis homeobox gene, ATHB16, regulates leaf development and the sensitivity to photoperiod in Arabidopsis. *Dev. Biol.* **2003**, *264*, 228–239. [CrossRef] [PubMed]
63. Lin, Z.F.; Hong, Y.G.; Yin, M.G.; Li, C.Y.; Zhang, K.; Grierson, D. A tomato HD-Zip homeobox protein, LeHB-1, plays an important role in floral organogenesis and ripening. *Plant J.* **2008**, *55*, 301–310. [CrossRef] [PubMed]
64. Fu, Y.; Liu, W.; Li, Q.; Li, J.; Wang, L.N.; Ren, Z.H. Comprehensive analysis of the homeodomain-leucine zipper IV transcription factor family in Cucumis sativus. *Genome* **2013**, *56*, 395–405. [CrossRef] [PubMed]
65. Ariel, F.D.; Manavella, P.A.; Dezar, C.A.; Chan, R.L. The true story of the HD-Zip family. *Trends Plant Sci.* **2007**, *12*, 419–426. [CrossRef] [PubMed]

66. Sakakibara, K.; Nishiyama, T.; Kato, M.; Hasebe, M. Isolation of homeodomain-leucine zipper genes from the moss Physcomitrella patens and the evolution of homeodomain-leucine zipper genes in land plants. *Mol. Biol. Evol.* **2001**, *18*, 491–502. [CrossRef] [PubMed]

67. Wang, C.; Tang, Y.F.; Li, Y.; Hu, C.; Li, J.Y.; Lyu, A. Genome-wide identification and bioinformatics analysis of the WD40 transcription factor family and candidate gene screening for anthocyanin biosynthesis in Rhododendron simsii. *BMC Genom.* **2023**, *24*, 488. [CrossRef] [PubMed]

68. Zhang, D.F. Transcriptomic profiling of sorghum leaves and roots responsive to drought stress at the seedling stage. *J. Integr. Agric.* **2021**, *20*, 1980–1995. [CrossRef]

69. Yan, H.P. *Study on Drought Resistence Functions of Two HD-Zip Transcription Factors Zmhdz13 and Zmhdz14 in Maize (Zea mays L.)*; Gansu Agricultural University: Lanzhou, China, 2016. (In Chinese)

70. Cabello, J.V.; Chan, R.L. The homologous homeodomain-leucine zipper transcription factors HaHB1 and AtHB13 confer tolerance to drought and salinity stresses via the induction of proteins that stabilize membranes. *Plant Biotechnol. J.* **2012**, *10*, 815–825. [CrossRef]

71. Wu, J.D.; Zhou, W.; Gong, X.F.; Cheng, B.J. Expression of ZmHDZ4, a Maize Homeodomain-Leucine Zipper I Gene, Confers Tolerance to Drought Stress in Transgenic Rice. *Plant Mol. Biol. Rep.* **2016**, *34*, 845–853. [CrossRef]

72. Goche, T.; Shargie, N.G.; Cummins, I.; Brown, A.P.; Chivasa, S.; Ngare, R. Comparative physiological and root proteome analyses of two sorghum varieties responding to water limitation. *Sci. Rep.* **2020**, *10*, 11835. [CrossRef]

73. Söderman, E.; Hjellström, M.; Fahleson, J.; Engstrom, P. The HD-Zip gene ATHB6 in Arabidopsis is expressed in developing leaves, roots and carpels and up-regulated by water deficit conditions. *Plant Mol. Biol.* **1999**, *40*, 1073–1083. [CrossRef]

74. Lechner, E.; Leonhardt, N.; Eisler, H.; Parmentier, Y.; Ailoua, M.; Jacquet, H.; Leung, J.; Genschik, P. MATH/BTB CRL3 receptors target the homeodomain-leucine zipper ATHB6 to modulate abscisic acid signaling. *Dev. Cell* **2011**, *21*, 1116–1128. [CrossRef]

75. Zhang, S.X.; Haider, I.; Kohlen, W.; Jiang, L.; Bouwmeester, H.; Meijer, A.H.; Schluepmann, H.; Liu, C.M.; Ouwerkerk, P.B.F. Function of the HD-Zip I gene OsHOX22 in ABA-mediated drought and salt tolerances in rice. *Plant Mol. Biol.* **2013**, *80*, 571–585. [CrossRef]

76. Zhao, Y.; Ma, Q.; Jin, X.L.; Peng, X.L.; Liu, J.Y.; Deng, L.; Yan, H.W.; Sheng, L.; Jiang, H.Y.; Cheng, B.J. A Novel Maize Homeodomain-Leucine Zipper (HD-Zip) I Gene, Zmhdz10, Positively Regulates Drought and Salt Tolerance in Both Rice and Arabidopsis. *Plant Cell Physiol.* **2014**, *55*, 1142–1156. [CrossRef]

77. Sessa, G.; Carabelli, M.; Sassi, M.; Ciolfi, A.; Possenti, M.; Mittempergher, F.; Becker, J.; Morelli, G.; Ruberti, I. A dynamic balance between gene activation and repression regulates the shade avoidance response in Arabidopsis. *Gene Dev.* **2005**, *19*, 2811–2815. [CrossRef]

78. Morelli, G.; Ruberti, I. Light and shade in the photocontrol of Arabidopsis growth. *Trends Plant Sci.* **2002**, *7*, 399–404. [CrossRef]

79. Steindler, C.; Matteucci, A.; Sessa, G.; Weimar, T.; Ohgishi, M.; Aoyama, T.; Morelli, G.; Ruberti, I. Shade avoidance responses are mediated by the ATHB-2 HD-zip protein, a negative regulator of gene expression. *Development* **1999**, *126*, 4235–4245. [CrossRef]

80. Rueda, E.C.; Dezar, C.A.; Gonzalez, D.H.; Chan, R.L. Hahb-10, a sunflower homeobox-leucine zipper gene, is regulated by light quality and quantity, and promotes early flowering when expressed in Arabidopsis. *Plant Cell Physiol.* **2005**, *46*, 1954–1963. [CrossRef]

81. Qin, Y.F.; Li, D.D.; Wu, Y.J.; Liu, Z.H.; Zhang, J.; Zheng, Y.; Li, X.B. Three cotton homeobox genes are preferentially expressed during early seedling development and in response to phytohormone signaling. *Plant Cell Rep.* **2010**, *29*, 1147–1156. [CrossRef]

82. Smith, Z.R.; Long, J.A. Control of Arabidopsis apical-basal embryo polarity by antagonistic transcription factors. *Nature* **2010**, *464*, 423–426. [CrossRef]

83. Emery, J.F.; Floyd, S.K.; Alvarez, J.; Eshed, Y.; Hawker, N.P.; Izhaki, A.; Baum, S.F.; Bowman, J.L. Radial patterning of Arabidopsis shoots by class III HD-ZIP and KANADI genes. *Curr. Biol.* **2003**, *13*, 1768–1774. [CrossRef]

84. Byrne, M.E. Shoot meristem function and leaf polarity: The role of class III HD-ZIP genes. *PLoS Gene* **2006**, *2*, 785–790. [CrossRef]

85. Singh, A.; Roy, S.; Singh, S.; Das, S.S.; Gautam, V.; Yadav, S.; Kumar, A.; Singh, A.; Sarkar, A.K. Phytohormonal crosstalk modulates the expression of miR166/165s, target Class III HD-ZIPs, and KANADI genes during root growth in Arabidopsis thaliana. *Sci. Rep.* **2017**, *7*, 3408. [CrossRef]

86. Williams, L.; Grigg, S.P.; Xie, M.T.; Christensen, S.; Fletcher, J.C. Regulation of Arabidopsis shoot apical meristem and lateral organ formation by microRNA miR166g and its AtHD-ZIP target genes. *Development* **2005**, *132*, 3657–3668. [CrossRef]

87. Guan, X.Y.; Li, Q.J.; Shan, C.M.; Wang, S.; Mao, Y.B.; Wang, L.J.; Chen, X.Y. The HD-Zip IV gene GaHOX1 from cotton is a functional homologue of the Arabidopsis GLABRA2. *Physiol. Plant.* **2008**, *134*, 174–182. [CrossRef]

88. Ito, M.; Sentoku, N.; Nishimura, A.; Hong, S.K.; Sato, Y.; Matsuoka, M. Position dependent expression of GL2-type homeobox gene, Roc1: Significance for protoderm differentiation and radial pattern formation in early rice embryogenesis. *Plant J.* **2002**, *29*, 497–507. [CrossRef]

89. Yu, L.H.; Chen, X.; Wang, Z.; Wang, S.M.; Wang, Y.P.; Zhu, Q.S.; Li, S.G.; Xiang, C.B. Arabidopsis enhanced drought tolerance1/HOMEODOMAIN GLABROUS11 confers drought tolerance in transgenic rice without yield penalty. *Plant Physiol.* **2013**, *162*, 1378–1391. [CrossRef]

90. Cao, Y.J.; Wei, Q.; Liao, Y.; Song, H.L.; Li, X.; Xiang, C.B.; Kuai, B.K. Ectopic overexpression of AtHDG11 in tall fescue resulted in enhanced tolerance to drought and salt stress. *Plant Cell Rep.* **2009**, *28*, 579–588. [CrossRef]

91. Ling, L.; Song, L.L.; Wang, Y.J.; Guo, C.H. Genome-wide analysis and expression patterns of the NAC transcription factor family in Medicago truncatula. *Physiol. Mol. Biol. Plants* **2017**, *23*, 343–356. [CrossRef]
92. Vernoud, V.; Laigle, G.; Rozier, F.; Meeley, R.B.; Perez, P.; Rogowsky, P.M. The HD-ZIP IV transcription factor OCL4 is necessary for trichome patterning and anther development in maize. *Plant J.* **2009**, *59*, 883–894. [CrossRef]
93. Henriksson, E.; Olsson, A.S.B.; Johannesson, H.; Hanson, J.; Engstrom, P.; Soderman, E. Homeodomain leucine zipper class I genes in Arabidopsis. Expression patterns and phylogenetic relationships. *Plant Physiol.* **2005**, *139*, 509–518. [CrossRef]
94. Agalou, A.; Purwantomo, S.; Overnas, E.; Johannesson, H.; Zhu, X.; Estiati, A.; de Kam, R.J.; Engstroem, P.; Slamet-Loedin, I.H.; Zhu, Z.; et al. A genome-wide survey of HD-Zip genes in rice and analysis of drought-responsive family members. *Plant Mol. Biol.* **2008**, *66*, 87–103. [CrossRef]
95. Cote, C.L.; Boileau, F.; Roy, V.; Ouellet, M.; Levasseur, C.; Morency, M.J.; Cooke, J.E.K.; Seguin, A.; MacKay, J.J. Gene family structure, expression and functional analysis of HD-Zip III genes in angiosperm and gymnosperm forest trees. *BMC Plant Biol.* **2010**, *10*, 273. [CrossRef]
96. Ambawat, S.; Sharma, P.; Yadav, N.R.; Yadav, R.C. MYB transcription factor genes as regulators for plant responses: An overview. *Physiol. Mol. Biol. Plants* **2013**, *19*, 307–321. [CrossRef]
97. Fang, Y.J.; Liao, K.F.; Du, H.; Xu, Y.; Song, H.Z.; Li, X.H.; Xiong, L.Z. A stress-responsive NAC transcription factor SNAC3 confers heat and drought tolerance through modulation of reactive oxygen species in rice. *J. Exp. Bot.* **2015**, *66*, 6803–6817. [CrossRef]
98. Baldoni, E.; Genga, A.; Cominelli, E. Plant MYB transcription factors: Their role in drought response mechanisms. *Int. J. Mol. Sci.* **2015**, *16*, 15811–15851. [CrossRef]
99. Scully, E.D.; Gries, T.; Sarath, G.; Palmer, N.A.; Baird, L.; Serapiglia, M.J.; Dien, B.S.; Boateng, A.A.; Ge, Z.X.; Funnell-Harris, D.L.; et al. Overexpression of SbMyb60 impacts phenylpropanoid biosynthesis and alters secondary cell wall composition in *Sorghum bicolor*. *Plant J.* **2016**, *85*, 378–395. [CrossRef]
100. Xiong, H.Y.; Li, J.J.; Liu, P.L.; Duan, J.Z.; Zhao, Y.; Guo, X.; Li, Y.; Zhang, H.L.; Ali, J.; Li, Z.C. Overexpression of OsMYB48-1, a novel MYB-related transcription factor, enhances drought and salinity tolerance in rice. *PLoS ONE* **2014**, *9*, e92913. [CrossRef]
101. Casaretto, J.A.; El-Kereamy, A.; Zeng, B.; Stiegelmeyer, S.M.; Chen, X.; Bi, Y.M.; Rothstein, S.J. Expression of OsMYB55 in maize activates stress-responsive genes and enhances heat and drought tolerance. *BMC Genom.* **2016**, *17*, 312. [CrossRef]
102. Tang, Y.H.; Bao, X.X.; Zhi, Y.L.; Wu, Q.; Guo, Y.R.; Yin, X.H.; Zeng, L.Q.; Li, J.; Zhang, J.; He, W.L.; et al. Overexpression of a MYB Family Gene, OsMYB6, Increases Drought and Salinity Stress Tolerance in Transgenic Rice. *Front. Plant Sci.* **2019**, *10*, 168. [CrossRef]
103. Dai, X.Y.; Xu, Y.Y.; Ma, Q.B.; Xu, W.Y.; Wang, T.; Xue, Y.B. Overexpression of an R1R2R3 MYB gene, OsMYB3R-2, increases tolerance to freezing, drought, and salt stress in transgenic Arabidopsis. *Plant Physiol.* **2007**, *143*, 1739–1751. [CrossRef]
104. Xiang, Y.; Sun, X.J.; Bian, X.L.; Wei, T.H.; Han, T.; Yan, J.W.; Zhang, A.Y. The transcription factor ZmNAC49 reduces stomatal density and improves drought tolerance in maize. *J. Exp. Bot.* **2021**, *72*, 1399–1410. [CrossRef]
105. Sanjari, S.; Shirzadian-Khorramabad, R.; Shobbar, Z.S.; Shahbazi, M. Systematic analysis of NAC transcription factors' gene family and identification of post-flowering drought stress responsive members in sorghum. *Plant Cell Rep.* **2019**, *38*, 361–376. [CrossRef]
106. Li, X.; Chang, Y.; Ma, S.Q.; Shen, J.Q.; Hu, H.H.; Xiong, L.Z. Genome-Wide Identification of SNAC1-Targeted Genes Involved in Drought Response in Rice. *Front. Plant Sci.* **2019**, *10*, 982. [CrossRef]
107. Hu, H.H.; You, J.; Fang, Y.J.; Zhu, X.Y.; Qi, Z.Y.; Qi, Z.Y.; Xiong, L.Z. Characterization of transcription factor gene SNAC2 conferring cold and salt tolerance in rice. *Plant Mol. Biol.* **2008**, *67*, 169–181, Erratum in *Plant Mol. Biol.* **2010**, *72*, 567–568. [CrossRef]
108. Pooam, M.; El-Ballat, E.M.; Jourdan, N.; Ali, H.M.; Hano, C.; Ahmad, M.; El-Esawi, M.A. SNAC3 Transcription Factor Enhances Arsenic Stress Tolerance and Grain Yield in Rice (*Oryza sativa* L.) through Regulating Physio-Biochemical Mechanisms, Stress-Responsive Genes, and Cryptochrome 1b. *Plants* **2023**, *12*, 2713. [CrossRef]
109. Tran, L.S.P.; Nakashima, K.; Sakuma, Y.; Osakabe, Y.; Maruyama, K.; Shinozaki, K.; Yamaguchi-Shinozaki, K. Role of the ZFHD1 and NAC transcription factors in drought-inducible expression of the early responsive to dehydration stress 1 (ERD1) gene of Arabidopsis. *Plant Cell Physiol.* **2006**, *47*, S226. (In Chinese)
110. Liu, Y.; Yao, X.Z.; Lv, L.T.; Lei, Y.T.; Dai, T.T.; Zhao, D.G. Cloning of SbSKIP Gene from Sorghum (*Sorghum bicolor*) and Analysis of Drought-resistant Function in Tobacco (*Nicotiana tabacum*). *J. Agric. Biotechnol.* **2016**, *24*, 1500–1511. (In Chinese) [CrossRef]
111. Wu, R.; Kong, L.X.; Wu, X.; Gao, J.; Niu, T.L.; Li, J.Y.; Li, Z.J.; Dai, L.Y. GsNAC2 gene enhances saline-alkali stress tolerance by promoting plant growth and regulating glutathione metabolism in *Sorghum bicolor*. *Funct. Plant Biol.* **2023**, *50*, 677–690. [CrossRef] [PubMed]
112. Han, Y.H.; Wang, Y.R.; Tao, Q.B. Advances of seed hormonal priming. *Pratacultural Sci.* **2017**, *33*, 2494–2502. (In Chinese) [CrossRef]

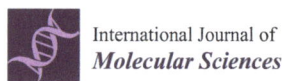

International Journal of
Molecular Sciences

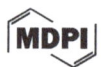

Article

Melatonin-Regulated Chaperone Binding Protein Plays a Key Role in Cadmium Stress Tolerance in Rice, Revealed by the Functional Characterization of a Novel Serotonin *N*-Acetyltransferase 3 (*SNAT3*) in Rice

Hyoung-Yool Lee and Kyoungwhan Back *

Department of Molecular Biotechnology, College of Agriculture and Life Sciences, Chonnam National University, Gwangju 61186, Republic of Korea; xanthine657@jnu.ac.kr
* Correspondence: kback@chonnam.ac.kr; Tel.: +82-62-530-2165

Abstract: The study of the mechanisms by which melatonin protects against cadmium (Cd) toxicity in plants is still in its infancy, particularly at the molecular level. In this study, the gene encoding a novel serotonin *N*-acetyltransferase 3 (*SNAT3*) in rice, a pivotal enzyme in the melatonin biosynthetic pathway, was cloned. Rice (*Oryza sativa*) OsSNAT3 is the first identified plant ortholog of archaeon *Thermoplasma volcanium* SNAT. The purified recombinant OsSNAT3 catalyzed the conversion of serotonin and 5-methoxytryptamine to *N*-acetylserotonin and melatonin, respectively. The suppression of *OsSNAT3* by RNAi led to a decline in endogenous melatonin levels followed by a reduction in Cd tolerance in transgenic RNAi rice lines. In addition, the expression levels of genes encoding the endoplasmic reticulum (ER) chaperones *BiP3*, *BiP4*, and *BiP5* were much lower in RNAi lines than in the wild type. In transgenic rice plants overexpressing *OsSNAT3* (SNAT3-OE), however, melatonin levels were higher than in wild-type plants. SNAT3-OE plants also tolerated Cd stress, as indicated by seedling growth, malondialdehyde, and chlorophyll levels. *BiP4* expression was much higher in the SNAT3-OE lines than in the wild type. These results indicate that melatonin engineering could help crops withstand Cd stress, resulting in high yields in Cd-contaminated fields.

Keywords: binding proteins; chaperone; cadmium tolerance; melatonin; serotonin *N*-acetyltransferase; transgenic rice

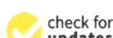

check for updates

Citation: Lee, H.-Y.; Back, K. Melatonin-Regulated Chaperone Binding Protein Plays a Key Role in Cadmium Stress Tolerance in Rice, Revealed by the Functional Characterization of a Novel Serotonin *N*-Acetyltransferase 3 (*SNAT3*) in Rice. *Int. J. Mol. Sci.* **2024**, *25*, 5952. https://doi.org/10.3390/ijms25115952

Academic Editors: Mateusz Labudda and Philippe Jeandet

Received: 1 May 2024
Revised: 27 May 2024
Accepted: 28 May 2024
Published: 29 May 2024

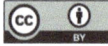
1. Introduction

Cadmium (Cd) is believed to act as one of the most harmful heavy metals for living organisms and is positioned 7th among the 20 most toxic metals; it is also a group 1 carcinogen [1]. In plants, Cd causes severe damage to growth and development, including by inhibiting photosynthesis [2,3], disrupting the ultrastructure of chloroplasts [4,5] and the endoplasmic reticulum (ER) [6], increasing the production of reactive oxygen species (ROS) [7], and disturbing cellular protein homeostasis [8]. To alleviate the adverse effects of Cd stress, plants have evolved a series of adaptative mechanisms against Cd toxicity. The first line of defense is the plant cell wall, which prevents Cd from entering cells by chelating it to cell wall components such as pectin and hemicellulose [9]. However, for Cd that invades inside cells, a number of defense responses are simultaneously induced to minimize Cd stress, such as Cd sequestration into vacuoles, Cd chelation by cytoplasmic organic acids or proteins, the enhanced production of antioxidant enzymes or other antioxidants, and the induction of heat shock proteins (HSPs) [5,8].

HSPs play a pivotal role in cellular protein homeostasis by acting as molecular chaperones of protein folding and hindering protein aggregation [10]. They are also induced in response to Cd, as well as other environmental stresses. In plants, there are five major classes of HSPs, identified based on their molecular masses: HSP60, HSP70, HSP90, HSP100, and small HSPs. HSP70 is highly conserved between bacteria and eukaryotes and is closely associated with the defense response in a wide range of plant species [11]. It maintains protein homeostasis by preventing the aggregation of stress-damaged proteins [12]. The rice genome contains 32 *HSP70* genes, whose protein products are localized in distinct subcellular compartments, including the cytoplasm, chloroplasts, and ER [12]. HSP70 proteins that reside in the ER are also referred to as binding proteins (BiPs). Like other HSP70 proteins, BiPs act as chaperones and interact with nascent immature proteins to facilitate their correct folding and assembly [13]. In the rice genome, there are at least five *BiP* genes, sharing >66% amino acid identity [14]. Among them, the expressions of *BiP4* and *BiP5* are positively correlated with the severity of ER stress [13], whereas *BiP1* expression plays a key role in the regulation of seed storage proteins [15]. While many environmental stresses, such as heat, salt, and drought, as well as heavy metal stress, evoke ER stress by causing dysfunctional protein folding [16–18], whether the amelioration of ER stress by *BiP* genes would improve plant growth and development remains elusive [18].

Melatonin is found in almost all living organisms, including animals, bacteria, archaea, and plants [19–22]. In animals, melatonin acts as a neurohormone, influencing circadian rhythms and seasonal reproduction [23]; other functions include energy metabolism, as well as anti-inflammatory, anti-cancer, and anti-aging effects [24]. In plants, however, melatonin does not function as a hormone, but rather as a signaling molecule, orchestrating a diverse array of physiological functions including growth and development, while also participating in defense responses against biotic and abiotic stresses [25] through protein quality control [26,27]. In plants, melatonin biosynthesis begins with the conversion of tryptophan into tryptamine in a reaction catalyzed by tryptophan decarboxylase, with intermediate serotonin—the last common substrate for melatonin biosynthesis in both animals and plants—produced through the enzymatic reaction of tryptamine 5-hydroxylase, located in the ER. Serotonin is converted into *N*-acetylserotonin or 5-methoxytryptamine by serotonin *N*-acetyltransferase (SNAT) or serotonin *O*-methyltransferase. The same enzymes catalyze the final steps that lead to melatonin biosynthesis [20]. Among these four enzymes, SNAT, as both the penultimate and final enzyme for melatonin biosynthesis depending on the substrate, has received considerable research attention due to its rate-limiting role in melatonin synthesis in animals and plants [19,28,29]. In plants, two *SNAT* isogenes, *SNAT1* and *SNAT2*, have been cloned and their respective proteins have been expressed in chloroplasts [30,31].

In this study, we cloned a third *SNAT* from rice (*Oryza sativa*), *OsSNAT3*, identified as an orthologous gene of the archaeon *Thermoplasma volcanium SNAT* [21]. In our experiments, we found that, in contrast to OsSNAT1 and OsSNAT2, OsSNAT3 is located in the cytoplasm. However, like *OsSNAT1* and *OsSNAT2*, the overexpression of *OsSNAT3* enhanced melatonin synthesis in transgenic rice, while its downregulation reduced it. It also conferred tolerance against Cd stress, while its downregulation increased the susceptibility of rice plants to Cd stress. These observations may be due to the differential expression of *BiP* genes. This is the first study to show that melatonin-regulated *BiP* regulation plays an important role in conferring Cd tolerance in rice, thus highlighting the close relationship between melatonin-induced *BiP* genes and Cd tolerance in plants.

2. Results

2.1. Rice (Oryza sativa) SNAT3 (OsSNAT3) Sequence Features, Bacterial Expression, and Purification of Recombinant OsSNAT3 Protein

A BLAST search showed that the rice gene with the highest homology to the archaeon *Thermoplasma volcanium* SNAT (TvSNAT) [21] is OsSNAT3, previously annotated as rice *N*-alpha-acetyltransferase 50 (OsNaa50). OsSNAT3 had a 36.25% protein-level identity with TvSNAT in its C-terminal 80 amino acids (Figure 1A). A Conserved Domain Database (CDD) search [32] showed that OsSNAT3 has a conserved acetyl CoA binding site made up of L96, G97, V98, G108, and S109, and that it harbors key residues for SNAT catalysis, including N123, D136, and Y142 [33]. OsSNAT3 has a high amino acid sequence identity

(51%) with human Naa50 [34], which also possesses SNAT activity [35]. In the rice genome, two SNAT isogenes, *SNAT1* and *SNAT2*, have been identified thus far. While both participate in melatonin biosynthesis, they differ in their downstream signaling responses in the brassinosteroid signaling pathway [20]. Phylogenetic analysis clearly indicated that *OsSNAT3* (or *OsNaa50*) is distantly related to the previously identified *SNAT* isogenes *OsSNAT1* and *OsSNAT2* (Figure 1B). To assess whether rice *OsSNAT3* harbors SNAT activity, recombinant OsSNAT3 was purified by expressing full-length *OsSNAT3* in *Escherichia coli*. As shown in Figure 1C, OsSNAT3 was expressed as a soluble protein and successfully purified on a Ni^{2+} affinity column.

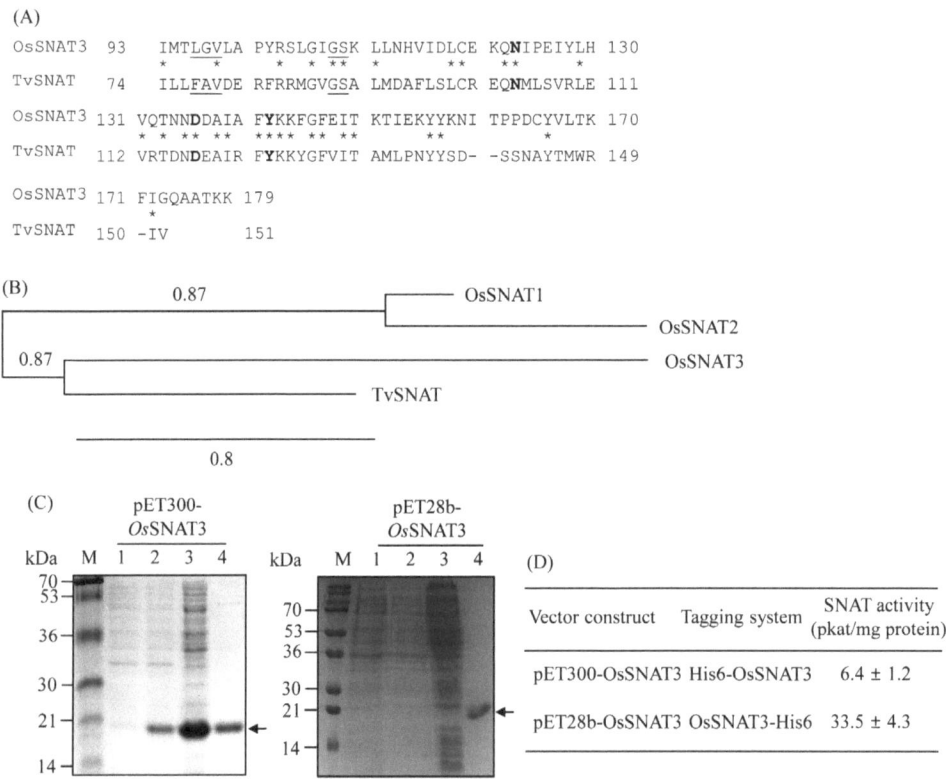

Figure 1. (A) Amino acid sequence alignment between archaeon TvSNAT and rice OsSNAT3. The conserved acetyl coenzyme A binding sites are underlined and key residues for SNAT activity are shown in bold. Stars indicate identical amino acids; dashes denote gaps. (B) Phylogenetic tree of *OsSNAT3* among multiple *SNAT* genes in rice. The scale bar represents 0.8 substitutions per site. GenBank accession numbers are NC_003413 (*TvSNAT*), AK059369 (*OsSNAT1*), AK068156 (*OsSNAT2*), and AK241100 (*OsSNAT3*). (C) Purification of His6-tagged OsSNAT3 proteins. *E. coli* BL21 (DE3) cells harboring pET300-OsSNAT3 and pET28b-OsSNAT3 plasmids were induced with isopropyl β-d-1-thiogalactopyranoside (IPTG) for 5 h at 28 °C. M, molecular mass standards. Lane 1, total proteins in 15 µL bacterial culture without IPTG; lane 2, total proteins in 15 µL bacterial culture with IPTG; lane 3, 30 µg soluble protein; lane 4, 5 µg affinity-chromatography-purified protein. (D) SNAT activity measured in purified N-terminal His6-tagged OsSNAT3 and purified C-terminal His6-tagged OsSNAT3. Protein samples were separated by SDS-PAGE on a 12% polyacrylamide gel and stained with Coomassie blue.

2.2. Characterization of OsSNAT3 Enzyme Kinetics

Two forms of the recombinant OsSNAT3 protein—N-terminal His-tagged OsSNAT3 (His6-OsSNAT3) and C-terminal His-tagged OsSNAT3 (OsSNAT3-His6)—were analyzed for SNAT activity using serotonin as the substrate. As shown in Figure 1D, the SNAT activity of the OsSNAT3-His6 protein was 5-fold higher than that of His6-OsSNAT3, indicating the inhibition of OsSNAT3-mediated catalysis by N-terminal His-tag sequences. The OsSNAT3-His6 recombinant protein was thus employed in further analyses of SNAT enzyme kinetics. Similar to TvSNAT, the optimum SNAT activity of OsSNAT3 was at pH 8.8 (Figure 2A). Peak OsSNAT3 activity was obtained at a temperature of 45 °C with a sharp decrease at 55 °C, in stark contrast to the many other plant SNAT proteins, whose peak activities were at 55 °C (Figure 2B) [29,35]. The K_m and V_{max} values of OsSNAT3 were 1152 μM and 4.8 nmol/min/mg protein, respectively, with serotonin as the substrate (Figure 2C), and 1587 μM and 12.6 nmol/min/mg protein, respectively, with 5-methoxytryptamine as the substrate (Figure 2D). The catalytic efficiency (V_{max}/K_m) of OsSNAT3 was 2-fold higher when 5-methoxytryptamine rather than serotonin served as the substrate. Based on K_m values for OsSNAT1 and OsSNAT2 of 270 μM and 371 μM, respectively, with serotonin as the substrate, it is likely that OsSNAT3 is functionally involved in melatonin biosynthesis under conditions of high serotonin levels, such as those induced by senescence and Cd stress [20].

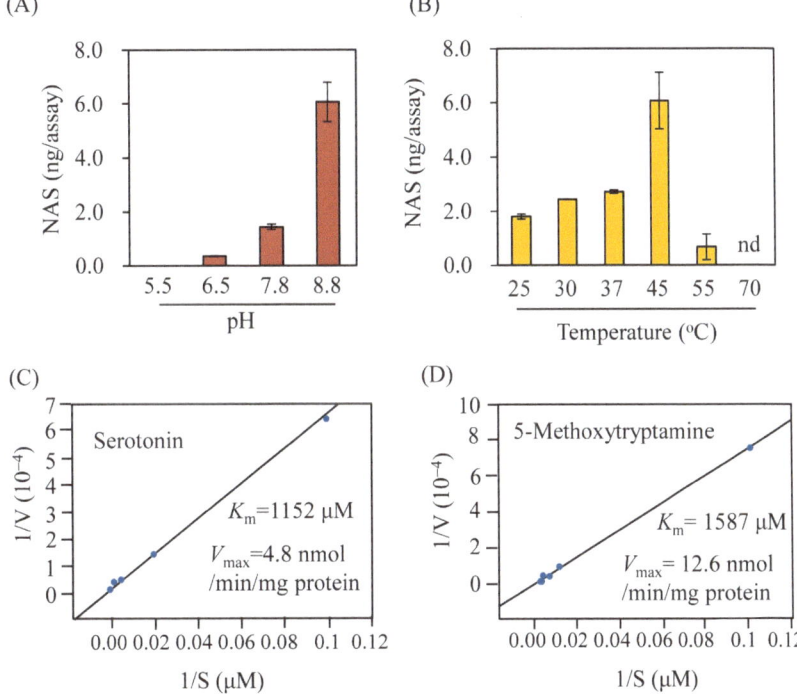

Figure 2. Enzyme kinetics of OsSNAT3. SNAT activity as a function of (**A**) pH and (**B**) temperature, and determination of K_m and V_{max} values of OsSNAT3 using (**C**) serotonin and (**D**) 5-methoxytryptamine (5-MT) as substrates. Recombinant purified OsSNAT3 (1 μg) was assayed in the presence of different serotonin and 5-MT concentrations for 1 h at different temperatures and pH values, followed by high-performance liquid chromatography detection of *N*-acetylserotonin (NAS) and melatonin. Kinetic values of K_m and V_{max} were determined using Lineweaver–Burk plots. Values are presented as the mean ± SD (*n* = 3). nd, not detected.

SNAT accepts multiple substrates, including tyramine, tryptamine, and polyamines [36]. As shown in Figure 3, the best substrates for OsSNAT3 were 5-methoxytryptamine (92.3 pkat/mg protein) and tyramine (92.2 pkat/mg protein), followed by tryptamine (46.9 pkat/mg protein) and serotonin (33.8 pkat/mg protein) (Figure 3B). Unlike TvSNAT, the activity of which is lowest when 5-methoxytryptamine is the substrate [21], OsSNAT3 activity peaked in response to this substrate. Both sheep SNAT and yeast SNAT also reach peak enzyme activity when provided with 5-methoxytryptamine [37]. In addition to the aforementioned arylalkylamines, other arylalkylamines (dopamine, octopamine, 2-phenylethylamine, and histamine) and polyamines (spermidine and putrescine) were tested for their acceptance as OsSNAT3 substrates. Due to the absence of respective standards, an SNAT inhibition assay (0.5 mM serotonin) was conducted in the presence of each potential substrate (0.5 mM) to determine its inhibitory effect on SNAT activity. Analogous to TvSNAT, OsSNAT3 activity was strongly inhibited by spermidine and octopamine (Figure 3C) and significantly inhibited by putrescine and dopamine. These data indirectly indicate that OsSNAT3 is able to acetylate dopamine, spermidine, putrescine, and octopamine, yielding *N*-acetyldopamine, *N*-acetylspermidine, *N*-acetylputrescine, and *N*-acetyloctopamine, respectively. These results suggest a broader substrate affinity of OsSNAT3 than TvSNAT. However, the relationship between acetylated polyamines and OsSNAT3, particularly with respect to stress defense responses in rice, remains to be studied in detail.

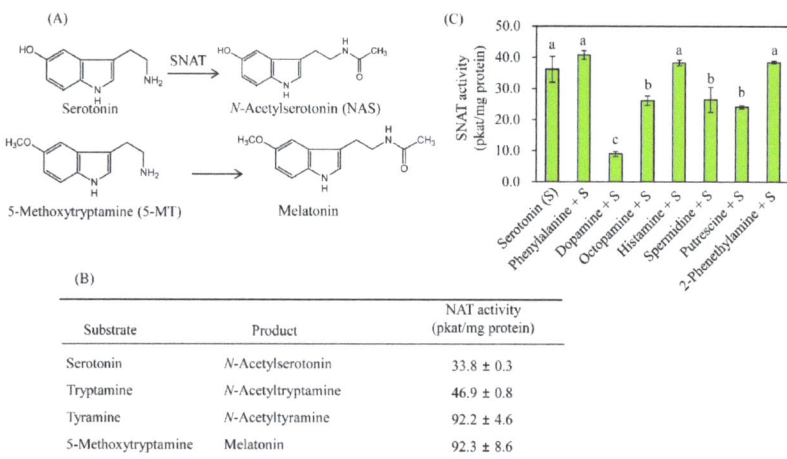

Figure 3. SNAT reactions and substrate preferences. (**A**) SNAT activity toward serotonin and 5-MT substrates. (**B**) SNAT activity toward other substrates. (**C**) Activity of recombinant purified OsSNAT3 toward serotonin (0.5 mM) and various amines (0.5 mM) at 55 °C and pH 8.8. Values are presented as the mean ± SD ($n = 3$). Different letters indicate significant differences vs. the wild type (Tukey's HSD; $p < 0.05$).

2.3. Subcellular Localization of OsSNAT3

The subcellular localization of OsSNAT3 was determined through in silico analysis. First, the possible presence of transit or signal sequences was examined in a TargetP analysis [38], followed by the use of cNLS Mapper to identify a nuclear localization signal (NLS) [39]. Although neither transit nor signal sequences are predicted by OsSNAT3 polypeptides, cNLS Mapper predicted two putative NLS sequences (LKKL-NTALEPVRYNEKYYHDTIASKEFS and DLCEKQNIPEIYLHVQTNNDDAIAFYKKFGFE) with scores of 3.2 and 4.3, implying both nuclear and cytoplasmic subcellular localization. In agreement with the cNLS prediction, an OsSNAT3-mCherry fusion protein was localized to the cytoplasm (Figure 4) when the fusion construct was transiently expressed in leaf epidermal cells of *Nicotiana benthamiana*, a native Australian tobacco species. While the subcellular localization of OsSNAT3 in the cytoplasm was predominantly observed in our experiments, the expression of OsSNAT3 in other subcellular compartments cannot be ruled out because the expression of *Arabidopsis thaliana* Naa50, an ortholog of OsSNAT3, in the nucleus, cytoplasm, and ER has been reported [40]. OsSNAT3 expression thus differs from that of OsSNAT1 and OsSNAT2, which have been localized to chloroplasts [30,31]. The location of SNAT protein isoforms—as key enzymes in melatonin biosynthesis in plants—in the cytoplasm, nucleus, chloroplasts, and mitochondria indicates the ubiquity of cellular melatonin biosynthesis [20,29,41,42].

(A) (B) (C)

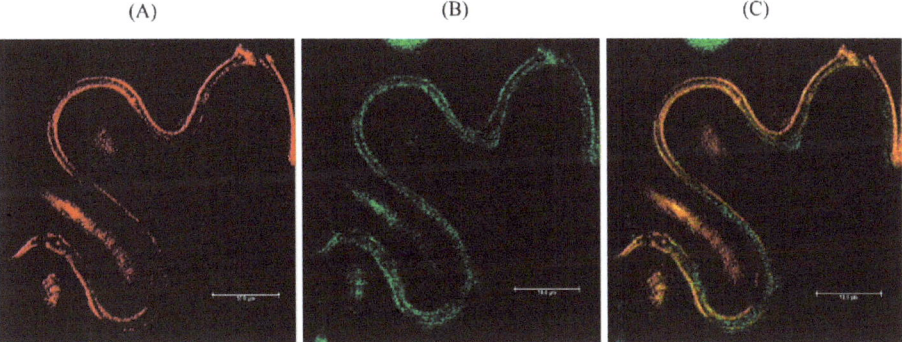

Figure 4. Subcellular localization of OsSNAT3. (**A**) Red fluorescence of OsSNAT3-mCherry. (**B**) Green fluorescence of cytoplasmic green fluorescent protein (GFP). (**C**) Merged fluorescence images (A + B). Thirty-day-old tobacco seedlings infiltrated with *Agrobacterium tumefaciens* (GV2260) containing XVE-inducible *OsSNAT3*-mCherry or constitutive 35S:GFP (cytosolic marker). Bars = 10 μm.

2.4. Reduced Synthesis of Melatonin in OsSNAT3-Suppressed Transgenic Rice Plants

From 14 T_0-independent transgenic lines generated via *Agrobacterium*-mediated rice transformation in vitro, 12 yielded T_1 seeds; the other two lines died during growth under field conditions. The obtained T_1 seeds, which exhibited hygromycin resistance and a sensitivity ratio of 3:1, were grown and three T_2 homozygous lines (lines 3, 6, and 9) were selected for further analyses (Figure 5). As shown in Figure 5B, the phenotypes of the 7-day-old *OsSNAT3* RNAi lines and wild-type seedlings did not significantly differ. However, in all three transgenic RNAi lines, *OsSNAT3* transcript levels were much lower than those of the wild type, thus confirming the successful generation of the *OsSNAT3* RNAi lines. *OsSNAT3* suppression did not affect the transcript levels of *OsSNAT1*, whereas those of *OsSNAT2* were slightly elevated, indicative of the feedback regulation between *OsSNAT2* and *OsSNAT3* transcripts. To determine the effect of *OsSNAT3* downregulation on melatonin levels, 7-day-old rice seedlings were challenged with 0.5 mM Cd for 3 days, after which melatonin induction was assessed by HPLC. As shown in Figure 5E, the average rate of melatonin production in wild-type seedlings was 195 ng/g fresh weight (FW) and that of the transgenic *OsSNAT3* RNAi lines was 77 ng/FW, a 2.5-fold difference. This result indicates that *OsSNAT3* mRNA is functionally coupled to in vivo melatonin synthesis in rice plants.

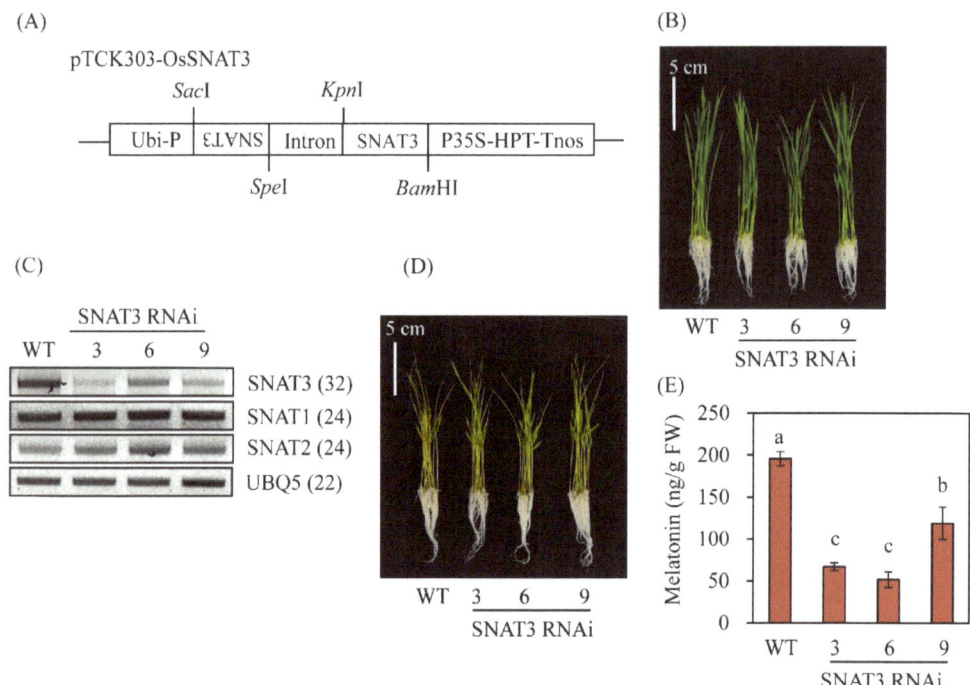

Figure 5. Generation of *OsSNAT3* RNAi transgenic rice and the melatonin content of rice seedlings. (**A**) RNAi binary vector used for *OsSNAT3* suppression. (**B**) Phenotypes of 7-day-old rice seedlings. (**C**) RT-PCR analyses of transgenic and wild-type 7-day-old rice seedlings. (**D**) Photograph of 7-day-old rice seedlings treated for 3 days with 0.5 mM CdCl$_2$. (**E**) Melatonin contents of 7-day-old rice seedlings treated for 3 days with 0.5 mM CdCl$_2$. *Ubi-P*, maize ubiquitin promoter; *HPT*, hygromycin phosphotransferase; WT, wild type; *UBQ5*, rice ubiquitin 5 gene. GenBank accession numbers of *SNAT1*, *SNAT2*, *SNAT3*, and *UBQ5* are AK059369, AK068156, AK241100, and AK061988, respectively. Different letters indicate significant differences vs. the wild type (Tukey's HSD; $p < 0.05$).

2.5. A Decrease in Endogenous Melatonin Aggravates Cd Toxicity

The enormous induction of endogenous melatonin biosynthesis by Cd in rice has been attributed to melatonin-mediated Cd tolerance [27]. When 7-day-old seedlings were challenged with Cd, as shown in Figure 5D, no significant differences in MDA levels between the wild-type and OsSNAT3 RNAi lines were observed. Thus, the effects of Cd response have been examined directly in MS medium in the presence of Cd (Figure 6). In this study, consistent with the reduced melatonin levels (Figure 6E), seedling growth in the *OsSNAT3* RNAi lines was strongly reduced compared to the wild type when dehusked rice seeds were grown for 7 days in half-strength MS medium containing 0.5 mM CdCl$_2$ (Figure 6A–C), with a much shorter root length (Figure 6C). In addition, the levels of malondialdehyde (MDA), a marker of lipid peroxidation and oxidative stress, were higher in *OsSNAT3* RNAi than in wild-type plants (Figure 6D). To identify the major genes responsible for the melatonin-regulated Cd response, we examined the expression of the antioxidant-related genes *SODA1* (encoding Mn-superoxide dismutase), *APX1* (ascorbate peroxidase), *GR2* (glutathione reductase), and *CatB* (catalase), and of the chaperone-related genes *PDIL1–1* (protein disulfide isomerase-like), *CNX* (calnexin), *BiP* (binding protein), and *SGT1* (suppressor of the G2 allele of skp1). In the *OsSNAT3* RNAi lines, among the antioxidant-related genes, only *CatB* expression was changed, with an increase compared to the wild type; there was no change in the expression levels of the other studied enzymes

(Figure 6F). Among the chaperone genes, *BiP3*, *BiP4*, and *BiP5* expressions were strongly downregulated while *BiP1*, *BiP2*, and *CNX* expressions were upregulated in the *OsSNAT3* RNAi lines, indicating the differential expression of *BiP* genes. A similar differential expression between *OsSNAT3* RNAi lines and the wild type was not observed for *PDIL1–1* and *SGT1*. These results indicate that *BiP3*, *BiP4*, and *BiP5* expressions are closely associated with the melatonin-mediated Cd susceptibility response.

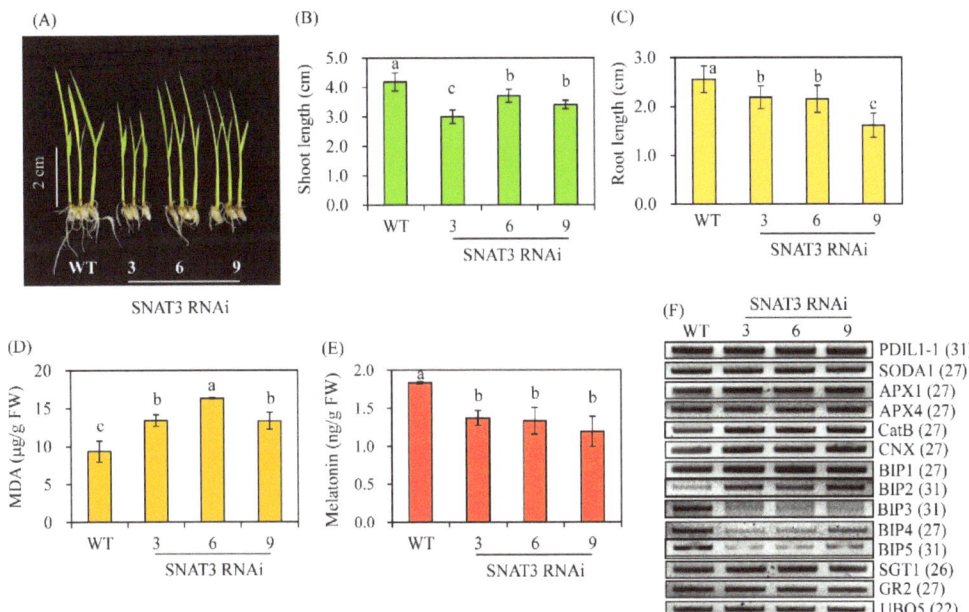

Figure 6. Enhanced Cd stress susceptibility in *OsSNAT3* RNAi transgenic rice plants. (**A**) Growth phenotype, (**B**) shoot length, (**C**) root length, (**D**) malondialdehyde (MDA) contents, and (**E**) melatonin content in 7-day-old rice seedlings. (**F**) Gene expression profiles determined by RT-PCR in Cd-stressed rice plants. Dehusked seeds were surface-sterilized and transferred for 7 days to half-strength Murashige Skoog (MS) medium containing 0.5 mM $CdCl_2$ under a 14 h light/10 h dark photoperiod and an incubation temperature of 28 °C/24 °C (day/night). Values are presented as the mean ± SD ($n = 3$). Different letters indicate significant differences vs. the wild type (Tukey's HSD; $p < 0.05$). GenBank accession numbers: *PDIL1–1* (AK068268), *SODA1* (AAA62657), *APX1* (AB050724), *APX4* (AK104490), *CatB* (AK069446), *CNX* (AK069118), *BiP1* (AK119653), *BiP2* (BAS86012), *BiP3* (BAS93656), *BiP4* (AK106696), *BiP5* (BAF23108), *SGT1* (BAF05534), *GR2* (BAF10399), and *UBQ5* (AK061988).

2.6. Increased Endogenous Melatonin Elevates Cd Tolerance in OsSNAT3-Overexpressing Lines

To examine the coupling of melatonin-regulated Cd tolerance to *BiP* expression, transgenic rice plants overexpressing *OsSNAT3* (SNAT3-OE) were generated (Figure 7A). From the 14 independent T_0 transgenic lines, three T_2 homozygous lines (lines 6, 8, and 10) overexpressing *SNAT3* (SNAT3-OE) were selected (Figure 7H). When SNAT3-OE seeds were grown for 7 days in MS medium containing 0.5 mM Cd, the seedlings exhibited enhanced growth compared to wild-type seedlings (Figure 7B–D). Chlorophyll levels were also higher in SNAT3-OE than in wild-type seedlings (Figure 7E), while MDA levels were reduced. These results indicate that greater melatonin production by the SNAT3-OE lines resulted in their better tolerance of Cd stress than wild-type seedlings (Figure 7G). *BiP4* was identified as the main gene responsible for conferring Cd tolerance in the SNAT3-OE lines, and its expression was accordingly higher than in wild-type plants, as shown by PCR and quantitative real-time PCR analyses (Figure 7H,I). The expressions of *BiP3* and *BiP5* did not differ between SNAT3-OE and wild-type plants.

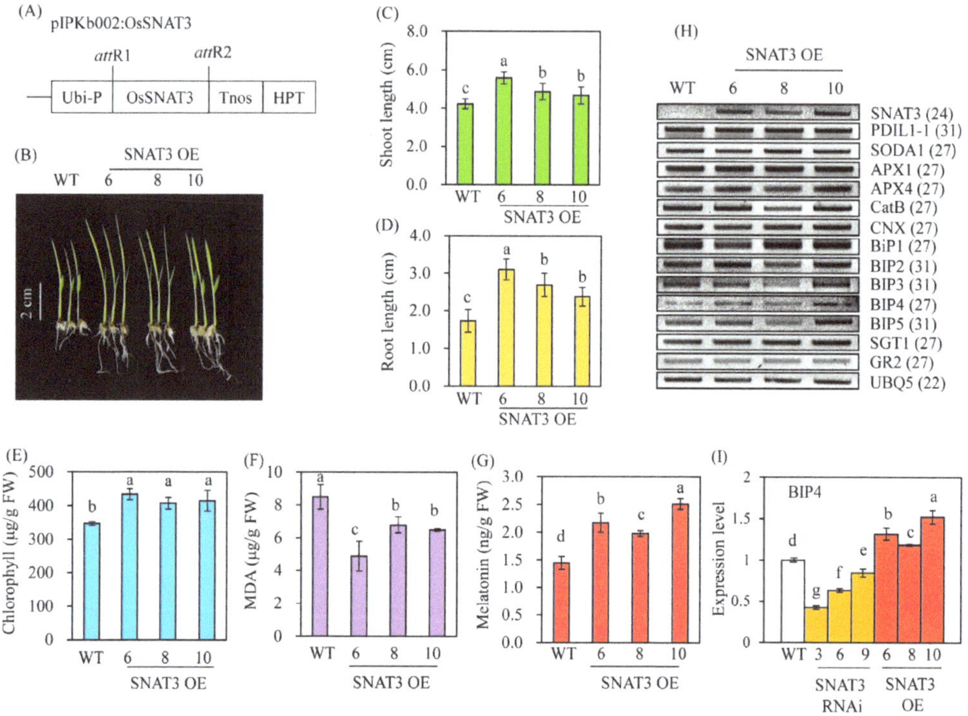

Figure 7. Enhanced Cd tolerance in *OsSNAT3*-overexpressing transgenic rice plants. (**A**) Schematic diagram of the binary vector for *OsSNAT3* overexpression. (**B**) Phenotype of Cd-treated 7-day-old rice seedlings. (**C**) Shoot length, (**D**) root length, and (**E**) chlorophyll, (**F**) MDA, and (**G**) melatonin contents in Cd-treated plants. (**H**) Gene expression profiles of Cd-treated rice plants, as determined by RT-PCR. (**I**) *BiP4* expression levels determined in a quantitative real-time PCR analysis of Cd-stressed rice plants. *OsSNAT3*, *Oryza sativa serotonin N-acetyltrasferase3*; *Ubi-P*, maize ubiquitin promoter; *HPT*, hygromycin phosphotransferase; WT, wild type; *UBQ5*, rice ubiquitin 5 gene. GenBank accession numbers are listed in Figure 6. Different letters indicate significant differences vs. the wild type (Tukey's HSD; $p < 0.05$).

3. Discussion

While many heavy metals, including copper, iron, zinc, cobalt, and manganese, are required as micronutrients for plant growth, Cd is toxic, causing severe damage to all living organisms, including plants and animals [43–45]. Among the many adverse effects of Cd on plant growth and development are the inhibition of root growth, leaf chlorosis, a reduction in photosynthesis, the inhibition of nutrient uptake and germination, and yield reduction [45]. To cope with Cd stress, plants have evolved a number of defense mechanisms, such as the chelation of Cd by metallothionein and phytochelatins, the regulation of heavy metal transporters, the induction of enzymatic and nonenzymatic antioxidants, and increased levels of plant hormones and HSPs [2,5,45].

Melatonin is a pleiotropic molecule found in all living organisms examined so far. It acts as a neurohormone in animals but as a signaling molecule in plants, although its potent antioxidant activity is common in all organisms [46,47]. Its antioxidant scavenging activity is directed against a diverse array of oxidants, including ROS and reactive nitrogen species, but as a signaling molecule melatonin also induces cellular antioxidant enzymes, such as catalase, APX1, and SOD [19,24,48]. Melatonin thus orchestrates the response to both biotic and abiotic stresses, including Cd stress in plants [25,27,49]. For instance, in rice seedlings treated with 1 µM melatonin in a hydroponic nutrient solution, Cd accumulation is efficiently alleviated by a mechanism involving enhanced hemicellulose levels in conjunction with decreased levels of transporter genes, thus lowering Cd intake [50]. In pepper seedlings, treatment with 5 µM melatonin enhances Cd stress tolerance by lowering leaf/root Cd concentrations and ROS contents while upregulating antioxidant genes encoding *SOD* and *APX* [7]. In *Wolffia arrhiza* exposed to 25 µM melatonin, Cd detoxification is increased via elevated phytochelatin and photosynthetic pigments [51]. In tomato seedlings exposed to Cd, melatonin treatment enhances the content of ascorbic acid and glutathione [52]. In Xing et al. [53], melatonin alleviated Cd-induced oxidative stress in tomato plants by increasing the ratio of reduced GSH to oxidized GSH and that of ascorbic acid to dehydroascorbic acid, in addition to inducing phytochelatin levels.

Rice is a major dietary crop capable of high levels of Cd adsorption [50], which together with its relatively high levels of melatonin production makes it well suited for the study of melatonin biosynthesis and Cd tolerance in plants [20]. Previous studies have shown that melatonin production is dramatically induced in Cd-treated rice plants [20,27,54]. Our findings of endogenous melatonin-mediated Cd tolerance by *BiP4* induction in rice, together with the studies summarized above, demonstrate the ability of melatonin to mitigate the negative effects of Cd stress through several different defense mechanisms. Therefore, melatonin is a pleiotropic molecule whose functions include protection against Cd stress in plants.

Heavy metal stresses inhibit cellular protein homeostasis by interfering with protein folding, resulting in the dysfunction of essential enzymes and other proteins. To maintain optimum protein homeostasis in the presence of heavy metal stress, plants induce the expression of HSPs, which assist in protein folding, prevent protein aggregation, and accelerate the degradation of aberrant proteins [8]. BiPs are HSP70 proteins residing in the ER [8]. They include *BiPD*, involved in drought tolerance in soybean and tobacco [55]; *BiP3*, associated with pathogen resistance in rice [56]; and *BiP1* and *BiP4*, involved in seed storage protein regulation [15], osmotic stress tolerance [27], and ER stress tolerance [13,27] in rice. However, while HSPs are well known to ameliorate the stress response in various plant species, endogenous melatonin-mediated *BiP4* expression in response to Cd stress has not been examined in plants.

SNAT is the penultimate or last enzyme for melatonin biosynthesis in animals and plants, catalyzing serotonin and 5-methoxytryptamine to yield *N*-acetylserotonin and melatonin, respectively [20]. Animals and humans possess a single copy of SNAT, but plants, including rice, harbor at least three isogenes, *SNAT1*, *SNAT2*, and *SNAT3*, with low amino acid identity among them. All three *SNAT* genes are functionally involved in melatonin synthesis, but their subcellular locations and physiological functions vary. Thus, both SNAT1 and SNAT2 localize in chloroplasts [29], while SNAT3 is found in the cytoplasm. *SNAT2*, but not *SNAT1*, is associated with brassinosteroid synthesis [57]. Importantly, *SNAT1* and *SNAT2* are specific to plants, whereas *SNAT3* orthologs are universally present in a diverse array of organisms, including rice (this report), archaea [21], humans [35], and *Escherichia coli* [22] (Figure 8). Our study identified rice *SNAT3* as a functional ortholog of archaeal *SNAT*. Its overexpression and downregulation were closely coupled with melatonin synthesis and the Cd stress response, with the latter involving the upregulated expression of the *BiP4* chaperone gene. Thus, it is tempting to speculate that melatonin-based Cd tolerance is one of many defense mechanisms by which rice and possibly other plants cope with Cd stress, with the induction of Cd intake-related genes [50], ROS detoxification genes [7,58], phytochelatin synthesis genes [53], and HSPs [8,27] among the others.

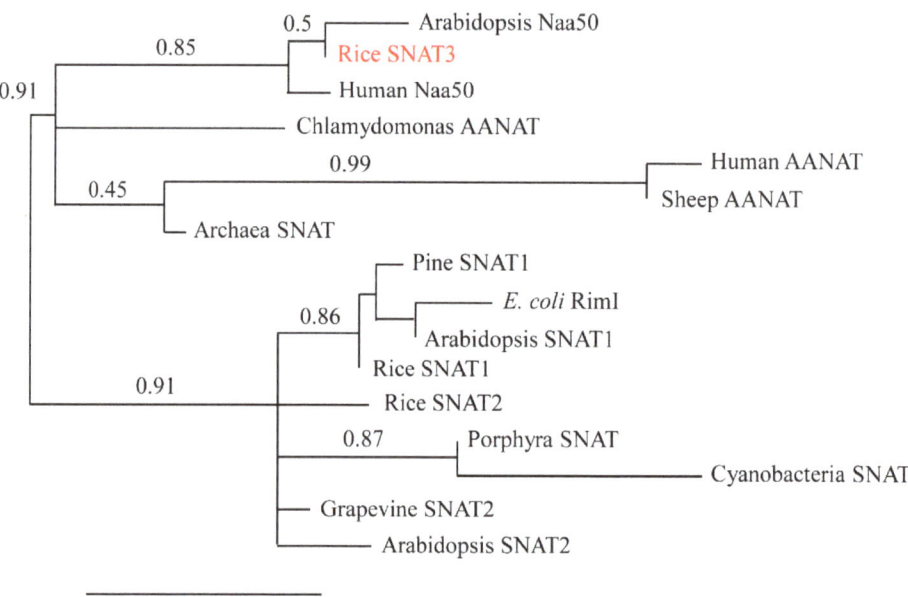

Figure 8. Phylogenetic tree of rice SNAT3 (OsSNAT3) shown as red words, an archaeal SNAT ortholog. The scale bar represents 0.3 substitutions per site. GenBank accession numbers are as follows: *Arabidopsis* Naa50 (NM_121172), rice SNAT3 (AK241100), human Naa50 (BAB14397), Chlamydomonas arylalkylamine *N*-acetyltransferase (AANAT) (AB474787), human AANAT (NP_001079), sheep AANAT (NP_001009461), archaea SNAT (NC_002689), pine SNAT1 (PSY00020345), *E. coli* RimI (WP_137442509), *Arabidopsis* SNAT1 (At1g32070), rice SNAT1 (AK059369), rice SNAT2 (AK068156), porphyra SNAT (NC_007932), cyanobacteria SNAT (NP_442603), grapevine SNAT2 (RVX06207), and *Arabidopsis* SNAT2 (At1g26220).

Our findings open a new window to crop improvement in areas with a high soil Cd content, by way of either classical breeding or genetic engineering strategies that increase melatonin synthesis.

4. Materials and Methods

4.1. Sequence Alignment and Phylogenetic Analysis

Full-length rice *SNAT3* cDNA (GenBank accession number AK241100) was kindly provided by the National Institute of Agrobiological Sciences [31,59,60]. The analysis of amino acid sequence homology was performed with the BLASTp tool (version 2.15.0) using the non-redundant protein sequences databases at the National Center for Biotechnology Information (http://www.ncbi.nlm.nih.gov/, accessed on 18 July 2019). The acetyl coenzyme A binding pocket was computed by the Conserved Domain Database (CDD), which is included in the National Center for Biotechnology Information (NCBL)'s online search services (accessed on 13 August 2019) [61]. We employed BLAST-Explorer [62] for phylogenetic trees analysis (accessed on 29 December 2022). TargetP analysis was used for the prediction of possible transit or signal sequences [38]. To predict the existence of nuclear localization signals (NLSs), the cNLS (calculating NLS scores) Mapper service was employed [39].

4.2. Escherichia coli Expression and Purification of Recombinant OsSNAT3 Protein

Two types of *Escherichia coli* expression vectors were used to express the full-length *OsSNAT3*. These two vectors were pET300 (Invitrogen, Carlsbad, CA, USA) and pET28b (Novagen, San Diego, CA, USA), which are designed to express *OsSNAT3* in either N-terminal- or C-terminal-hexahistidine tagged form. As for the pET300 vector, full-length *OsSNAT3* cDNA was amplified by PCR by using a primer set (*OsSNAT3* forward primer, 5′-AAA AAG CAG GCT CCA TGG GCG CCG GGG AAG-3′; *OsSNAT3* reverse primer, 5′-AGA AAG CTG GGT TCA TTT CTT TGT AGC-3′) with a template plasmid containing *OsSNAT3* cDNA provided by the National Institute of Agrobiological Sciences. The first PCR product was used for the template of the second PCR using the *attB* primer set, as described previously [22]. The second *OsSNAT3* PCR product was cloned using gateway recombination reactions in the pDONR221 vector (Invitrogen, Carlsbad, CA, USA) to generate pDONR221-OsSNAT3 plasmid, and then recombined into the destination vector pET300/NT-DEST (Invitrogen) resulting in the pET300-OsSNAT3 plasmid, according to the manufacturer's procedure. As for the pET28b vector, the full-length *OsSNAT3* was amplified by PCR with *Nco*I forward primer (5′-ACC ATG GGC GCC GGG GAA GGG-3′) and *Xho*I reverse primer (5′-CTC GAG TTT CTT TGT AGC AGC CTG ACC-3′). The resulting *OsSNAT3* PCR product was first cloned into a TA cloning vector (RBC Bioscience, New Taipei City, Taiwan) followed by *Nco*I and *Xho*I digestion. The *Nco*I and *Xho*I inserts of *OsSNAT3* were then ligated into the same restriction endonuclease sites of the pET28b vector. Both pET300-OsSNAT3 and pET28b-OsSNAT3 plasmids were transformed into *E. coli* BL21 (DE3) strains (Invitrogen) using the heat shock method. Bacterial culture and recombinant protein purification procedures were performed according to the manufacturer's recommendations (Qiagen, Tokyo, Japan).

4.3. Measurement of SNAT Enzyme Kinetics

The purified recombinant OsSNAT3 protein (0.5 µg) was assayed in the presence of 0.5 mM acetyl-CoA and varying concentrations of serotonin (or other substrates) in 100 mM potassium phosphate (pH 8.8 or varying pH) at 45 °C (or other temperatures) for 30 min. The in vitro enzymatic reaction products and endogenous melatonin contents in the transgenic rice seedlings were quantified by high-performance liquid chromatography (HPLC), as described previously [21]. Lineweaver–Burk plots were generated for calculating substrate affinity (K_m) and the maximum reaction rate (V_{max}) with the OsSNAT3 recombinant protein (0.25 µg) after 20 mins of enzymatic reaction. Protein levels were determined using the Bradford method and a protein assay dye (Bio-Rad, Hercules, CA, USA). The analysis was performed in triplicate.

4.4. Subcellular Localization of OsSNAT3

The pER-mCherry binary vector was generously provided by Dr. H.G. Kang (Texas State University, San Marcos, TX, USA). The full-length of *OsSNAT3* cDNA was amplified by PCR using a primer set containing *Asc*I sites (*Asc*I forward primer 5′-GGC GCG CCA TGG GCG CCG GGG AAG GGG AT-3′; *Asc*I reverse primer, 5′-GGC GCG CCG TTT CTT TGT AGC AGC CTG-3′) with a template plasmid cDNA (GenBank accession number AK241100). The resulting *OsSNAT3* PCR product was initially ligated into the TA vector (RBC Bioscience) followed by *Asc*I restriction endonuclease enzyme digestion. The purified *Asc*I insert of *OsSNAT3* was then introduced into the *Asc*I site of the binary vector pER8-mCherry containing the estrogen-inducible XVE promoter (Pxve), resulting in pER8-OsSNAT3-mCherry. The pER8-OsSNAT3-mCherry plasmid construct was transformed into the *Agrobacterium tumefaciens* GV2260 strain using the freeze–thaw method. The *Agrobacterium*-mediated transient expression of OsSNAT3-mCherry fusion protein was identified and confocal microscope analysis (TCS-SP5; Leica, Wetzlar, Germany) was performed, as described previously [30].

4.5. Transgenic Rice Plants either Downregulating or Overexpressing OsSNAT3

The pTCK303 RNAi binary vector was utilized to knockdown the expression of the rice *OsSNAT3* gene, as previously described [57]. In brief, a 290-bp *OsSNAT 3* cDNA fragment positioned in the middle region of the *SNAT3* cDNA was amplified by polymerase chain reaction (PCR) with the following primer set: *OsSNAT3* forward 5'-<u>ACT AGT</u> AAC ACG GCG CTC TTC CCC GTC-3' (*Spe*I site underlined) and *OsSNAT3* reverse 5'-<u>GAG CTC</u> AGC AAT GGC ATC ATC GTT GTT-3' (*Sac*I site underlined). The amplified *OsSNAT3* PCR product was first cloned into the T&A cloning vector (T&A: OsSNAT3; RBC Bioscience), from which the Os*SNAT3* insert (antisense) was acquired by the digestion of *Sac*I and *Spe*I restriction enzymes, while the sense *OsSNAT3* insert was obtained by *Kpn*I and *Bam*HI digestion. The antisense *OsSNAT3* was first ligated into the pTCK303 vector, which was predigested by the same restriction enzymes. Thereafter, the sense fragment of the *OsSNAT3* insert was further ligated into the pTCK303 vector harboring the antisense DNA fragment. The resulting pTCK303:OsSNAT3 RNAi binary vector was transformed into *Agrobacterium tumefaciens* strain LBA4404, followed by rice transformation to the Korean Japonica cultivar Dongjin. The transgenic rice plants were regenerated from calli in the presence of hygromycin via a somatic embryogenesis process, as previously described [57]. As for the *OsSNAT3* overexpression vector construct, the pIPKb002 binary vector [63], which is designed to overexpress the transgene *OsSNAT3* under the control of maize ubiquitin promoter, was used. The pDONR221-OsSNAT3 plasmid was recombined with the pIPKb002 destination vector using the LR clonase enzyme (Invitrogen) to yield the pIPKb002-OsSNAT3 binary plasmid. The pIPKb002-OsSNAT3 binary vector was transformed into *Agrobacterium tumefaciens* LBA4404 and rice, as described above.

4.6. RNA Extraction and Reverse Transcription–Polymerase Chain Reaction (RT-PCR) Analysis

Total RNA from rice seedlings was isolated using a NucleoSpin RNA Plant Kit (Macherey-Nagel, Düren, Germany). First-strand cDNA was synthesized from 2 μg of total RNA using EcoDry^{TM} Premix (Takara Bio USA, Inc., Mountain View, CA, USA). The conditions of RT-PCR were begun with initial denaturation at 95 °C (3 min) followed by varying cycles of denaturation at 95 °C (30 s), annealing at 56 °C (30 s), and extension at 72 °C (30 s) in 30 μL of master mix (Takara Bio Inc., Kusatsu, Shiga, Japan). The primer sequences for *OsSNAT3* were forward primer (5'-ATG GGC GCC GGG GAA GGG GAT-3') and reverse primer (5'-TTT CTT TGT AGC AGC CTG-3'). The other primer sequences were as described in previous reports [14,22,40]. Quantitative real-time PCR was carried out as described previously [35].

4.7. Cadmium Treatment and Melatonin Measurement

Dehusked rice seeds were sterilized with 2% NaOCl for 50 min, after which they were thoroughly rinsed with sterile distilled water and sown on half-strength Murashige and Skoog (MS) medium under cool daylight fluorescent lamps (60 μmol m^{-2} s^{-1}) (Philips, Amsterdam, The Netherlands) under a 14 h light/10 h dark photoperiod at 28 °C/24 °C (day/night). The 7-day-old seedlings collected from MS medium were incubated in 50 mL polypropylene conical tubes containing 30 mL water and 0.5 mM CdCl$_2$ (Sigma-Aldrich, St. Louis, MO, USA) and incubated for 7 days for melatonin quantification. As for the cadmium response experiment, the surface-sterilized rice seeds were sown and grown on half-strength MS medium containing a 0.5 mM concentration of cadmium for 7 days, as described above. Melatonin contents were measured from frozen samples (0.1 g), which were pulverized to a powder in liquid nitrogen using the TissueLyser II (Qiagen, Tokyo, Japan). The sample powders were then extracted with 1 mL chloroform followed by centrifugation for 10 min at 12,000 rpm, and then the supernatants (200 μL) were evaporated and dissolved in 0.1 mL of 40% methanol. The resulting 10 μL aliquots were subjected to high-performance liquid chromatography (HPLC) using a fluorescence detector system (Waters, Milford, MA, USA), as described previously [30].

Int. J. Mol. Sci. **2024**, *25*, 5952

4.8. Measurements of Chlorophyll and Malondialdehyde

The powder of the rice seedlings (100 mg) was extracted with 1 mL of 0.1 mM NH_4OH (containing 80% acetone). Chlorophyll concentrations were determined at wavelengths of 647, 644, and 750 nm using a spectrophotometer (MicroDigital Nabi, GyungGi, Republic of Korea) according to Porra et al. [64]. As for measuring the malondialdehyde (MDA) levels, the powder (50 mg) was extracted with 1.5 mL of reaction buffer containing 0.5% thiobarbituric acid and 20% trichloroacetic acid. The supernatants decanted from centrifugation at $12,000 \times g$ for 15 min were boiled at 95 °C for 25 min and placed on ice for 5 min. MDA content was recorded at wavelengths of 440, 532, and 600 nm using a spectrophotometer (MicroDigital Nabi) with a molar extinction coefficient of 156/nmol/L/cm.

4.9. Statistical Analysis

The data were evaluated by analysis of variance using IBM SPSS Statistics 25 software (IBM Corp. Armonk, NY, USA). Different letters above the histograms indicate significantly different values at $p < 0.05$ according to Tukey's post hoc honestly significant difference (HSD) test. Data are presented as means $\pm$ standard deviations.

5. Conclusions

Elucidating Cd tolerance mechanisms in plants is the first step toward generating Cd-tolerant crops by either classical breeding or genetic engineering strategies. SNAT is the rate-limiting enzyme for melatonin biosynthesis in plants and animals. This report describes the cloning and characterization of the *SNAT3* gene from rice, a functional ortholog of archaeal *SNAT*. The downregulation of *SNAT3* resulted in reduced melatonin synthesis and an enhanced susceptibility to Cd stress, whereas its overexpression increased melatonin synthesis and improved Cd tolerance through a mechanism involving the BiP4 chaperone, an ER-resident HSP, although conclusions about the relationship between OsSNAT3 and BIP4 need more evidence. These results suggest that the adoption by the agriculture industry of melatonin engineering and/or exogenous melatonin application could allow crops to withstand Cd stress, thus improving yields and allowing the harvesting of safe food in Cd-contaminated fields.

Author Contributions: Conceptualization, K.B.; Investigation, K.B. and H.-Y.L.; Writing—original draft, K.B.; Funding acquisition, K.B.; Formal analysis, K.B. and H.-Y.L. All authors have read and agreed to the published version of the manuscript.

Funding: This research was supported by grants from the Basic Science Research Program of the National Research Foundation of Korea (NRF-2021R1I1A2042237), funded by the Ministry of Education.

Institutional Review Board Statement: Not applicable.

Informed Consent Statement: Not applicable.

Data Availability Statement: Data are contained within the article.

Conflicts of Interest: The authors declare no conflicts of interest.

References

1. Jaishankar, M.; Tseten, T.; Anbalagan, N.; Mathew, B.B.; Beeregowda, K.N. Toxicity, mechanism and health effects of some heavy metals. *Interdiscip. Toxicol.* **2014**, *7*, 60. [CrossRef] [PubMed]
2. Fan, P.; Wu, L.; Wang, Q.; Wang, Y.; Luo, H.; Song, J.; Yang, M.; Yao, H.; Chen, S. Physiological and molecular mechanisms of medicinal plants in response to cadmium stress: Current status and future perspective. *J. Hazard. Mater.* **2023**, *450*, 131008. [CrossRef] [PubMed]
3. Saqib, M.; Shahzad, U.; Zulfiqar, F.; Tiwari, R.K.; Lal, M.K.; Naz, S.; Jahan, M.S.; Awan, Z.A.; El-Sheikh, M.A.; Altaf, M.A. Exogenous melatonin alleviates cadmium-induced inhibition of growth and photosynthesis through upregulating antioxidant defense system in strawberry. *S. Afr. J. Bot.* **2023**, *157*, 10–18. [CrossRef]
4. Bora, M.S.; Sarma, K.P. Anatomical and ultrastructural alterations in *Ceratopteris pteridoies* under cadmium stress: A mechanism of cadmium tolerance. *Ecotoxicol. Environ. Saf.* **2021**, *218*, 112285. [CrossRef] [PubMed]

5. Zulfiqar, U.; Jiang, W.; Xiukang, W.; Hussain, S.; Ahmad, M.; Maqsood, M.F.; Ali, N.; Ishfaq, M.; Kaleem, M.; Haider, U.; et al. Cadmium phytotoxicity, tolerance, and advanced remediation approaches in agricultural soils; a comprehensive review. *Front. Plant Sci.* **2022**, *13*, 773815. [CrossRef] [PubMed]
6. Lee, H.Y.; Back, K. Cadmium disrupts subcellular organelles, including chloroplasts, resulting in melatonin induction in plants. *Molecules* **2017**, *22*, 1791. [CrossRef] [PubMed]
7. Altaf, M.A.; Hao, Y.; Shu, H.; Mumtaz, M.A.; Cheng, S.; Alyemeni, M.N.; Ahmad, P.; Wang, Z. Melatonin enhanced the heavy metal-stress tolerance of pepper by mitigating the oxidative damage and reducing the heavy metal accumulation. *J. Hazard. Mater.* **2023**, *454*, 131468. [CrossRef] [PubMed]
8. Hasan, M.K.; Cheng, Y.; Kanwar, M.K.; Chu, X.-Y.; Ahammed, G.J.; Qi, Z.-Y. Responses of plant proteins to heavy metal stress-a review. *Front. Plant Sci.* **2017**, *8*, 1492. [CrossRef] [PubMed]
9. Xiao, Y.; Wu, X.; Liu, D.; Yao, J.; Liang, G.; Song, H.; Ismail, A.M.; Luo, J.S.; Zhang, Z. Cell wall polysaccharide-mediated cadmium tolerance between two *Arabidopsis thaliana* ecotypes. *Front. Plant Sci.* **2020**, *11*, 473. [CrossRef]
10. Wang, W.; Vinocur, B.; Shoseyov, O.; Altman, A. Role of plant heat-shock proteins and molecular chaperones in the abiotic stress response. *Trends Plant Sci.* **2004**, *9*, 244–252. [CrossRef]
11. Usman, M.G.; Rafli, M.Y.; Martini, M.Y.; Yusuff, O.A.; Ismail, M.R.; Miah, G. Molecular analysis of Hsp70 mechanisms in plants and their function in response to stress. *Biotechnol. Genet. Eng. Rev.* **2017**, *33*, 26–39. [CrossRef] [PubMed]
12. Sarkar, N.K.; Kundnani, P.; Grover, A. Functional analysis of Hsp70 superfamily proteins of rice (*Oryza sativa*). *Cell Stress Chaperones* **2013**, *18*, 427–437. [CrossRef] [PubMed]
13. Wakasa, Y.; Hayashi, S.; Takaiwa, F. Expression of OsBiP4 and OsBiP5 is highly correlated with the endoplasmic reticulum stress response in rice. *Planta* **2012**, *236*, 1519–1527. [CrossRef] [PubMed]
14. Hayashi, S.; Wakasa, Y.; Takahashi, H.; Kawakatsu, T.; Takaiwa, F. Signal transduction by IRE1-mediated splicing of bZIP50 and other stress sensors in the endoplasmic reticulum stress response of rice. *Plant J.* **2012**, *69*, 946–956. [CrossRef] [PubMed]
15. Wakasa, Y.; Yasuda, H.; Oono, Y.; Kawakatsu, T.; Hirose, S.; Takahashi, H.; Hayashi, S.; Yang, L.; Takaiwa, F. Expression of ER quality control-related genes in response to changes in BiP1 levels in developing rice endosperm. *Plant J.* **2011**, *65*, 675–689. [CrossRef] [PubMed]
16. Gao, H.; Brandizzi, F.; Benning, C.; Larkin, R.M. A membrane-tethered transcription factor defines a branch of the heat stress response in *Arabidopsis thaliana*. *Proc. Natl. Acad. Sci. USA* **2008**, *105*, 16398–16403. [CrossRef] [PubMed]
17. Howell, S.H. Endoplasmic reticulum stress responses in plants. *Annu. Rev. Plant Biol.* **2013**, *64*, 477–499. [CrossRef] [PubMed]
18. Simoni, E.B.; Oliveira, C.C.; Fraga, O.T.; Reis, P.A.B.; Fontes, E.P.B. Cell death signaling from endoplasmic reticulum stress: Plant-specific and conserved features. *Front. Plant Sci.* **2022**, *13*, 835738. [CrossRef] [PubMed]
19. Zhao, D.; Yu, Y.; Shen, Y.; Liu, Q.; Zhao, Z.; Sharma, R.; Reiter, R.J. Melatonin synthesis and function: Evolutionary history in animals and plants. *Front. Endocrinol.* **2019**, *10*, 249. [CrossRef] [PubMed]
20. Back, K. Melatonin metabolism, signaling and possible roles in plants. *Plant J.* **2021**, *105*, 376–391. [CrossRef]
21. Lee, K.; Choi, G.H.; Back, K. Functional characterization of serotonin N-acetyltransferase in archaeon *Thermoplasma volcanium*. *Antioxidants* **2022**, *11*, 596. [CrossRef] [PubMed]
22. Lee, K.; Back, K. *Escherichia coli* RimI encodes serotonin N-acetyltransferase activity and its overexpression leads to enhanced growth and melatonin biosynthesis. *Biomolecules* **2023**, *13*, 908. [CrossRef] [PubMed]
23. Reiter, R.J.; Tan, D.X.; Sharma, R. Historical perspective and evaluation of the mechanisms by which melatonin mediates seasonal reproduction in mammals. *Melatonin Res.* **2018**, *1*, 59–77. [CrossRef]
24. Tan, D.X.; Reiter, R.J.; Zimmerman, S.; Hardeland, R. Melatonin: Both a messenger of darkness and a participant in the cellular actions of non-visible solar radiation of near infrared light. *Biology* **2023**, *12*, 89. [CrossRef] [PubMed]
25. Arnao, M.B.; Hernández-Ruiz, J. Melatonin: A new plant hormone and/or a plant master regulator? *Trends Plant Sci.* **2019**, *24*, 38–48. [CrossRef] [PubMed]
26. Lee, H.Y.; Back, K. Melatonin regulates chloroplast protein quality control via a mitogen-activated protein kinase signaling pathway. *Antioxidants* **2021**, *10*, 511. [CrossRef] [PubMed]
27. Lee, H.Y.; Hwang, O.J.; Back, K. Phytomelatonin as a signaling molecule for protein quality control via chaperone, autophagy, and ubiquitin–proteasome systems in plants. *J. Exp. Bot.* **2022**, *73*, 5863–5873. [CrossRef] [PubMed]
28. Klein, D.C. Arylalkylamine N-acetyltransferase: "the timezyme". *J. Biol. Chem.* **2007**, *282*, 4233–4237. [CrossRef]
29. Lee, H.Y.; Hwang, O.J.; Back, K. Functional characterization of tobacco (*Nicotiana benthamiana*) serotonin N-acetyltransferases (*NbSNAT1* and *NbSNAT2*). *Melatonin Res.* **2021**, *4*, 507–521.
30. Byeon, Y.; Lee, H.Y.; Lee, K.; Park, S.; Back, K. Cellular localization and kinetics of the rice melatonin biosynthetic enzymes SNAT and ASMT. *J. Pineal Res.* **2014**, *56*, 107–114. [CrossRef]
31. Byeon, Y.; Lee, H.Y.; Back, K. Cloning and characterization of the serotonin N-acetyltransferase-2 gene (SNAT2) in rice (*Oryza sativa*). *J. Pineal Res.* **2016**, *61*, 198–207. [CrossRef] [PubMed]
32. Yu, Y.; Bian, L.; Jiao, Z.; Keke, Y.; Wan, Y.; Zhang, G.; Guo, D. Molecular cloning and characterization of a grapevine (*Vitis vinifera* L.) serotonin N-acetyltransferase (*VvSNAT2*) gene involved in plant defense. *BMC Genom.* **2019**, *20*, 880. [CrossRef] [PubMed]
33. Liao, L.; Zhou, Y.; Xu, Y.; Zhang, Y.; Liu, X.; Liu, B.; Chen, X.; Guo, Y.; Zeng, Z.; Zhao, Y. Structural and molecular dynamics analysis of plant serotonin N-acetyltransferase reveal an acid/base-assisted catalysis in melatonin biosynthesis. *Angew. Chem. Int. Ed.* **2021**, *60*, 12020–12026. [CrossRef] [PubMed]

34. Neubauer, M.; Innes, R.W. Loss of the acetyltransferase NAA50 induces endoplasmic reticulum stress and immune responses and suppresses growth. *Plant Physiol.* **2020**, *183*, 1838–1854. [CrossRef] [PubMed]
35. Lee, K.; Back, K. Human *Naa50* harbors serotonin *N*-acetyltransferase activity and its overexpression enhances melatonin biosynthesis resulting in osmotic stress tolerance in rice. *Antioxidants* **2023**, *12*, 319. [CrossRef] [PubMed]
36. Falcón, J.; Coon, S.L.; Besseau, L.; Cazamea-Catalan, D.; Fuentes, M.; Magnanou, E.; Paulin, C.H.; Boeuf, G.; Sauzet, S.; Jorgensen, E.H.; et al. Drastic neofunctionalization associated with evolution of the timezyme AANAT 500 Mya. *Proc. Natl. Acad. Sci. USA* **2014**, *111*, 314–319. [CrossRef] [PubMed]
37. Ganguly, S.; Mummaneni, P.; Steinbach, P.J.; Klein, D.C.; Coon, S.L. Characterization of the *Saccharomyces cerevisiae* homolog of the melatonin rhythm enzyme arylalkylamine *N*-acetyltransferase (EC 2.3.1.87). *J. Biol. Chem.* **2001**, *276*, 47239–47247. [CrossRef] [PubMed]
38. Emanuelsson, O.; Nielsen, H.; Brunak, S.; Heijne, G. Predicting subcellular localization of proteins based on their N-terminal amino acid sequence. *J. Mol. Biol.* **2000**, *300*, 1005–1016. [CrossRef] [PubMed]
39. Kosugi, S.; Hasebe, M.; Tomita, M.; Yanagawa, H. Systematic identification of yeast cell cycle-dependent nucleocytoplasmic shuttling proteins by prediction of composite motifs. *Proc. Natl. Acad. Sci. USA* **2009**, *106*, 10171–10176. [CrossRef]
40. Armbruster, L.; Linster, E.; Boyer, J.P.; Brünje, A.; Eirich, J.; Stephan, I.; Bienvenut, W.V.; Weidenhausen, J.; Meinnel, T.; Hell, R.; et al. NAA50 is an enzymatically active N^α-acetyltransferase that is crucial for development and regulation of stress responses. *Plant Physiol.* **2020**, *183*, 1502–1516. [CrossRef]
41. Wang, L.; Feng, C.; Zheng, X.; Guo, Y.; Zhou, F.; Shan, D.; Liu, X.; Kong, J. Plant mitochondria synthesize melatonin and enhance the tolerance of plants to drought stress. *J. Pineal Res.* **2017**, *63*, e12429. [CrossRef] [PubMed]
42. Zhou, W.; Yang, S.; Zhang, Q.; Xiao, R.; Li, B.; Wang, D.; Niu, J.; Wang, S.; Wang, Z. Functional characterization of serotonin *N*-acetyltransferase genes (SNAT1/2) in melatonin biosynthesis of *Hypericum perforatum*. *Front. Plant Sci.* **2021**, *12*, 781717. [CrossRef] [PubMed]
43. Arif, N.; Yadav, V.; Singh, S.; Singh, S.; Ahmad, P.; Mishra, R.; Sharma, S.; Tripathi, D.K.; Dubey, N.K.; Chauhan, D.K. Influence of high and low levels of plant-beneficial heavy metal ions on plant growth and development. *Front. Environ. Sci.* **2016**, *4*, 69. [CrossRef]
44. Cao, Z.; Fang, Y.; Lu, Y.; Tan, D.; Du, C.; Li, Y.; Ma, Q.; Yu, J.; Chen, M.; Zhou, C.; et al. Melatonin alleviates cadmium-induced liver injury by inhibiting the TXNIP-NLRP3 inflammasome. *J. Pineal Res.* **2017**, *62*, e12389. [CrossRef] [PubMed]
45. Haider, F.U.; Liqun, C.; Coulter, J.A.; Cheema, S.A.; Wu, J.; Zhang, R.; Wenjun, M.; Farooq, M. Cadmium toxicity in plants: Impacts and remediation strategies. *Ecotoxicol. Environ. Saf.* **2021**, *211*, 111887. [CrossRef] [PubMed]
46. Arnao, M.B.; Cano, A.; Hernández-Ruiz, J. Phytomelatonin: An unexpected molecule with amazing performance in plants. *J. Exp. Bot.* **2022**, *73*, 5779–5800. [CrossRef] [PubMed]
47. Kuwabara, W.M.T.; Gomes, P.R.L.; Andrade-Silva, J.; Soares, J.M., Jr.; Amaral, F.G.; Cipolla-Neto, J. Melatonin and its ubiquitous effects on cell function and survival: A review. *Melatonin Res.* **2022**, *5*, 192–208. [CrossRef]
48. Corpas, F.J.; Rodríguez-Ruiz, M.; Muñoz-Vargas, M.A.; González-Gordo, S.; Reiter, R.J.; Palma, J.M. Interaction of melatonin, reactive oxygen species, and nitric oxide during fruit ripening: An update and prospective view. *J. Exp. Bot.* **2022**, *73*, 5947–5960. [CrossRef]
49. Muhammad, I.; Ahmad, S.; Shen, W. Melatonin-mediated molecular responses in plants: Enhancing stress tolerance and mitigating environmental challenges in cereal crop production. *Int. J. Mol. Sci.* **2024**, *25*, 4551. [CrossRef]
50. Huang, J.; Jing, H.K.; Zhang, Y.; Chen, S.Y.; Wang, H.Y.; Cao, Y.; Zhang, Z.; Lu, Y.H.; Zheng, Q.S.; Shen, R.F.; et al. Melatonin reduces cadmium accumulation via mediating the nitric oxide accumulation and increasing the cell wall fixation capacity of cadmium in rice. *J. Hazard. Mater.* **2023**, *445*, 130529. [CrossRef]
51. Chmur, M.; Bajguz, A. Melatonin involved in protective effects against cadmium stress in *Wolffia arrhiza*. *Int. J. Mol. Sci.* **2023**, *24*, 1178. [CrossRef] [PubMed]
52. Xu, J.; Wei, Z.; Lu, X.; Liu, Y.; Yu, W.; Li, C. Involvement of nitric oxide and melatonin enhances cadmium resistance of tomato seedlings through regulation of the ascorbate-glutathione cycle and ROS metabolism. *Int. J. Mol. Sci.* **2023**, *24*, 9526. [CrossRef]
53. Xing, Q.; Hasan, M.K.; Li, Z.; Yang, T.; Jin, W.; Qi, Z.; Yang, P.; Wang, G.; Ahammed, G.J.; Zhou, J. Melatonin-induced plant adaptation to cadmium stress involves enhanced phytochelatin synthesis and nutrient homeostasis in *Solanum lycopersicum* L. *J. Hazard. Mater.* **2023**, *456*, 131670. [CrossRef] [PubMed]
54. Ye, T.; Yin, X.; Yu, L.; Zheng, S.J.; Cai, W.J.; Wu, Y.; Feng, Y.Q. Metabolic analysis of the melatonin biosynthesis pathway using chemical labeling coupled with liquid chromatography-mass spectrometry. *J. Pineal Res.* **2019**, *66*, e12531. [CrossRef] [PubMed]
55. Valente, M.A.S.; Faria, J.A.Q.A.; Soares-Ramos, J.R.L.; Reis, P.A.B.; Pinheiro, G.L.; Piovesan, N.D.; Morais, A.T.; Menezes, C.C.; Cano, M.A.O.; Fietto, L.G.; et al. The ER luminal binding protein (BiP) mediates an increase in drought tolerance in soybean and tobacco. *J. Exp. Bot.* **2008**, *60*, 533–546. [CrossRef] [PubMed]
56. Park, C.J.; Bart, R.; Chern, M.; Canlas, P.E.; Bai, W.; Ronald, P.C. Overexpression of the endoplasmic reticulum chaperone BiP3 regulates XA21-mediated innate immunity in rice. *PLoS ONE* **2010**, *5*, e9262. [CrossRef] [PubMed]
57. Hwang, O.J.; Back, K. Melatonin deficiency confers tolerance to multiple abiotic stresses in rice via decreased brassinosteroid levels. *Int. J. Mol. Sci.* **2019**, *20*, 5173. [CrossRef] [PubMed]

58. Zhang, T.; Wang, Y.; Ma, X.; Ouyang, Z.; Deng, L.; Shen, S.; Dong, X.; Du, N.; Dong, H.; Guo, Z.; et al. Melatonin alleviates copper toxicity via improving ROS metabolism and antioxidant defense response in tomato seedlings. *Antioxidants* **2022**, *11*, 758. [CrossRef]
59. Kikuchi, S.; Satoh, K.; Nagata, T.; Kawagashira, N.; Doi, K.; Kishimoto, N.; Yazaki, J.; Ishikawa, M.; Yamada, H.; Ooka, H.; et al. Collection, mapping, and annotation of over 28,000 cDNA clones from japonica rice. *Science* **2003**, *301*, 376–379. [CrossRef]
60. Satoh, K.; Doi, K.; Nagata, T.; Kishimoto, N.; Suzuki, K.; Otomo, Y.; Kawai, J.; Nakamura, M.; Hirozane-Kishikawa, T.; Kanagawa, S.; et al. Gene organization in rice revealed by full-length cDNA mapping and gene expression analysis through microarray. *PLoS ONE* **2007**, *2*, e1235. [CrossRef]
61. Marchler-Bauer, A.; Bo, Y.; Han, L.; He, J.; Lanczycki, C.J.; Lu, S.; Chitsaz, F.; Derbyshire, M.K.; Geer, R.C.; Gonzales, N.R.; et al. CDD/SPARCLE: Functional classification of proteins via subfamily domain architectures. *Nucleic Acids Res.* **2017**, *45*, D200–D2003. [CrossRef] [PubMed]
62. Dereeper, A.; Audic, S.; Claverie, J.M.; Blanc, G. BLAST-EXPLORER helps you building datasets for phylogenetic analysis. *BMC Evol. Biol.* **2020**, *10*, 8. [CrossRef] [PubMed]
63. Himmelbach, A.; Zierold, U.; Hensel, G.; Riechen, J.; Douchkov, D.; Schweizer, P.; Kumlehn, J. A set of modular binary vectors for transformation of cereals. *Plant Physiol.* **2007**, *145*, 1192–1200. [CrossRef] [PubMed]
64. Porra, R.J.; Thompson, W.A.; Kriedmann, P.E. Determination of accurate extinction coefficients and simultaneous equations for assaying chlorophylls a and b extracted with four different solvents: Verification of the concentration of chlorophyll standards by atomic absorption spectroscopy. *Biochim. Biophys. Acta* **1989**, *975*, 384–394. [CrossRef]

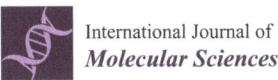

International Journal of
Molecular Sciences

MDPI

Article

Physiological and Proteomic Responses of the Tetraploid *Robinia pseudoacacia* L. to High CO$_2$ Levels

Jianxin Li [1,2,†], **Subin Zhang** [2,†], **Pei Lei** [1], **Liyong Guo** [2], **Xiyang Zhao** [1,3,*] and **Fanjuan Meng** [1,3,*]

1   College of Forestry and Grassland, Jilin Agriculture University, Changchun 130118, China; ljxin1022@163.com (J.L.); 18800465845@163.com (P.L.)
2   College of Life Science, Northeast Forestry University, Harbin 150040, China; zhbin972@163.com (S.Z.); 18512231143@163.com (L.G.)
3   Jilin Provincial Key Laboratory of Tree and Grass Genetics and Breeding, Changchun 130118, China
*   Correspondence: zhaoxyphd@163.com (X.Z.); mfjtougao@163.com (F.M.)
†   These authors contributed equally to this work.

Abstract: The increase in atmospheric CO$_2$ concentration is a significant factor in triggering global warming. CO$_2$ is essential for plant photosynthesis, but excessive CO$_2$ can negatively impact photosynthesis and its associated physiological and biochemical processes. The tetraploid *Robinia pseudoacacia* L., a superior and improved variety, exhibits high tolerance to abiotic stress. In this study, we investigated the physiological and proteomic response mechanisms of the tetraploid *R. pseudoacacia* under high CO$_2$ treatment. The results of our physiological and biochemical analyses revealed that a 5% high concentration of CO$_2$ hindered the growth and development of the tetraploid *R. pseudoacacia* and caused severe damage to the leaves. Additionally, it significantly reduced photosynthetic parameters such as Pn, Gs, Tr, and Ci, as well as respiration. The levels of chlorophyll (Chl a and b) and the fluorescent parameters of chlorophyll (Fm, Fv/Fm, qP, and ETR) also significantly decreased. Conversely, the levels of ROS (H$_2$O$_2$ and O$_2{}^{·-}$) were significantly increased, while the activities of antioxidant enzymes (SOD, CAT, GR, and APX) were significantly decreased. Furthermore, high CO$_2$ induced stomatal closure by promoting the accumulation of ROS and NO in guard cells. Through a proteomic analysis, we identified a total of 1652 DAPs after high CO$_2$ treatment. GO functional annotation revealed that these DAPs were mainly associated with redox activity, catalytic activity, and ion binding. KEGG analysis showed an enrichment of DAPs in metabolic pathways, secondary metabolite biosynthesis, amino acid biosynthesis, and photosynthetic pathways. Overall, our study provides valuable insights into the adaptation mechanisms of the tetraploid *R. pseudoacacia* to high CO$_2$.

Keywords: *Robinia pseudoacacia* L.; high CO$_2$; photosynthesis; respiration; proteomic; stomatal

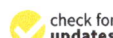

check for
updates

Citation: Li, J.; Zhang, S.; Lei, P.; Guo, L.; Zhao, X.; Meng, F. Physiological and Proteomic Responses of the Tetraploid *Robinia pseudoacacia* L. to High CO$_2$ Levels. *Int. J. Mol. Sci.* **2024**, *25*, 5262. https://doi.org/10.3390/ijms25105262

Academic Editors: Philippe Jeandet and Mateusz Labudda

Received: 28 March 2024
Revised: 6 May 2024
Accepted: 9 May 2024
Published: 11 May 2024

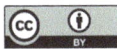
1. Introduction

CO$_2$ is a crucial substrate for plant photosynthesis. The levels of atmospheric CO$_2$ have a significant impact on plant growth, development, and biomass [1]. Since the industrial era, atmospheric CO$_2$ concentrations have increased by more than 40%, and the current ambient CO$_2$ concentrations exceed 417 ppm [2]. The rise in CO$_2$ concentration has resulted in significant alterations in global temperatures, intensifying the greenhouse effect and exposing plants to elevated CO$_2$ levels, higher temperatures, and drought. Consequently, this poses a considerable challenge to plant growth and reproduction. The impact of CO$_2$ enrichment on growth and yield for C3 plants can vary and may be influenced by species-specific factors [3].

Previous studies have consistently shown that higher levels of CO$_2$ have a significant impact on the physiological functioning of plants [4–6]. On the one hand, elevated CO$_2$ directly affects plant photosynthesis. Increased atmospheric CO$_2$ concentrations lead to a higher number of leaves, longer branches, and greater biomass while also causing a decrease in stomatal density. Additionally, it can result in visible symptoms such as wilting and drooping leaves [3,7]. According to previous studies, the net photosynthetic rate and water use efficiency (WUE) of *A. marina* and *R. stylosa* increased when exposed to a slight elevation in CO_2 concentration. These findings suggest that the promotion of photosynthesis was facilitated by the elevated CO_2 concentration [7]. Furthermore, it has been observed that rising CO_2 concentrations contribute to an increase in phytoplankton growth rate and lipid productivity [8]. Another study found that corn exhibits higher biomass and leaf area, as well as enhanced starch synthesis, when exposed to elevated CO_2 concentrations [9]. The Rubisco content and light-saturated photosynthetic rate in plant leaves were observed to be significantly reduced in a high CO_2 environment [10]. Similarly, when *Pinus sylvestris* was exposed to this environment for an extended period, both the stomatal conductance and total stomatal number showed a significant decrease [11]. On the other hand, in *Allium sativum* L., the elevated CO_2 atmosphere had a contrasting effect, significantly enhancing the activity of pyruvate decarboxylase (PDC) and alcohol dehydrogenase (ADH). This, in turn, caused a substantial increase in the content of alcohols, aldehydes, and phenols, resulting in toxic effects [12]. On the contrary, research has demonstrated that high CO_2 levels can also actually mitigate ozone-induced oxidative damage in wheat [8]. Additionally, the impact of CO_2 concentrations varies depending on the plant species. For example, in the case of reticulated melons, low CO_2 has been found to increase both the initial and maximum photosynthetic efficiency. However, when exposed to high CO_2, the maximum photosynthetic efficiency of reticulated melons actually declines [13].

On the other hand, previous studies have demonstrated that CO_2-induced stomatal closure is dependent on Ca^{2+} and that elevated CO_2 levels stimulate an increase in free Ca^{2+} concentration in defense cells [14–17]. Stomata, which are small pores on the leaf surface, play a crucial role in regulating the uptake of carbon dioxide for photosynthesis and the loss of water through transpiration [18]. The movement of stomata is influenced by various environmental factors, including CO_2 concentration. Stomatal opening is promoted by low concentrations of CO_2, while stomatal closure is induced by high concentrations of CO_2. In the guard cells of *Arabidopsis thaliana*, the carbonic anhydrases βCA1 and βCA4 are involved in mediating CO_2-controlled stomatal movement and development [19]. Additionally, BIG proteins play a critical role in inhibiting stomatal opening and promoting stomatal closure in response to CO_2 [20]. Reactive oxygen species (ROS) and nitric oxide (NO) are important signaling molecules that regulate stomatal movement in plants [21]. It has been shown that CO_2-mediated stomatal closure requires the generation of ROS, which has an important role in the regulation of stomatal aperture [22,23]. NO plays a role in both abscisic acid (ABA)- and Ca^{2+}-mediated stomatal closure and is located downstream of ROS, an important participant in the stomatal closure process [24,25]. In *A. thaliana*, ROS are mainly produced by NADPH oxidase and peroxidase at the plasma membrane [26,27], while NO is mainly produced by nitrate reductase (NR) and NOA1 and induces stomatal closure [28].

Plant respiration is a significant metabolic process on a global scale, accounting for approximately 40–60% of the rate of carbon assimilation [29]. Mitochondria, which are essential organelles involved in cellular material and energy metabolism, possess two respiratory pathways on their inner mitochondrial membrane [30]. There are two pathways involved in respiration: the cytochrome pathway, which is found in nearly all organisms, and the alternate respiration pathway. The alternate respiration pathway is activated when the cytochrome pathway experiences stress conditions like low temperature, drought, ozone, and high salinity soils [31]. The impact of CO_2 on mitochondrial respiration is of great significance in the investigation of plant respiratory metabolism. Previous studies have demonstrated that there exists an alternate respiration pathway, which is insensitive to cyanide (CN) but sensitive to SHAM and is facilitated by alternate oxidase (AOX) [32–34]. Additionally, pyruvate, a crucial metabolite in organisms, has been found to have a notable enhancing effect on the activity of AOX [35–37].

The respiration rate serves as a primary indicator of plant respiratory metabolism. By examining the respiration rate of plants, we can directly observe the impact of high CO_2 concentration on plant respiratory metabolism. However, the effect of elevated CO_2 concentration on the plant respiration rate varies depending on the specific plants and environmental conditions. It has been discovered that elevated CO_2 concentrations resulted in an 8.4% decrease in the daily respiration rate of wheat and sunflower, as well as a 16.2% decrease in the respiration rate during darkness. This could be attributed to the reduction in leaf nitrogen content and the downregulation of photosynthesis caused by elevated CO_2 concentrations, which subsequently leads to a decrease in plant respiration rate [38]. However, previous studies have demonstrated that elevated CO_2 concentrations have the potential to enhance respiratory substrate utilization, upregulate respiratory genes, and increase the number of mitochondria. As a result, this leads to an overall increase in the rate of plant respiration [39,40].

The tetraploid *R. pseudoacacia* L. is a deciduous ornamental tree species belonging to the genus *R. pseudoacacia* in the family Leguminosae. It has four sets of chromosomes (4n = 44) and was created through the application of colchicine to the diploid *R. pseudoacacia* (2n = 22) of a homologous species. This tetraploid species was introduced to China from South Korea [41]. Compared to the diploid *R. pseudoacacia*, the tetraploid *R. pseudoacacia* is considered an excellent variety due to its higher yield, faster growth rate, larger leaves, and numerous outstanding characteristics such as drought resistance, saline resistance, low-temperature resistance, and heat resistance [42–45]. The tetraploid *R. pseudoacacia* exhibits a robust root system, strong adaptability to various environments, and a high capacity for photosynthetic carbon sequestration [46]. In light of prevalent environmental pollution and global climate change, it is imperative to investigate the effects of high CO_2 levels on the physiological processes of the tetraploid *R. pseudoacacia*.

Plants display distinct physiological and biochemical traits when subjected to prolonged exposure to elevated CO_2 concentrations. This study focuses on the tetraploid *R. pseudoacacia* as the experimental material to examine the stomatal movement pattern and physiological alterations in photosynthesis and respiration in response to high CO_2 conditions. Additionally, a proteomic approach was employed to identify crucial regulatory networks and proteins associated with the response of the tetraploid *R. pseudoacacia* to high CO_2 treatment. The objective of this research is to gain insights into the mechanisms by which plants respond to high CO_2 environments.

2. Results

2.1. Response of Morphological and Gas Exchange Parameters of Tetraploid R. pseudoacacia to High CO_2

Under normal CO_2 conditions, the growth of the tetraploid *R. pseudoacacia* was uniform and healthy (CK-H_2O). When the respiratory inhibitor SHAM was added (CK-SHAM), the REC increased, and the RWC of the leaves decreased. However, supplementation with the respiratory enhancer PA (CK-PA) did not cause significant changes in REC and RWC compared to the control. After 9 days of treatment with a 5% CO_2 concentration, the leaves exhibited wilting, drooping, yellowing, and even abscission at the apex (T-H_2O). The yellowing and abscission of leaves worsened with the addition of SHAM (T-SHAM), while the wilting was alleviated with the addition of PA (T-PA) (Figure 1a). After 6 days of treatment, the REC of the CO_2-treated leaves significantly increased by 34.2%, 27.2%, and 52.2% in T-H_2O, T-PA, and T-SHAM, respectively (Figure 1b). However, the RWC of T-H_2O, T-PA, and T-SHAM significantly decreased by 7.6%, 5.3%, and 8.4%, respectively, after 9 days of CO_2 treatment (Figure 1c).

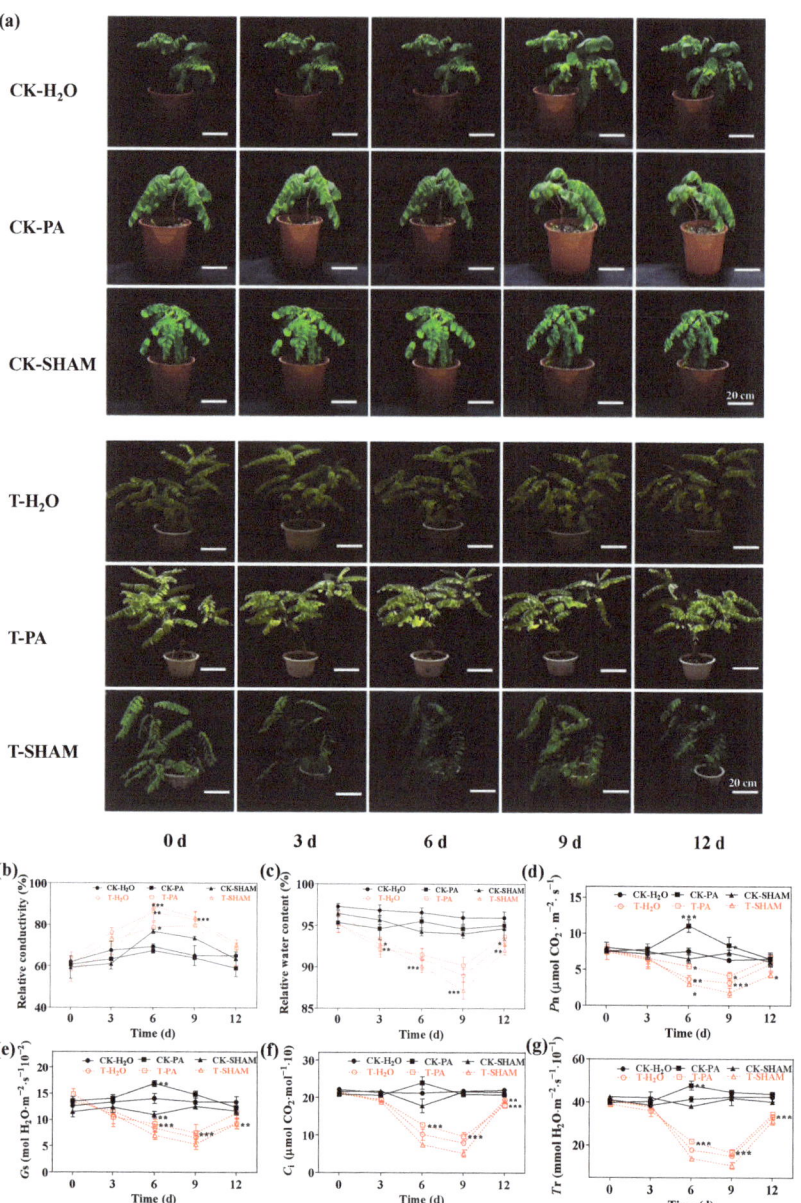

Figure 1. Physiological response of the tetraploid *R. pseudoacacia* to high CO_2 concentrations. (**a**) Phenotypes of *R. pseudoacacia* under CO_2 treatment. Plants were exposed to CO_2 stress for 9 days and then recovered to air CO_2 levels for 3 days. CK-H_2O: control; CK-PA: pyruvic acid-treated; CK-SHAM: salicylhydroxamic acid-treated; T-H_2O: CO_2-treated; T-PA: co-treated with CO_2 and PA; and T-SHAM: co-treated with CO_2 and SHAM. Bar: 20 cm. Effect of high CO_2 concentrations on relative electrical conductivity (**b**), relative water content (**c**), net photosynthetic rate (*Pn*) (**d**), stomatal conductance (*Gs*) (**e**), intercellular CO_2 concentration (*Ci*) (**f**), and transpiration rate (*Tr*) (**g**). Six biological replicates were analyzed, and the error bars represent the SE. Asterisks indicate significant differences as determined by Dunnett's test. (* $p \leq 0.05$; ** $p \leq 0.01$; *** $p \leq 0.001$).

Under normal CO_2 conditions, the presence of PA did not have a significant effect on the photosynthetic parameters (*Pn*, *Gs*, *Ci*, and *Tr*) of the tetraploid *R. pseudoacacia*'s leaves compared to the control (CK-H_2O). However, after supplementation with SHAM on the 6th day, there was a slight fluctuation and decrease in *Pn*, *Gs*, and *Tr* (excluding *Ci*) compared to the control. When exposed to high CO_2, the photosynthetic parameters of the leaves (*Pn*, *Gs*, *Ci*, and *Tr*) significantly decreased compared to the control (CK-H_2O), reaching the lowest values on the 9th day. *Pn*, *Gs*, *Ci*, and *Tr* were 49.5%, 50.5%, 63%, and 63.7% lower than the control, respectively. After the high CO_2 treatment, *R. pseudoacacia* showed some recovery for three days under normal CO_2 conditions, with an increase in the photosynthetic parameters. However, these parameters were consistently lower than the control (Figure 1d–g). In conclusion, the results indicate that the photosynthetic gas parameters of *R. pseudoacacia* leaves significantly decreased after exposure to high CO_2. The addition of the respiration enhancer PA mitigated the inhibition of photosynthesis caused by high CO_2, while the addition of the respiration inhibitor SHAM enhanced the inhibition of photosynthesis by high CO_2.

2.2. Response of Antioxidant System of Tetraploid R. pseudoacacia to High CO_2

To investigate the impact of high CO_2 on the antioxidant system of the tetraploid *R. pseudoacacia*, we initially measured the levels of H_2O_2 and $O_2{}^{\cdot-}$. Under normal CO_2 conditions, the levels of H_2O_2 and $O_2{}^{\cdot-}$ decreased after PA treatment compared to CK-H_2O, whereas the levels of H_2O_2 and $O_2{}^{\cdot-}$ increased after SHAM supplementation. After 6 days of high CO_2 treatment, the levels of H_2O_2 and $O_2{}^{\cdot-}$ in the leaves were significantly higher than in CK-H_2O. Furthermore, after SHAM supplementation, the levels of H_2O_2 and $O_2{}^{\cdot-}$ were further increased compared to T-H_2O. On the other hand, after PA treatment, the levels of H_2O_2 and $O_2{}^{\cdot-}$ were slightly decreased compared to T-H_2O but were still higher than CK-H_2O (Figure 2c,f). In addition, there was no significant difference in the staining intensity of DAB and NBT on the leaves before CO_2 treatment. However, after 6 days of high CO_2 treatment, the mean staining intensities of DAB and NBT on the leaves were significantly higher compared to CK-H_2O. Similarly, the SHAM treatment increased the mean staining intensity, while PA treatment decreased it compared to T-H_2O (Figure 2a–f).

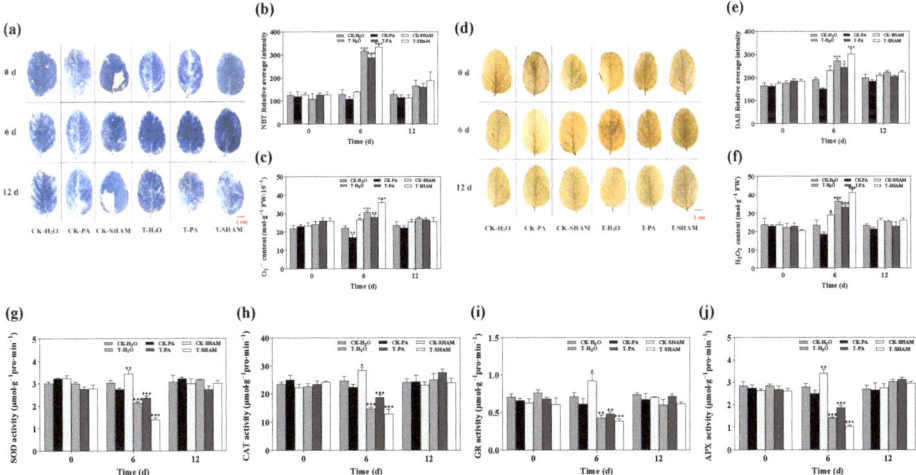

Figure 2. Effect of high CO_2 on NBT staining of the fresh leaves (**a,b**), $O_2{}^{\cdot-}$ level (**c**), DAB staining of the fresh leaves (**d,e**), H_2O_2 content (**f**), SOD (**g**), CAT (**h**), GR (**i**), and APX (**j**). Bar: 1 cm. Six biological replicates were analyzed, and the error bars represent the SE. Asterisks indicate significant differences as determined by Dunnett's test. (* $p \leq 0.05$; ** $p \leq 0.01$; *** $p \leq 0.001$).

SOD and CAT are considered the most significant enzymes in the plant antioxidant system, as their activity levels indicate the extent of damage caused by external factors. Meanwhile, GR and APX play a crucial role in maintaining the balance of the ASA-DHA cycle. APX functions to eliminate the excessive accumulation of H_2O_2 in a plant, while GR is primarily responsible for converting oxidized glutathione to reduced glutathione. When CO_2 conditions are normal, the addition of SHAM slightly enhances the activities of SOD, CAT, GR, and APX. On the other hand, the supplementation of PA does not lead to any significant changes in the activities of these enzymes. However, under high CO_2 levels, the activities of SOD, CAT, GR, and APX decrease. Specifically, in T-H_2O, T-PA, and T-SHAM, SOD activity decreased by 29.7%, 22.4%, and 54.3%, respectively, CAT activity decreased by 40.3%, 24.1%, and 47.8%, respectively, GR activity decreased by 39.6%, 32.6%, and 46%, respectively, and APX activity decreased by 49.2%, 32.8%, and 62.7%, respectively (Figure 2g–j).

2.3. Changes in Chlorophyll Levels and Fluorescence Parameters

Under normal CO_2 conditions, there were no significant differences in the content of Chl a and Chl b, as well as the ratio of Chl a/b, among the CK-H_2O, CK-PA, and CK-SHAM groups. However, in the high CO_2 treatment group, the levels of Chl a and Chl b increased, but the ratio of Chl a/b decreased compared to CK-H_2O after 3 days. In the CK-PA and CK-SHAM groups, there was a significant decrease in the levels of Chl a and Chl b, while the ratio of Chl a/b significantly increased after 6–9 days. Interestingly, the T-SHAM group had lower levels of Chl a and Chl b, whereas the T-PA group had higher levels of Chl a and Chl b (Figure 3a–c).

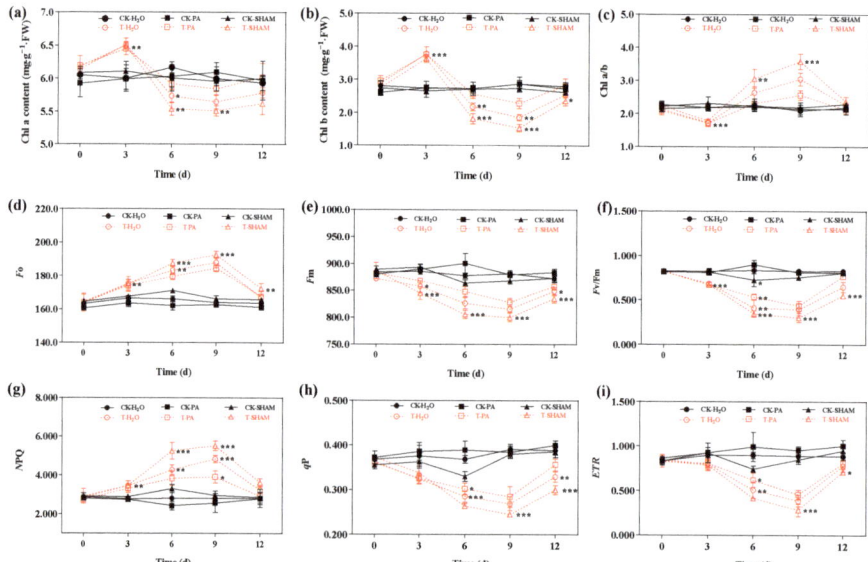

Figure 3. Effect of high CO_2 concentration on chlorophyll content and chlorophyll fluorescence parameters in *R. pseudoacacia*. Chl a content (**a**), Chl b content (**b**), Chl a/b (**c**), minimal fluorescence (*Fo*) (**d**), maximal fluorescence (*Fm*) (**e**), primary light energy conversion efficiency of PSII (*Fv/Fm*) (**f**), nonphotochemical quenching (NPQ) (**g**), photochemical quenching (*q*P) (**h**), and relative electron transport rate (*ETR*) (**i**). Six biological replicates were analyzed, and the error bars represent the SE. Asterisks indicate significant differences as determined by Dunnett's test. (* $p \leq 0.05$; ** $p \leq 0.01$; *** $p \leq 0.001$).

Under normal CO_2 conditions, the leaf chlorophyll fluorescence parameters did not show a significant response to supplementation with SHAM and PA compared to the control. However, after 9 days of high CO_2 treatment, Fo and NPQ increased by 15.6% and 63.4%, respectively. Fo and NPQ were higher than in T-H_2O after supplementation with SHAM but lower than in T-H_2O after supplementation with PA. Upon restoration of normal CO_2 conditions, Fo and NPQ returned to the control values (Figure 3d,g). During the high CO_2 treatment, Fm, Fv/Fm, qP, and ETR exhibited a decreasing trend and were significantly different compared to CK-H_2O. On day 9 of treatment, Fm, Fv/Fm, qP, and ETR decreased by 7.3%, 51.3%, 31% and 56.5%, respectively. Fm, Fv/Fm, qP, and ETR showed a more significant decrease with SHAM supplementation compared to T-H_2O, while the addition of the accelerator increased Fm, Fv/Fm, qP, and ETR (Figure 3e,f,h,i). These results indicate that high CO_2 has a severe impact on the chlorophyll levels and fluorescence parameters of the tetraploid *R. pseudoacacia*.

2.4. Effect of High CO_2 on Leaf Respiration Parameters

Under normal CO_2 conditions, the presence of PA contributed to an increase in V_{alt} and V_t, while the addition of SHAM inhibited the increase in V_{cyt}, V_{alt}, and V_t. After 6 days of high CO_2 treatment, there was a rapid increase in Valt but a significant decrease in V_{cyt} and V_t compared to CK-H_2O. When compared to T-H_2O, V_{cyt}, V_{alt}, and V_t increased with PA supplementation but decreased with SHAM supplementation. Upon restoring normal CO_2 conditions, there were no significant differences in V_{cyt}, V_{alt}, and V_t compared to the control (Figure 4a–c).

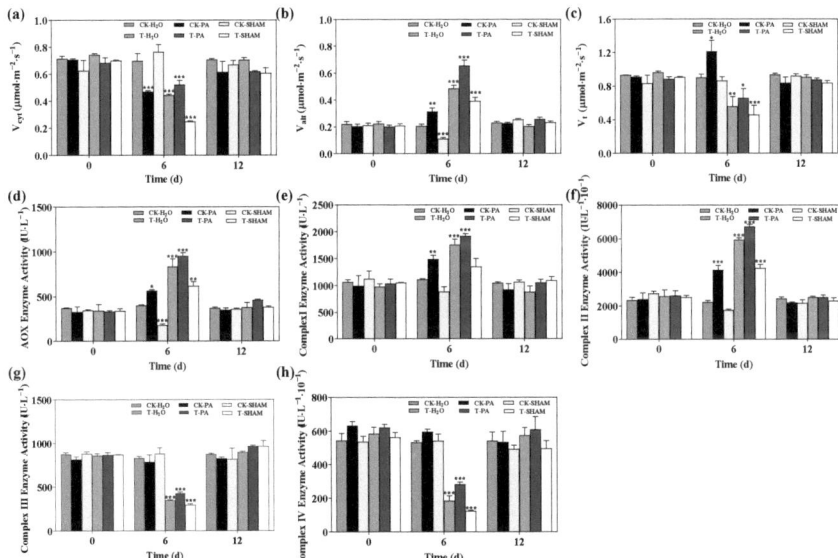

Figure 4. Effect of high CO_2 concentration on respiratory parameters and mitochondrial electron transport chain complex enzyme activities in *R. pseudoacacia*. Cytochrome pathway capacity (V_{cyt}) (**a**), alternative pathway capacity (V_{alt}) (**b**), total respiration (V_t) (**c**), AOX enzyme activity (**d**), complex I enzyme activity (**e**), complex II enzyme activity (**f**), complex III enzyme activity (**g**), and complex IV enzyme activity (**h**). Six biological replicates were analyzed, and the error bars represent the SE. Asterisks indicate significant differences as determined by Dunnett's test. (* $p \leq 0.05$; ** $p \leq 0.01$; *** $p \leq 0.001$).

The enzyme activities of AOX, complex I, and complex II were increased by PA compared to CK-H_2O. No significant changes in the enzyme activities of AOX, complex

I, and complex II were observed after supplementation with SHAM under normal CO_2 conditions. However, the enzyme activities of AOX, complex I, and complex II were significantly increased under high CO_2 treatment. Furthermore, PA supplementation led to a more significant increase in the enzyme activities of AOX, complex I, and complex II compared to T-H_2O, while the SHAM treatment also resulted in a significant increase in the enzyme activities of AOX, complex I, and complex II (Figure 4d–f). There were no significant changes in the enzyme activities of complexes III and IV, including after PA and SHAM supplementation, under normal CO_2 conditions. However, under high CO_2 conditions, the enzyme activities of complexes III and IV were significantly reduced. PA increased the enzyme activities of complexes III and IV compared to T-H_2O, while SHAM decreased the enzyme activities of complexes III and IV. After restoration of normal CO_2 conditions, the mitochondrial electron transport chain enzyme activities were not significantly different from those of the control (Figure 4g,h).

2.5. Effect of High CO_2 on Leaf Stomatal Movement

To investigate the movement of stomata in the tetraploid *R. pseudoacacia* under high CO_2 conditions, we conducted observations on stomatal morphology and counted the stomatal apertures. When exposed to normal CO_2 levels, SHAM caused stomata closure, while PA had a lesser effect on the stomata and did not significantly change the stomatal aperture compared to CK-H_2O. However, under the high CO_2 treatment, T-H_2O showed a 67.9% reduction in stomatal apertures compared to CK-H_2O. Additionally, supplementation with SHAM further decreased the stomatal apertures by 30% compared to T-H_2O, whereas supplementation with PA increased the stomatal apertures by 81.7% (Figure 5).

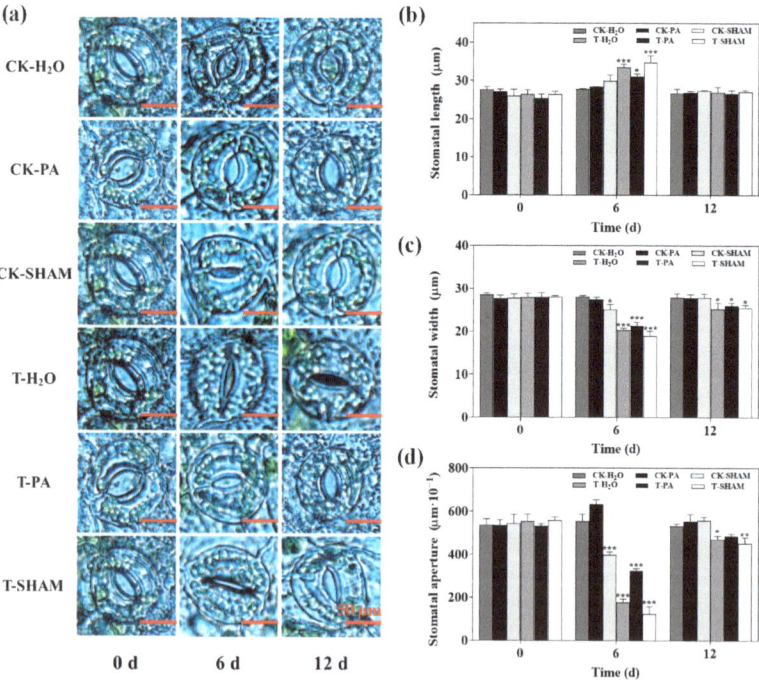

Figure 5. Effects of high CO_2 concentration on stomatal morphology (**a**), stomatal length (**b**), stomatal width (**c**), and stomatal aperture of plant (**d**). Bar: 50 μm. Six biological replicates were analyzed, and the error bars represent the SE. Asterisks indicate significant differences as determined by Dunnett's test. (* $p \leq 0.05$; ** $p \leq 0.01$; *** $p \leq 0.001$).

The fluorescence staining intensity of the guard cells was significantly enhanced after high CO_2 treatment, as observed through the use of the fluorescent probes H_2DCF-DA and DAF-2DA. This indicates that high CO_2 treatment increased the accumulation of ROS and NO in the guard cells. Supplementation with SHAM further increased the fluorescence staining intensity, suggesting an increase in the accumulation of ROS and NO. On the other hand, supplementation with PA decreased the fluorescence staining intensity, indicating a decrease in the accumulation of ROS and NO in the guard cells (Figure 6). In conclusion, the tetraploid *R. pseudoacacia* regulates stomatal closure in response to a high CO_2 environment by inducing the accumulation of ROS and NO in the guard cells.

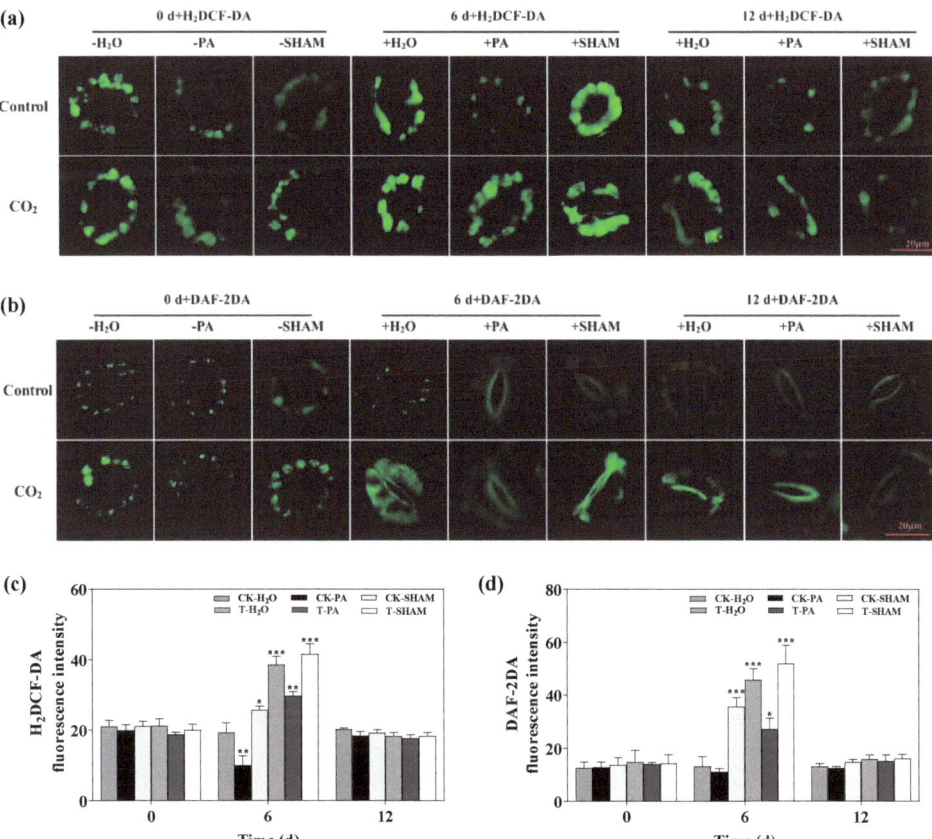

Figure 6. $2',7'$-Dichlorodihydrofluorescein diacetate (H_2DCF-DA) (**a,c**) and 5,6-Diaminofluorescein diacetate (DAF-2DA) (**b,d**) staining of guard cells under high CO_2 conditions. Ten biological replicates were analyzed, and the error bars represent the SE. Asterisks indicate significant differences as determined by Dunnett's test. (* $p \leq 0.05$; ** $p \leq 0.01$; *** $p \leq 0.001$).

2.6. Proteomic Analysis of Tetraploid R. pseudoacacia Based on High CO_2 Conditions

To investigate the response of the tetraploid *R. pseudoacacia* to high CO_2 levels, we conducted a proteomic analysis on six groups of *R. pseudoacacia* leaves (CK-H_2O, CK-PA, CK-SHAM, T-H_2O, T-PA, and T-SHAM). The quality of the samples was confirmed by analyzing the total ion chromatograms, which showed uniform peaks (Figure S1). Additionally, the PCA analysis indicated low variability among samples within each group, as the distribution of the three biological replicates was relatively concentrated. Two-dimensional plots demonstrated significant differences in the principal components between the high CO_2 treatment groups and the groups under normal CO_2 conditions (Figure S2). A total of 1652 proteins were quantified below the protein threshold of the 1.0% FDR criterion. Furthermore, we randomly selected six DAPs from the proteome sequencing data and examined the variations in their transcript levels using qRT-PCR. The results showed that the abundance variations of the six candidate proteins under high CO_2 treatment were consistent with the trend of transcriptional expression (Figure S6).

After conducting a one-way ANOVA test, we screened the differential protein data using Fold Change in Expression (FC) $\geq$ 1.5-fold as a criterion. To investigate the response mechanism of the tetraploid *R. pseudoacacia* under high CO_2 treatment, we performed a systematic clustering analysis of the differentially abundant proteins (DAPs) (Figure S4). The results revealed a significant change in the expression of DAPs under high CO_2 treatment. Under normal CO_2 conditions, in the CK-PA/CK-H_2O group, we found 50 DAPs, with 11 proteins' abundances increased and 39 proteins' abundances decreased (Figure 7b). Similarly, in the CK-SHAM/CK-H_2O group, we observed 194 DAPs, with 82 proteins' abundances increased and 112 proteins' abundances decreased (Figure 7c). In the T-H_2O/CK-H_2O group, we identified 504 DAPs, out of which 142 proteins were in elevated abundance, including 3-hydroxybutyryl-CoA dehydrogenase (I3SLI5), glutamine synthetase (I3T8A0), and cytochrome c oxidase subunit Vb (I3SVI7), while 362 proteins were reduced in abundance, including calnexin homolog (I3SD49), glutathione transferase (I3T7D8), and the NAD-dependent epimerase/dehydratase domain-containing protein (I3SMX7) (Figure 7a). In the T-PA/CK-H_2O group, we detected 522 DAPs, with 351 proteins, including aquaporin PIP13 (A0A0U2BZJ5), photosystem II protein D1 (A0A1C7D3T6), and class V chitinase CHIT5 (A0A1B1J8Z2), showing a significant reduction in abundance. On the other hand, xylose isomerase (I3S153), NADH-ubiquinone oxidoreductase chain 5 (G9JLS7), cytochrome c oxidase subunit 3 (G9JLU6), and 171 other proteins exhibited a significant increase in abundance (Figure 7d). In the T-SHAM/CK-H_2O group, a total of 506 DAPs were identified. Among these, the abundance of 155 proteins, including ATP synthase β-subunit (Q9FUC8), 3-hydroxybutyryl-CoA dehydrogenase (I3SLI5), and 15-cis-phytoene synthase (I3SHI7), was significantly reduced. On the other hand, the relative abundance of 351 proteins, including peroxidase (I3SDX6), ribonuclease T (I3SNB3), and the prolyl 4-hydroxylase alpha subunit domain-containing protein (I3SZ73), was significantly increased (Figure 7e). In the T-PA/T-H_2O group, there were a total of 37 DAPs, with 20 proteins' abundances increased and 17 proteins' abundances decreased (Figure 7f). Similarly, in the T-SHAM/T-H_2O group, there were 35 DAPs, with 16 being upregulated and 19 being downregulated (Figure 7g).

Under normal CO_2 conditions, the comparison of CK-PA/CK-H_2O and CK-SHAM/CK-H_2O revealed 26 overlapping DAPs (Figure S3A). However, under high CO_2 treatment, there was a significant increase in the number of DAPs in the tetraploid *R. pseudoacacia*, with a total of 388 overlapping DAPs in T-PA/CK-H_2O and T-SHAM/CK-H_2O (Figure S3B). When comparing T-PA/T-H_2O and T-SHAM/T-H_2O to T-H_2O, there were only 19 overlapping DAPs after PA and SHAM treatments at high CO_2 concentrations (Figure S3C).

2.7. KOG Functional Annotation and GO Enrichment Analysis of Tetraploid R. pseudoacacia DAPs' Response to High CO_2

The distribution of KOG functions was analyzed, and the results showed that, under high CO_2 treatment, the most abundant functions in T-H_2O/CK-H_2O (52 DAPs) were posttranslational modification, protein turnover, and chaperones; nucleotide transport and metabolism, translation, ribosomal structure and biogenesis, and energy production and conversion included 48, 41, and 35 DAPs, respectively (Figure 8a). In the case of normal CO_2 treatment, the DAPs in CK-PA/CK-H_2O were mainly associated with general function prediction only, lipid transport and metabolism, posttranslational modification, protein turnover, and chaperones (Figure 8b), whereas the DAPs in CK-SHAM/CK-H_2O were mainly distributed in translation, ribosomal structure and biogenesis, posttranslational modification, protein turnover, and energy production and conversion (Figure 8c). Under high CO_2 treatment, the DAPs in T-PA/CK-H_2O were mainly associated with general function prediction only, posttranslational modification, protein turnover, chaperones, and energy production and conversion (Figure 8d). Similarly, the DAPs in T-SHAM/CK-H_2O were mainly related to general function prediction only, posttranslational modification, protein turnover, chaperones, intracellular trafficking, secretion, and vesicular transport (Figure 8e). There was no significant difference in the distribution of KOG function between T-PA/T-H_2O and T-SHAM/T-H_2O after supplementation with PA and SHAM under high CO_2 treatment (Figure 8f,g).

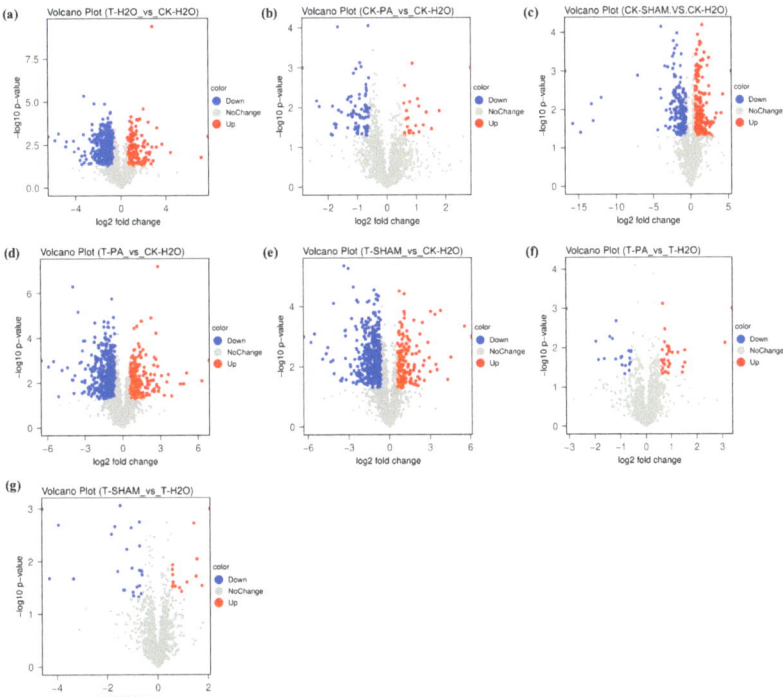

Figure 7. Volcano maps of differentially expressed proteins (DEPs) in *R. pseudoacacia* under CO_2 treatment. The horizontal coordinate is log2 (fold change), and the vertical coordinate is the negative logarithm of the *p*-value of the *t*-test significance test −log10 (padj). (**a**) T-H_2O vs. CK-H_2O; (**b**) CK-PA vs. CK-H_2O; (**c**) CK-SHAM vs. CK-H_2O; (**d**) T-PA vs. CK-H_2O; (**e**) T-SHAM vs. CK-H_2O; (**f**) T-PA vs. T-H_2O; and (**g**) T-SHAM vs. T-H_2O. Red represents upregulated proteins, blue represents downregulated proteins, grey represents proteins with no differential change, and the dotted grey line in the middle represents the threshold line for the DAP screening criteria.

In the GO enrichment analysis, DAPs were categorized into three groups: biological processes, molecular functions, and cellular components. Under normal CO_2 conditions, there were fewer DAPs in the CK-PA/CK-H_2O group with no significant differential enrichment (Figure S5a). For the CK-SHAM/CK-H_2O group, the most enriched biological processes were cellular (128 DAPs) and metabolic (118 DAPs) processes; the most enriched molecular functions were catalytic activity (107 DAPs) and binding (99 DAPs); and the most enriched cellular components were cell parts (142 DAPs) and intracellular parts (135 DAPs) (Figure S5c). Under high CO_2 treatment, the most responsive biological processes were cellular (287 DAPs) and metabolic (252 DAPs) processes in the T-H_2O/CK-H_2O group; the most responsive molecular functions were catalytic activity (259 DAPs) and binding (259 DAPs); and the most responsive cellular components were cell parts (327 DAPs) and intracellular parts (309 DAPs) (Figure S5b). The significantly enriched categories of each GO classification in the T-PA/CK-H$_2$O and T-SHAM/T-H$_2$O groups largely overlapped with those in the T-H$_2$O/CK-H$_2$O group (Figure S5d,e). These results indicate a significant increase in GO-enriched DAPs under high CO$_2$ treatment.

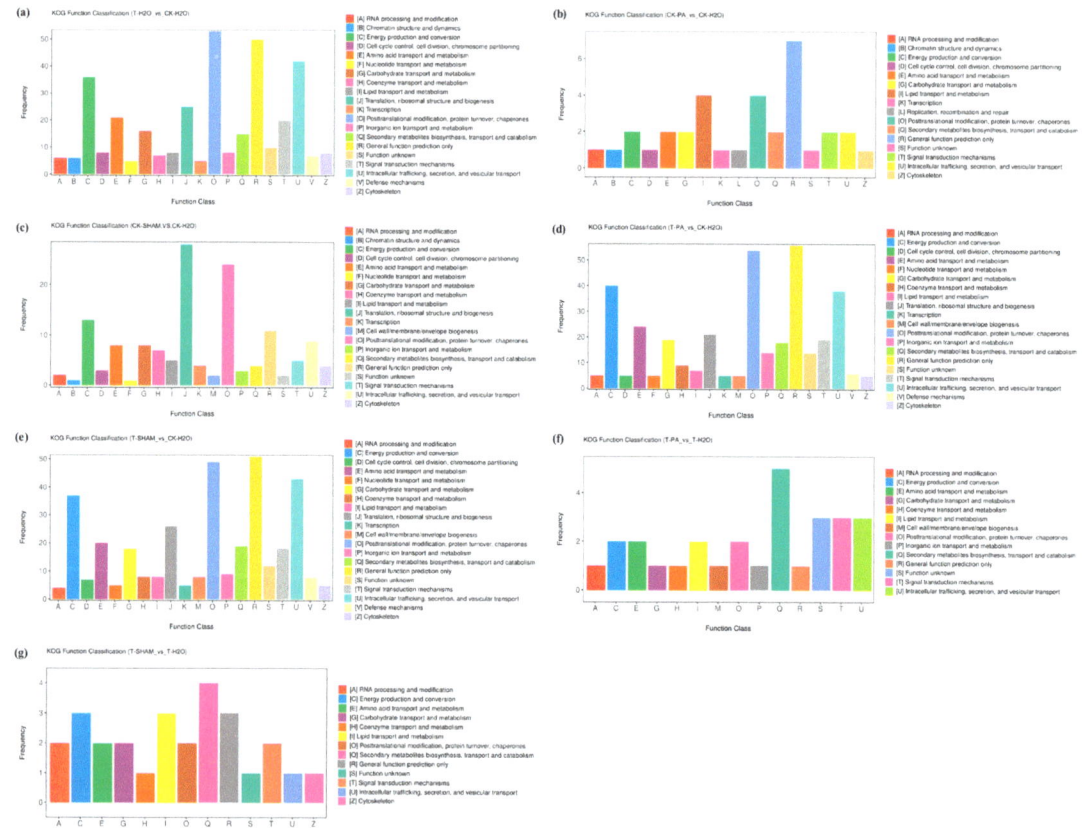

Figure 8. Cluster analysis of orthologous groups (KOG/COG) of DEPs in *R. pseudoacacia* under CO$_2$ treatment. (**a**) T-H$_2$O vs. CK-H$_2$O; (**b**) CK-PA vs. CK-H$_2$O; (**c**) CK-SHAM vs. CK-H$_2$O; (**d**) T-PA vs. CK-H$_2$O; (**e**) T-SHAM vs. CK-H$_2$O; (**f**) T-PA vs. T-H$_2$O; and (**g**) T-SHAM vs. T-H$_2$O.

2.8. Pathway Analysis of DAPs in Tetraploid R. pseudoacacia under High CO$_2$ Treatment

To further elucidate the metabolic pathways involved in the DAPs of the tetraploid *R. pseudoacacia*, DAPs were analyzed for KEGG enrichment. Under normal CO$_2$ conditions, the DAPs in the CK-PA/CK-H$_2$O group were mainly enriched in fatty acid biosynthesis, fatty acid metabolism, and biotin metabolism (Figure 9b). In the CK-SHAM/CK-H$_2$O group, the DAPs were mainly enriched in metabolic pathways, the biosynthesis of secondary metabolites, glutathione metabolism, and carotenoid biosynthesis (Figure 9c). Under high CO$_2$ treatment, the DAPs in the T-H$_2$O/CK-H$_2$O group were significantly enriched in metabolic pathways, carbon metabolism, the biosynthesis of secondary metabolites, the biosynthesis of amino acids, and photosynthesis (Figure 9a). The DAPs in the T-PA/CK-H$_2$O and T-SHAM/CK-H$_2$O groups were significantly enriched in metabolic pathways, the biosynthesis of secondary metabolites, the biosynthesis of amino acids, phenylalanine metabolism, phenylacetone biosynthesis, and glutathione metabolism (Figure 9d,e). Finally, the DAPs in the T-PA/T-H$_2$O and T-SHAM/T-H$_2$O groups were mainly enriched in phenylalanine metabolism, metabolic pathways, the biosynthesis of secondary metabolites, and phenylpropanoid biosynthesis (Figure 9f,g).

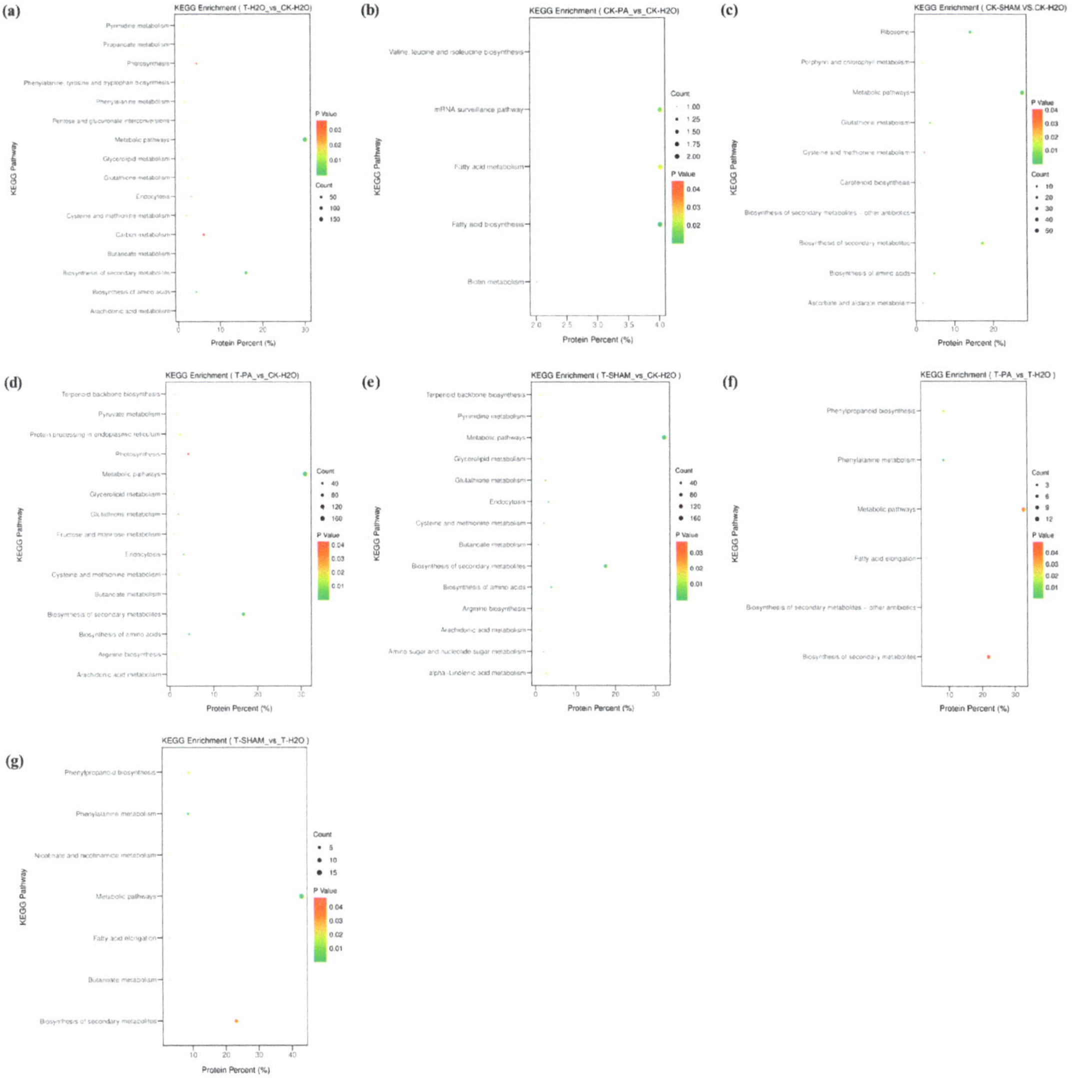

Figure 9. KEGG enrichment analysis of DEPs identified in *R. pseudoacacia* under CO_2 treatment. (**a**) T-H_2O vs. CK-H_2O; (**b**) CK-PA vs. CK-H_2O; (**c**) CK-SHAM vs. CK-H_2O; (**d**) T-PA vs. CK-H_2O; (**e**) T-SHAM vs. CK-H_2O; (**f**) T-PA vs. T-H_2O; and (**g**) T-SHAM vs. T-H_2O. The *x*-axis represents the enrichment factor, and the *y*-axis represents the pathway of enrichment. Larger orange points represent major pathway enrichment and higher pathway impact values, respectively.

3. Discussion

Short-term CO_2 enrichment has been found to alleviate the impact of abiotic stresses, such as drought and salt, on plants [47,48]. In the tetraploid *R. pseudoacacia*, prolonged exposure to high CO_2 resulted in a gradual decrease in the relative water content of its leaves over time, ultimately leading to the inhibition of its growth and development. In the present study, we observed the yellowing, wilting, and abscission of leaves, as well as a decrease in the relative water content in the tetraploid *R. pseudoacacia* at high CO_2 concentrations (Figure 1a). This phenomenon could be attributed to a reduction in water flux caused by high CO_2 and weakened upward water transport due to a decreased transpiration rate [49,50]. These factors contribute to the recovery of plants once the CO_2 concentration is restored (Figure 1c). The magnitude of the REC can indicate the condition of the plant membrane system. When plants face adversity or injuries, the cell membrane may rupture, causing a leakage of cytoplasmic cytosol and consequently increasing the conductivity. The substantial increase in REC observed at high CO_2 concentrations suggests that the plant experienced stress injury and cell damage (Figure 1b). PA, known as a facilitator of the alternate respiration pathway, and SHAM, an inhibitor [32,33,35], have shown contrasting effects on the stress symptoms of the tetraploid *R. pseudoacacia*. PA supplementation alleviated the stress response of the tetraploid *R. pseudoacacia* to high CO_2, whereas SHAM supplementation exacerbated this stress response (Figure 1).

Photosynthesis involves important physiological indicators used to study the impact of abiotic stress on plants. High levels of CO_2 can reduce the photosynthetic capacity of plants. This reduction is mainly seen through decreased CO_2 assimilation capacity and photochemical activities [10,13,51]. In our study, we observed a decrease in photosynthetic parameters in the tetraploid *R. pseudoacacia*'s leaves when exposed to high CO_2, indicating the inhibition of photosynthetic performance. However, after treatment with PA, the photosynthetic performance showed signs of recovery. After SHAM treatment, photosynthesis in the tetraploid *R. pseudoacacia* was found to be even more inhibited (Figure 1e–g). This could be due to a decrease in photosynthetic parameters resulting from a reduction in the amount and activity of Rubisco, stomatal conductance, and photorespiration [52,53].

A high concentration of CO_2 induces an accumulation of ROS in plants [54,55]. Previous studies have shown that an excessive accumulation of electrons in the PSII leads to an over-reduction in electrons, which in turn causes the electron transport chain to become highly reduced, resulting in the formation of ROS. This oxidative stress not only causes damage to plants but also triggers retrograde signals to the nucleus, leading to responses at the gene expression level [56,57]. In the tetraploid *R. pseudoacacia*, there was a significant increase in ROS levels compared to the control group under high CO_2. This change in ROS levels was observed when the AOX pathway was stimulated or inhibited (Figure 2a–c), which aligns with Dinakar's study [58]. Algae have developed various antioxidant defense mechanisms to mitigate the oxidative stress caused by H_2O_2. These mechanisms include enzymatic processes involving the ascorbate–glutathione cycle, glutathione S-transferase (GST), glutathione peroxidase (GPX), and CAT. Additionally, nonenzymatic mechanisms related to carotenoids and glutathione also play a role [59–61]. Most ROS-scavenging enzymes, such as CAT, SOD, and APX, are predominantly bound to cystoid membranes and exhibit similarities. When plants experience stress, they promptly remove ROS to prevent toxicity caused by ROS diffusion into the matrix [61]. To maintain ROS homeostasis, the activity of antioxidant enzymes is typically enhanced to eliminate excess ROS, thus safeguarding the plant from oxidative damage and enhancing its stress tolerance [62,63]. However, this mechanism is effective against mild oxidative damage, and if the damage surpasses the plant's tolerance threshold, the inability to eliminate ROS will hinder the functioning of antioxidant enzymes [64,65]. In this study, high concentrations of CO_2 led to a significant increase in ROS levels in the tetraploid *R. pseudoacacia*, exceeding the capacity of the antioxidant system and resulting in the suppression of SOD, CAT, GR, and APX activities, ultimately causing damage to the plant (Figure 2d–f).

Chlorophyll content can have a direct impact on a plant's capacity to capture light energy. The decrease in chlorophyll content can be attributed to two factors: the blockage of chlorophyll synthesis and the degradation of chlorophyll [66]. In our study, we observed that the levels of both Chl a and b initially increased and then decreased under high CO_2 treatments (Figure 3a,b). This finding aligns with previous research and suggests that high concentrations of CO_2 may inhibit chlorophyll synthesis [67]. We investigated the impact of an elevated CO_2 concentration on the activity of PSII using the chlorophyll fluorescence technique. The intensity of chlorophyll fluorescence is an indicator of the redox state of the main receptor Q in PSII [68]. Our findings revealed that the treatment with high CO_2 levels resulted in an increase in *Fo* but a significant decrease in Fm and *Fv/Fm* in the tetraploid *R. pseudoacacia* (Figure 3d–f). This suggests that the activity of PSII was hindered, leading to an excessive accumulation of electrons in PSII. Additionally, *q*P and NPQ represent the capacities for photochemical and nonphotochemical excitation quenching, respectively, and the quantum yields of these two types of fluorescence quenching are interconnected [69]. A decrease in *ETR* signifies a decline in photosynthetic activity. In the tetraploid *R. pseudoacacia*, photosynthesis is hindered, disrupting the balance of the system. When the plant is under stress, PSII is inhibited (Figure 3), resulting in the generation of a chlorophyll triplet state and singlet oxygen ($^1O_2$), which ultimately leads to the accumulation of ROS.

The regulation of the mitochondrial electron transport chain, which includes the cytochrome respiratory (COX) and AOX respiratory pathways, is influenced by abiotic stress. Under high CO_2 conditions, AOX respiration is upregulated in plant mitochondria to support normal plant physiological activities [70]. Research has demonstrated the significance of the AOX pathway in *A. thaliana* in response to elevated CO_2 [71]. It was observed that the rate of cytochrome respiration in the tetraploid *R. pseudoacacia* decreased, while the rate of AOX respiration increased under high CO_2 stress. However, overall respiration was inhibited. AOX respiration, which is a SHAM-sensitive type of respiration, was stimulated by PA treatment and had a significant effect on AOX [32,33,35]. PA treatment notably enhanced the AOX respiration pathway, while the response of AOX respiration in the tetraploid *R. pseudoacacia* to high CO_2 was inhibited by SHAM (Figure 4d). In contrast, the mitochondrial transfer chain (ETC) complexes (I, II, III, and IV) exhibited distinct responses under high CO_2. The activities of complexes I and II were decreased, while the activities of complexes III and IV were downregulated (Figure 4e–h). This alteration in activity levels could be attributed to mitochondrial damage resulting from the accumulation of ROS.

Low CO_2 promotes stomatal opening, while high CO_2 induces stomatal closure. Stomata, which serve as the primary site for gas exchange, can adjust the pore size in response to changes in the external environment. Studies have shown that high CO_2 stimulates an increase in the concentration of free Ca^{2+} in guard cells, leading to the induction of stomatal closure [14–17]. Transient changes in the pH and membrane potential of guard cells occur alongside stomatal closure when the CO_2 concentration is increased [72]. Stomata control the size of pores in the leaf in response to CO_2 concentration, and elevated CO_2 also inhibits stomatal development [73,74]. Previous studies have demonstrated that high levels of CO_2 can induce stomatal closure, with ROS playing a crucial role in this regulatory process [22,75]. NO plays a role in both ABA- and Ca^{2+}-mediated stomatal closure, which is an important participant in the stomatal closure process [24,25,76]. When compared with normal CO_2, high CO_2 significantly induces stomatal closure. PA alleviates this process, while SHAM exacerbates the degree of closure. Additionally, SHAM also causes a slight closure of stomata at normal CO_2 concentrations. Through fluorescence staining, it was observed that CO_2-induced stomatal closure is accompanied by a large accumulation of H_2O_2 and NO in the guard cells (Figures 5 and 6). This provides evidence for the crucial role of ROS and NO in the stomatal closure of the tetraploid *R. pseudoacacia* in response to high CO_2 stress.

Quantitative proteomics analysis is a crucial technology in proteomics research [77]. We employed DIA quantitative proteomic analysis to investigate protein alterations in the tetraploid *R. pseudoacacia* under high CO_2 treatment. The identified proteins were found to be involved in significant pathways, including metabolic pathways, carbon metabolism, the biosynthesis of secondary metabolites, the biosynthesis of amino acids, and photosynthesis (Figures 7–9). Additionally, we screened several key proteins in all DAPs in response to high CO_2, including ribulose diphosphate carboxylase-related subunits (A0A0F6Y5S8,

C0J370), photosystems I-II-related proteins (A0A898CWR3, A0A898CTK1, A0A898CW46, A0A898CTN3, A0A898CW14), antioxidant-related proteins (I1KP94, A0A0R4J3P1, K7KDM7, A0A0R0ERX9), cytochrome-related proteins (A0A898CTT0, I1MWP7, A0A0R0H975), and NADPH-related proteins (A0A0R4J3V9, I1LT63) (Table S2).

In C3 plants, glucose is primarily biosynthesized through the Calvin cycle. A crucial step in this process is the formation of glycerate-3-phosphate (3PGA) through the action of 1,5-bisphosphate ribulose carboxylase using CO_2 [28]. Rubiscos, which are photosynthetic CO_2-fixing enzymes, are activated by Rubisco activase (Rcas). However, if the N-terminus of the large subunit is missing, Rubiscos are not activated [78]. The involvement of carbon dioxide is also essential for the activation of Rubiscos [79]. In this study, we observed a significant downregulation of many 1,5-bisphosphate ribulose carboxylase-related subunits (I6QMJ2, A0A0F6Y5S8, C0J370, A0A898CTM2) under high CO_2 treatment. This downregulation resulted in the inability of Rubiscos to be activated under light and CO_2 conditions, leading to a decrease in the photosynthesis rate. Furthermore, the inhibition of photosynthesis was also attributed to the impact on photosystem protein synthesis, electron transfer between photosystems, and chlorophyll binding [80–82]. Pigment–protein complexes CP43 and CP47 are known to transfer excitation energy from the outer antenna of photosystem II to the photochemical reaction center, as well as being involved in the process of water oxidation [83,84]. The excess energy absorbed by the photosystem I complex is transferred to P700 via chlorophyll, thus protecting the pigment–protein complex from photodestruction [85]. The photosystem II D1/D2 complex proteins catalyze the oxidation of water due to a high REDOX potential [86]. Light trapping and the conversion of light energy to chemical energy occur through the iron–sulfur center in photosystem I [87,88]. In our study, we observed a significant downregulation of various photosystem constitutive proteins in the tetraploid *R. pseudoacacia*. These proteins include photosystem II CP43/47 reaction center proteins (A0A6H0EHP1, A0A1C7D4D5), photosystem I P700 chlorophyll a apoprotein A1/A2 (A0A1C7D3U7, A0A1C7D4C6, A0A6H0EHR0), photosystem I reaction center subunit II (I3STB2), photosystem II D1/D2 proteins (A0A1C7D3T6, A0A1C7D3V4), electron-transfer-mediating protein cytochrome f (A0A1C7D3W5), plastoquinone–plastocyanin reductase (I3RZ73, I1LUB3), the photosystem I iron–sulfur center (A0A1C7D3Z6), and the chlorophyll a–b binding protein (I3SIW2). This downregulation resulted in the inhibition of electron transfer and light capture, ultimately leading to the blockage of photosynthesis in the tetraploid *R. pseudoacacia*.

Glutathione (GSH) plays a crucial role in various biological processes. When GSH is oxidized to oxidized glutathione (GSSG) by GPX, it catalyzes the reduction of H_2O_2. Additionally, GR helps in regenerating GSH. Furthermore, GSH has been found to effectively increase the antioxidant capacity of plants and enhance the activity of respiratory enzymes [89]. In certain studies, advanced GSH treatment has proven to be effective in preventing broccoli fermentation in a high CO_2 atmosphere. This is achieved by promoting the AsA–GSH cycle and the electron (ETC) pathway [78]. Exogenous PA can maintain intracellular glutathione levels in H_2O_2-treated cells and enhance their antioxidant capacity [90]. The presence of GSH is vital for copepods in defending against seawater acidification induced by varying CO_2 concentrations [91]. In this study, the expression of GPX (I3SK85, I1KP94, I1MX60, C6SY48) was significantly decreased by high CO_2 treatment. However, this decrease was reversed when PA was applied, indicating that the antioxidant capacity of the tetraploid *R. pseudoacacia* was restored. The decrease in GPX expression resulted in the accumulation of ROS. GR plays a crucial role in the interconversion between oxidized and reduced glutathione, facilitating the recirculation of GSH. In soybeans, enhancing GR can effectively improve the removal of ROS [92]. In the context of this experiment, high CO_2 levels led to the downregulation of GR and diminished the regeneration ability of GSH. However, the application of PA facilitated the conversion between GSH and GSSG under high CO_2 conditions, which enhanced the scavenging of H_2O_2 and alleviated oxidative damage.

4. Materials and Methods

4.1. Plant Materials and Stress Treatment

The plant materials comprised the tetraploid *R. pseudoacacia*, which was two years old. In the spring, bare-root seedlings were planted in uniform-sized pots (diameter × height × bottom diameter = 20 × 28 × 20 cm), and seedlings with uniform growth were chosen for CO_2 treatment after 2 months of growth under normal conditions. The potted seedlings were placed in a light incubator for 3 days for pre-cultivation to acclimate to the new environment. The soil moisture was maintained at 70% throughout, and the culture conditions were as follows: 16 h of light, 8 h of darkness, temperature set at 25 °C, air humidity at 70%, and light intensity at 6000 Lux. The seedlings undergoing the high CO_2 treatment were divided into a control group (natural conditions, a CO_2 concentration of about 0.031%) and treatment groups (a CO_2 concentration of 5%), and the seedlings were subjected to high CO_2 treatment for 9 days before being incubated again under normal CO_2 concentration for 3 days. On day 6 of CO_2 treatment, a respiration accelerator (pyruvic acid, 0.1 mM) and a respiration inhibitor (salicylhydroxamic acid, 1 mM) were sprayed on the leaves of the tetraploid *R. pseudoacacia* every 3 h. Morphological observations on leaves were made after 0 d, 3 d, 6 d, 9 d, and 12 d. For each treatment, leaves were collected for physiological and proteomic measurements, with three or six biological replicates.

Here, $CK-H_2O$: untreated control group; CK-PA: pyruvic acid-treated group; CK-SHAM: salicylhydroxamic acid-treated group; $T-H_2O$: CO_2-treated group; T-PA: CO_2 co-treated with PA; and T-SHAM: CO_2 co-treated with SHAM.

4.2. Determination of Relative Water Content and Relative Electrical Conductivity

After 0.5 g of fresh leaves (FWs) moistened in distilled water for 4 h, the surface water was removed, weighed, and recorded as TW, and then the leaves were dried in a drying oven and recorded as DW. Relative water content: RWC (%) = (FW − DW)/(TW − DW) × 100.

A total of 0.1 g of evenly chopped leaves were poured in 5 mL of ddH_2O and shaken at 160 rpm for 1 h. The electrical conductivity was measured and recorded as L2 using a DDS-IIA conductivity meter (INESA Scientific Instruments Co., Shanghai, China), and the control of ddH_2O was recorded as L1. After cooling to ambient temperature, the samples were immersed in a boiling water bath for 15 min, and the electrical conductivity was measured and recorded as L3. Relative electrical conductivity (%) = (L2 − L1)/(L3 − L1) × 100.

4.3. Determination of Chlorophyll Content and Photosynthetic and Fluorescence Parameters

The chlorophyll content of the fourth and fifth leaves from the end, located in the middle of the acacia branches, was determined. A total of 0.2 g of leaves were immersed in the extraction solution (80% acetone/ethanol/ddH_2O = 4.5:4.5:1). The leaves were then kept in the dark for 24 h. The optical density at wavelengths of 470 nm, 645 nm, and 663 nm was measured. Chlorophyll a (Chl a) = $12.72A_{663} - 2.59A_{645}$; chlorophyll b (Chl b) = $22.88A_{645} - 4.67A_{663}$; and Chl a/b = chlorophyll a/b.

The photosynthetic parameters of leaves were determined using a Li-COR 6400 photosynthesis system (LI-COR, Lincoln, NE, USA). Six leaves per group were analyzed, and the measurements were repeated three times. These parameters included the net photosynthetic rate (*Pn*), the transpiration rate (*Tr*), the intercellular carbon dioxide concentration (*Ci*), and the stomatal conductance (*Gs*). The measurements were conducted under specific conditions, including a temperature of 24 °C, a photon flux density (PFD) of 90 $\mu mol\ m^{-2} \cdot s^{-1}$, a relative humidity of 70%, and an ambient CO_2 concentration of 400 $\mu mol\ CO_2\ mol^{-1}$.

The chlorophyll fluorescence parameters of leaves were measured using an FC800-O fluorescence imaging system (FluorCam, Drásov, Czech Republic) [93]. The leaves were dark-adapted for 30 min, following the previously described method. The data collected included initial fluorescence yield (*Fo*), maximum fluorescence yield (*Fm*), photochemical quenching (*qP*), the maximum photochemical efficiency of photosystem II (PSII) (*Fv/Fm*), nonphotochemical quenching (NPQ), and the relative electron transfer rate (ETR). A total of six leaves were measured for each treatment group.

4.4. Determination of Leaf Respiration Parameters

The leaf respiration rate was determined using the OXYTHE-RM oxygen electrode. The total respiration rate (V_t) was determined by incubating 0.1 g leaves of *R. pseudoacacia* from the same location in a reaction medium containing 2 mM HEPES, 10 mM MES (pH 10.7), and 2 mM $CaCl_2$ for 30 min in the dark. To determine the residual respiration (V_{res}), SHAM (200 mM) and KCN (200 mM) were added to the assay. V_{res} was then subtracted from the respiratory activity observed when SHAM was added alone to obtain the activity of the major cytochrome pathway (V_{cyt}). Similarly, V_t was subtracted from the respiratory activity observed when SHAM was added alone to obtain the actual activity of the alternative pathway (V_{alt}).

The activity of mitochondrial electron transport chain complex I-IV (complex I-IV) and AOX was measured in the central leaves of *R. pseudoacacia* using the Plant Mitochondrial Respiratory Chain Complex I-IV and Plant AOX Activity Kit (Hengyuan Biologicals, Shanghai, China).

4.5. Stomatal Movement

Under controlled light and temperature conditions, fresh leaves were collected from plants grown under normal conditions and with high CO_2 treatments. The upper epidermis and leaf pulp of both the proximal and distal axes of the leaf blades were gently scraped. Stomatal morphology was then observed randomly using a microscope. More than 100 stomata were selected for each treatment sample. The length and width of the stomatal images were measured using ImageJ v1.8.0 to calculate the stomatal openness.

4.6. Fluorescent Probe Staining

Fresh leaves were collected from plants under both normal conditions and high CO_2 treatments after 0, 6, and 12 days. Leaf blades, excluding the main veins, were cut into 1 cm pieces. These pieces were then immersed in 50 mM H_2DCF-DA or 0.1 mM DAF-2DA for 30 min in the absence of light. Subsequently, they were photographed using a fluorescence microscope in 10 randomly selected fields of view. The average fluorescence intensity was calculated using ImageJ.

4.7. Histochemical Staining

The leaves were fully immersed in a staining solution containing 10 mg·mL^{-1} DAB and NBT. To eliminate air bubbles, a vacuum pump was used for 30 min. Subsequently, the leaves were stained under dark conditions for 24 h. Chlorophyll was completely removed by submerging the leaves in a decolorizing solution. The leaves were then photographed and recorded, and the average fluorescence intensity was measured using ImageJ.

4.8. Determination of H_2O_2 and $O_2^{·-}$ Content

A total of 0.5 g of leaves were homogenized in 0.1% TCA in an ice bath. The homogenate was then centrifuged at 12,000 rpm for 10 min. The extract was mixed with phosphate buffer solution (PBS) (pH 7.5) and KI (1 M). The absorbance of the mixture was measured at 390 nm.

Similarly, a total of 0.5 g of leaves were homogenized in hydroxylamine hydrochloride in an ice bath and then centrifuged at 12,000 rpm for 10 min. The supernatant obtained was incubated with 1-Naphthylamine and aminobenzenesulfonic acid for 2 min at room temperature. Subsequently, the absorbance of the solution was measured at 520 nm [94].

4.9. Determination of Antioxidant Enzyme Activity

Crude enzyme extract was prepared by grinding 0.5 g of leaves in liquid nitrogen and centrifuging in PBS at 12,000 rpm for 10 min. A mixture of 20 µL of extract, 50 mM

PBS (pH 7.8), 100 μM ethylene diamine tetraacetic acid (EDTA), and 10 mM pyrogallic acid was thoroughly mixed. Superoxide dismutase (SOD) activity was measured by UV spectrophotometry at 420 nm. Another mixture of 0.2 mL of extract, 50 mM PBS, and ddH$_2$O was thoroughly mixed, and the reaction was carried out in a water bath at 25 °C for 10 min; catalase (CAT) activity was measured at 240 nm. Additionally, 0.05 mL of extract, PBS, and 5 mM ASA were mixed thoroughly. This mixture was then followed by the addition of 0.1 mM H$_2$O$_2$, and the activity of ascorbate peroxidase (APX) was measured at 290 nm. Furthermore, a mixture of 10 μL of extract, 100 mM PBS, 2 mM EDTA, and 0.5 mM glutathione was mixed thoroughly. This mixture was then followed by the addition of 0.2 mM NADPH, and the activity of glutathione reductase (GR) was detected at 340 nm [45].

4.10. Quantitative Proteomics Analysis

Six sets of samples were pretreated using the iST Sample Pretreatment Kit (PreOmics, Planegg, Germany) and stored at −80 °C under vacuum conditions. The samples were crushed in liquid nitrogen and then mixed with buffer (1:10) and protease inhibitors. After vortexing for 10 min, the samples were vortexed for another 10 min with an equal volume of Tris-saturated phenol (pH 8.0). Subsequently, they were centrifuged at 12,000 rpm for 20 min at 4 °C, and the phenol phase was combined with buffer and vortexed before centrifugation. The precipitate was then treated with pre-cooled ammonium acetate–methanol solution, precipitated overnight at −20 °C, and finally centrifuged at 12,000 rpm for 20 min at 4 °C. The supernatant was discarded, and the precipitate was washed twice with 90% acetone. The precipitate was then suspended in an appropriate volume of lysate to solubilize the sample proteins, followed by centrifugation at 12,000 rpm for 20 min at 4 °C to collect the supernatant. This step was repeated to ensure maximum collection of the supernatant. Each sample was then suspended in 30 μL of solvent A, and 1 μL of 10×iTR peptide was added to 9 μL of each sample. After thorough mixing, the samples were subjected to nanoliquid chromatography. For tandem mass spectrometry analysis, 4 μL of the samples were taken. The separation of the sample occurred over a 90 min gradient with a column flow rate of 600 nL·min^{-1} and a column temperature of 55 °C. The gradient started at 4% B-phase and was equilibrated for 4 min, followed by a nonlinear gradient increase to 30% over 80 min. Subsequently, the gradient increased to 90% in 2 min and was held for 8 min.

The mass spectrometry conditions were as follows: (1) MS: scan range (m/z): 350–1500; resolution: 120,000; normalized AGC target: 100%; and maximum injection time: 50 ms; (2) HCD-MS/MS: resolution: 30,000; normalized AGC target: 600%; maximum injection time: 90 ms; and collision energy: 35; (3) variable window acquisition was used with 60 windows set up, and overlapping serial ports were set up with 1 m·z^{-1} overlap per window.

Data analysis: DIA data were analyzed using Spectronaut 15.0 default parameters (Omicsolution Co., Ltd., Shanghai, China). The sequence database used was the uniprot-robinioid clade database, and trypsin enzymatic digestion was applied. The search library parameters included a fixed modification, carbamidomethyl (C), and a variable modification, methionine oxidation. The criteria for protein characterization were a precursor threshold of 1.0% false discovery rate (FDR) and a protein threshold of a 1.0% FDR. To generate the decoy database, a mutation strategy was employed, similar to perturbing a random number of amino acid sequences. Spectronaut 15.0 performed auto-correction, and a local normalization strategy was implemented for data normalization. Protein group quantification was conducted by calculating the average of the peak areas of the first 3 peptides below 1.0% FDR. For differential screening, proteins with a p adj value < 0.05 and | fold change | > 1.5 were considered significant after analysis by a one-way ANOVA test.

4.11. Functional Annotation and Cluster Analysis

An unsupervised principal component analysis (PCA) was conducted on the entire dataset to provide a comprehensive overview of the quantitative proteomics data, assessing its relevance and reproducibility. Volcano plots were then analyzed using a one-way ANOVA test, with a significance threshold of a p adj value < 0.05. To identify differentially abundant proteins (DAPs), we considered a fold change greater than 1.5. For the functional annotation and enrichment analysis of the DAPs, we utilized the GO (Gene Ontology), KOG (Eukaryotic Orthologous Groups), and KEGG (Kyoto Encyclopedia of Genes and Genomes) databases, which helped us understand the functions, distributions, and pathways associated with these DAPs.

4.12. Data Submission

MS data were translated to PRIDE XML using the PRIDE Submission Tool Version 2.7.3. A total of 34 PRIDE XML files were submitted to the ProteomeXchange repository following the ProteomeXchange submission guidelines [95]. The data were deposited under the identifier PXD047363.

4.13. Quantitative Real-Time Polymerase Chain Reaction (qRT-PCR)

Samples were ground to powder in liquid nitrogen, and total RNA was isolated using the Omega Plant RNA Kit (Shanghai Yuanmu Biotechnology Co., Shanghai, China) following the manufacturer's instructions. cDNA was prepared with the PrimeScript Reverse Transcriptase Kit (Takara, Shiga, Japan). qPCR was performed in a LightCycler 480 System (Roche, Indianapolis, IN, USA) with LightCycler 480 SYBR Green I Master Mix and specific primers (Supplementary Table S1). Three biological replicates were used for each sample. The *18SRNA* gene was used as an internal control. Relative gene expression levels were calculated using the $\Delta\Delta C_t$ method after normalization to the reference gene *18SRNA*.

4.14. Statistical Analysis

All experiments were performed with at least three to six biological replicates; experimental data were analyzed with SPSS 25.0; and to determine statistical significance, asterisks indicated significant differences (Student's *t*-test; * $p \leq 0.05$; ** $p \leq 0.01$; *** $p \leq 0.001$).

5. Conclusions

In conclusion, this study investigated the response mechanism of the tetraploid *R. pseudoacacia* to high CO_2 concentrations through physiology and proteomics. The findings indicate that high CO_2 had a negative impact on the normal growth of the tetraploid *R. pseudoacacia*. Specifically, the photosynthesis and respiration of the tetraploid *R. pseudoacacia*'s leaves decreased under the high CO_2 treatment compared to normal conditions, leading to an excessive accumulation of ROS. Additionally, the activities of the antioxidant enzymes SOD, CAT, GR, and APX were reduced, and the levels of chlorophyll and chlorophyll fluorescence parameters were significantly diminished. Furthermore, the accumulation of ROS and NO in guard cells induced stomatal closure. The proteomic analysis revealed that the DAPs were primarily enriched in metabolic pathways, the biosynthesis of secondary metabolism, and amino acid biosynthesis pathways under high CO_2 treatment. Notably, the key DAPs were primarily associated with ribulose diphosphate carboxylase-related subunits, photosystem I-II-related proteins, antioxidant-related proteins, and cytochrome-related proteins. Overall, this study provides valuable insights into the adaptation of the tetraploid *R. pseudoacacia* to high CO_2 environments. However, further research is required to validate the target proteins.

Supplementary Materials: The supporting information can be downloaded at https://www.mdpi.com/article/10.3390/ijms25105262/s1.

Author Contributions: Conceptualization, J.L. and F.M.; methodology, J.L.; validation, J.L. and S.Z.; formal analysis, P.L. and L.G.; data curation, S.Z.; writing—original draft preparation, J.L. and S.Z.; writing—review and editing, F.M.; funding acquisition, X.Z. and F.M. All authors have read and agreed to the published version of the manuscript.

Funding: This research was funded by the National Natural Science Foundation of China, grant numbers 32071728 and 31170568.

Data Availability Statement: MS data were translated to PRIDE XML using the PRIDE Submission Tool Version 2.7.3. A total of 34 PRIDE XML files were submitted to the ProteomeXchange repository following the ProteomeXchange submission guidelines. The data were deposited under the identifier PXD047363.

Acknowledgments: The authors would like to acknowledge the technical support from the Analysis and Testing Center of Northeast Forestry University.

Conflicts of Interest: The authors declare no conflicts of interest.

References

1. Zhang, H.; Zhang, S.K.; Song, W.Q.; Tigabu, M.; Fu, M.; Xue, H.F.; Sun, A.R.; Zhao, M.H.; Cai, K.W.; Li, Y.; et al. Climate response of radial growth and early selection of *Larix olgensis* at four trials in northeast China. *Dendrochronologia* **2022**, *73*, 125955. [CrossRef]
2. Cubasch, U.; Wuebbles, D.; Chen, D.; Facchini, M.C.; Frame, D.; Mahowald, N.; Winther, J.G. Introduction. In *Climate Change 2013: The Physical Science Basis. Contribution of Working Group I to the Fifth Assessment Report of the Intergovernmental Panel on Climate Change*; Cambridge University Press: Cambridge, UK; New York, NY, USA, 2013; pp. 95–123.
3. Morin, F.; André, M.; Betsche, T. Growth Kinetics, Carbohydrate, and Leaf Phosphate Content of Clover (*Trifolium subterraneum* L.) after Transfer to a High CO_2 Atmosphere or to High Light and Ambient Air 1. *Plant Physiol.* **1992**, *99*, 89–95. [CrossRef]
4. Siriphanich, J.; Kader, A.A. Changes in Cytoplasmic and Vacuolar pH in Harvested Lettuce Tissue as Influenced by CO_2. *J. Am. Soc. Hortic. Sci.* **1986**, *111*, 73–77. [CrossRef]
5. Larrigaudiere, C.; Pintoó, E.; Lentheric, S.; Vendrell, M. Involvement of oxidative processes in the development of core browning in controlled-atmosphere stored pears. *J. Hortic. Sci. Biotechnol.* **2001**, *76*, 157–162. [CrossRef]
6. Shuyun, Y.; Qingguo, Z.; Yuelin, J.; Fengwen, W.; Xiaofei, Z. Effect of high CO_2 density on photosynthesis speed of *Pinus massoniana*. *J. Anhui Agric. Univ.* **2006**, *33*, 100–104.
7. Jacotot, A.; Marchand, C.; Gensous, S.; Allenbach, M. Effects of elevated atmospheric CO_2 and increased tidal flooding on leaf gas-exchange parameters of two common mangrove species: *Avicennia marina* and *Rhizophora stylosa*. *Photosynth. Res.* **2018**, *138*, 249–260. [CrossRef] [PubMed]
8. Rao, M.V.; Hale, B.A.; Ormrod, D.P. Amelioration of Ozone-Induced Oxidative Damage in Wheat Plants Grown under High Carbon Dioxide (Role of Antioxidant Enzymes). *Plant Physiol.* **1995**, *109*, 421–432. [CrossRef]
9. Maroco, J.P.; Edwards, G.E.; Ku, M.S. Photosynthetic acclimation of maize to growth under elevated levels of carbon dioxide. *Planta* **1999**, *210*, 115–125. [CrossRef] [PubMed]
10. Tomimatsu, H.; Sakata, T.; Fukayama, H.; Tang, Y. Short-term effects of high CO_2 accelerate photosynthetic induction in *Populus koreana × trichocarpa* with always-open stomata regardless of phenotypic changes in high CO_2 growth conditions. *Tree Physiol.* **2019**, *39*, 474–483. [CrossRef]
11. Zhou, Y.; Han, S.; Liu, Y.; Jia, X. Stomatal response of *Pinus sylvestriformis* to elevated CO_2 concentrations during the four years of exposure. *J. For. Res.* **2005**, *16*, 15–18.
12. Chen, J.; Hu, Y.; Yan, R.; Hu, H. Effect of high carbon dioxide injury on the physiological characteristics of fresh-cut garlic scapes. *Sci. Hortic.* **2019**, *250*, 359–365. [CrossRef]
13. Niu, Q.; Huang, D.; Aierken, Y.; Chen, C. Effects of CO_2 and Temperature on Canopy Photosynthesis of Muskmelon. *Acta Hortic. Sin.* **2006**, *33*, 272–277.
14. Schulze, S.; Dubeaux, G.; Ceciliato, P.H.O.; Munemasa, S.; Nuhkat, M.; Yarmolinsky, D.; Aguilar, J.; Diaz, R.; Azoulay-Shemer, T.; Steinhorst, L.; et al. A role for calcium-dependent protein kinases in differential CO_2- and ABA-controlled stomatal closing and low CO_2-induced stomatal opening in Arabidopsis. *New Phytol.* **2020**, *229*, 2765–2779. [CrossRef] [PubMed]
15. Schwartz, A. Role of Ca^{2+} and EGTA on Stomatal Movements in *Commelina communis* L. *Plant Physiol.* **1985**, *79*, 1003–1005. [CrossRef] [PubMed]
16. Schwartz, A.; Ilan, N.; Grantz, D.A. Calcium Effects on Stomatal Movement in *Commelina communis* L. *Plant Physiol.* **1988**, *87*, 583–587. [CrossRef] [PubMed]
17. Webb, A.A.R.; Mcainsh, M.R.; Mansfield, T.A.; Hetherington, A.M. Carbon dioxide induces increases in guard cell cytosolic free calcium. *Plant J.* **2010**, *9*, 297–304. [CrossRef]
18. Haworth, M.; Killi, D.; Materassi, A.; Raschi, A. Coordination of stomatal physiological behavior and morphology with carbon dioxide determines stomatal control. *Am. J. Bot.* **2015**, *102*, 677–688. [CrossRef] [PubMed]
19. Ries, A.B. Carbonic anhydrases function as mediators of CO-induced stomatal movements and regulators of stomatal development in Arabidopsis thaliana. *Diss. Theses-Gradworks* **2009**, *59*, 253–257.
20. He, J.; Zhang, R.X.; Peng, K.; Tagliavia, C.; Li, S.; Xue, S.; Liu, A.; Hu, H.; Zhang, J.; Hubbard, K.E.; et al. The BIG protein distinguishes the process of CO_2-induced stomatal closure from the inhibition of stomatal opening by CO_2. *New Phytol.* **2018**, *218*, 232–241. [CrossRef]
21. Muhlemann, J.K.; Younts, T.L.B.; Muday, G.K. Flavonols control pollen tube growth and integrity by regulating ROS homeostasis during high-temperature stress. *Proc. Natl. Acad. Sci. USA* **2018**, *115*, E11188–E11197. [CrossRef]
22. Sierla, M.; Waszczak, C.; Vahisalu, T.; Kangasjärvi, J. Reactive Oxygen Species in the Regulation of Stomatal Movements. *Plant Physiol.* **2016**, *171*, 1569–1580. [CrossRef] [PubMed]

23. He, J.J.; Zhang, R.X.; Kim, D.S.; Sun, P.; Liu, H.G.; Liu, Z.M.; Hetherington, A.M.; Liang, Y.K. ROS of Distinct Sources and Salicylic Acid Separate Elevated CO_2-Mediated Stomatal Movements in Arabidopsis. *Front. Plant Sci.* **2020**, *11*, 542. [CrossRef] [PubMed]

24. Yang, J.; Matsumoto, Y.; Etoh, T.; Iwai, S. Nitric oxide (NO)-dependent and NO-independent signaling pathways act in ABA-inhibition of stomatal opening. *Plant Signal. Behav.* **2008**, *3*, 131–132. [CrossRef] [PubMed]

25. Liu, X.; Zhang, S.; Lou, C. Involvement of Ca^{2+} in Stomatal Movements of *Vicia faba* L. Regulated by Nitric Oxide. *J. Plant Physiol. Mol. Biol.* **2003**, *29*, 342–346.

26. Song, Y.; Miao, Y.; Song, C.-P. Behind the scenes: The roles of reactive oxygen species in guard cells. *New Phytol.* **2014**, *201*, 1121–1140. [CrossRef] [PubMed]

27. Singh, R.; Parihar, P.; Singh, S.; Mishra, R.K.; Singh, V.P.; Prasad, S.M. Reactive oxygen species signaling and stomatal movement: Current updates and future perspectives. *Redox Biol.* **2017**, *11*, 213–218. [CrossRef] [PubMed]

28. Waheeda, K.; Kitchel, H.; Wang, Q.; Chiu, P.L. Molecular mechanism of Rubisco activase: Dynamic assembly and Rubisco remodeling. *Front. Mol. Biosci.* **2023**, *10*, 1125922. [CrossRef]

29. Loughran, T.F.; Boysen, L.; Bastos, A.; Hartung, K.; Havermann, F.; Li, H.; Nabel, J.; Obermeier, W.A.; Pongratz, J. Past and Future Climate Variability Uncertainties in the Global Carbon Budget Using the MPI Grand Ensemble. *Glob. Biogeochem. Cycles* **2021**, *35*, e2021GB007019. [CrossRef]

30. Ikkonen, E.N.; Shibaeva, T.G.; Sherudilo, E.G.; Titov, A.F. Effect of Continuous Lighting on Mitochondrial Respiration in Solanacea Plants. *Russ. J. Plant Physiol.* **2022**, *69*, 114. [CrossRef]

31. McDonald, A.E. Unique opportunities for future research on the alternative oxidase of plants. *Plant Physiol.* **2023**, *191*, 2084–2092. [CrossRef]

32. Torrentino-Madamet, M.; Almeras, L.; Travaille, C.; Sinou, V.; Pophillat, M.; Belghazi, M.; Fourquet, P.; Jammes, Y.; Parzy, D. Proteomic analysis revealed alterations of the Plasmodium falciparum metabolism following salicylhydroxamic acid exposure. *Res. Rep. Trop. Med.* **2011**, *2*, 109–119. [CrossRef] [PubMed]

33. Mallo, N.; Lamas, J.; Leiro, J.M. Evidence of an Alternative Oxidase Pathway for Mitochondrial Respiration in the Scuticociliate Philasterides dicentrarchi. *Protist* **2013**, *164*, 824–836. [CrossRef] [PubMed]

34. Kirimura, K.; Yoda, M.; Shimizu, H.; Sugano, S.; Mizuno, M.; Kino, K.; Usami, S. Contribution of cyanide-insensitive respiratory pathway, catalyzed by the alternative oxidase, to citric acid production in *Aspergillus niger*. *Biosci. Biotechnol. Biochem.* **2000**, *64*, 2034–2039. [CrossRef]

35. Onda, Y.; Kato, Y.; Abe, Y.; Ito, T.; Ito-Inaba, Y.; Morohashi, M.; Ito, Y.; Ichikawa, M.; Matsukawa, K.; Otsuka, M.; et al. Pyruvate-sensitive AOX exists as a non-covalently associated dimer in the homeothermic spadix of the skunk cabbage, *Symplocarpus renifolius*. *Febs Lett.* **2007**, *581*, 5852–5858. [CrossRef]

36. Umbach, A.L.; Wiskich, J.T.; Siedow, J.N. Regulation of alternative oxidase kinetics by pyruvate and intermolecular disulfide bond redox status in soybean seedling mitochondria. *FEBS Lett.* **1994**, *348*, 181–184. [CrossRef] [PubMed]

37. Carré, J.E.; Affourtit, C.; Moore, A.L. Interaction of purified alternative oxidase from thermogenic Arum maculatum with pyruvate. *Febs Lett.* **2011**, *585*, 397–401. [CrossRef] [PubMed]

38. Sun, Y.R.; Ma, W.T.; Xu, Y.N.; Wang, X.M.; Li, L.; Tcherkez, G.; Gong, X.Y. Short- and long-term responses of leaf day respiration to elevated atmospheric CO_2. *Plant Physiol.* **2023**, *191*, 2204–2217. [CrossRef]

39. Tjoelker, M.G.; Oleksyn, J.; Lorenc-Plucinska, G.; Reich, P.B. Acclimation of respiratory temperature responses in northern and southern populations of Pinus banksiana. *New Phytol.* **2009**, *181*, 218–229. [CrossRef] [PubMed]

40. Li, X.; Zhang, G.Q.; Sun, B.; Zhang, S.; Zhang, Y.Q.; Liao, Y.W.K.; Zhou, Y.H.; Xia, X.J.; Shi, K.; Yu, J.Q. Stimulated Leaf Dark Respiration in Tomato in an Elevated Carbon Dioxide Atmosphere. *Sci. Rep.* **2013**, *3*, 3433. [CrossRef]

41. Zhang, G.; Li, Y.; Li, F.; Xu, Z.; Sun, Y. Effects of root age on biomass and leaf nutrition in tetraploid *Robinia pseudoacacia*. *J. Beijing For. Univ.* **2009**, *31*, 37–41.

42. Tan, X.; Peng, Z.; Jia, Z.; Ma, L. Influence of air temperatures on photosynthetic light-response curves of *Robinia pseudoacacia* L. *J. Beijing For. Univ.* **2010**, *32*, 64–68.

43. Meng, F.J.; Pang, H.Y.; Huang, F.L.; Liu, L.; Wang, Y.J. Tetraploid black locust *Robinia pseudoacacia* L. Increased salt tolerance by activation of the antioxidant system. *Biotechnol. Biotechnol. Equip.* **2012**, *26*, 3351–3358. [CrossRef]

44. Zhang, Y.; Luo, X.; Shen, Y. Dynamic changes of anti-oxidation system in new cultvars of *Robinia pseudoacacia* under gradual drought stress of soil. *J. Zhejiang For. Coll.* **2005**, *22*, 166–169.

45. Liu, J.; Zhang, Z.; Li, Y.; Han, J.; Si, H.; Mi, Y.; Wang, S.; Wei, X.; Yang, H.; Sun, Y.; et al. Effects of the vegetative propagation method on juvenility in *Robinia pseudoacacia* L. *For. Res.* **2022**, *2*, 17. [CrossRef]

46. Xu, F.; Jiang, M.; Meng, F. Short-term effect of elevated CO_2 concentration (0.5%) on mitochondria in diploid and tetraploid black locust *Robinia pseudoacacia* L. *Ecol. Evol.* **2017**, *7*, 4651–4660. [CrossRef] [PubMed]

47. AbdElgawad, H.; Zinta, G.; Hornbacher, J.; Papenbrock, J.; Markakis, M.N.; Asard, H.; Beemster, G.T.S. Elevated CO_2 mitigates the impact of drought stress by upregulating glucosinolate metabolism in *Arabidopsis thaliana*. *Plant Cell Environ.* **2023**, *46*, 812–830. [CrossRef] [PubMed]

48. Maurer, R.; Tapia, M.E.; Shor, A.C. Exogenous Root Uptake of Glycine Betaine Mitigates Improved Tolerance to Salinity Stress in *Avicenna germinans* under Ambient and Elevated CO_2 Conditions. *FASEB J.* **2020**, *34*, 1–1. [CrossRef]

49. Cohen, I.; Lichston, J.E.; de Macêdo, C.E.C.; Rachmilevitch, S. Leaf coordination between petiole vascular development and water demand in response to elevated CO_2 in tomato plants. *Plant Direct* **2022**, *6*, e371. [CrossRef] [PubMed]

50. Souza, J.P.; Melo, N.M.J.; Pereira, E.G.; Halfeld, A.D.; Gomes, I.N.; Prado, C. Responses of woody Cerrado species to rising atmospheric CO_2 concentration and water stress: Gains and losses. *Funct. Plant Biol.* **2016**, *43*, 1183–1193. [CrossRef]
51. Silvola, J.; Ahlholm, U. Photosynthesis in willows (*Salix × dasyclados*) grown at different CO_2 concentrations and fertilization levels. *Oecologia* **1992**, *91*, 208–213. [CrossRef]
52. Ellsworth, D.S.; Reich, P.B.; Naumburg, E.S.; Koch, G.W.; Kubiske, M.E.; Smith, S.D. Photosynthesis, carboxylation and leaf nitrogen responses of 16 species to elevated pCO_2 across four free-air CO_2 enrichment experiments in forest, grassland and desert. *Glob. Chang. Biol.* **2004**, *10*, 2121–2138. [CrossRef]
53. Nowak, R.S.; Ellsworth, D.S.; Smith, S.D. Functional responses of plants to elevated atmospheric CO_2—Do photosynthetic and productivity data from FACE experiments support early predictions? *New Phytol.* **2004**, *162*, 253–280. [CrossRef]
54. Li, C.T.; Trigani, K.; Zuñiga, C.; Eng, R.; Chen, E.; Zengler, K.; Betenbaugh, M.J. Examining the impact of carbon dioxide levels and modulation of resulting hydrogen peroxide in *Chlorella vulgaris*. *Algal Res.-Biomass Biofuels Bioprod.* **2021**, *60*, 102492. [CrossRef]
55. Ezraty, B.; Chabalier, M.; Ducret, A.; Maisonneuve, E.; Dukan, S. CO_2 exacerbates oxygen toxicity. *Embo Rep.* **2011**, *12*, 321–326. [CrossRef] [PubMed]
56. Gollan, P.J.; Tikkanen, M.; Aro, E.M. Photosynthetic light reactions: Integral to chloroplast retrograde signalling. *Curr. Opin. Plant Biol.* **2015**, *27*, 180–191. [CrossRef]
57. Foyer, C.H. Reactive oxygen species, oxidative signaling and the regulation of photosynthesis. *Environ. Exp. Bot.* **2018**, *154*, 134–142. [CrossRef]
58. Dinakar, C.; Vishwakarma, A.; Raghavendra, A.S.; Padmasree, K. Alternative Oxidase Pathway Optimizes Photosynthesis During Osmotic and Temperature Stress by Regulating Cellular ROS, Malate Valve and Antioxidative Systems. *Front. Plant Sci.* **2016**, *7*, 171347. [CrossRef]
59. Mallick, N.; Mohn, F.H. Reactive oxygen species: Response of algal cells. *J. Plant Physiol.* **2000**, *157*, 183–193. [CrossRef]
60. del Río, L.A.; Sandalio, L.M.; Corpas, F.J.; Palma, J.M.; Barroso, J.B. Reactive oxygen species and reactive nitrogen species in peroxisomes.: Production, scavenging, and role in cell signaling. *Plant Physiol.* **2006**, *141*, 330–335. [CrossRef]
61. Asada, K. Production and scavenging of reactive oxygen species in chloroplasts and their functions. *Plant Physiol.* **2006**, *141*, 391–396. [CrossRef]
62. Zhu, L.; Wu, J.; Li, M.; Fang, H.; Zhang, J.; Chen, Y.; Chen, J.; Cheng, T. Genome-wide discovery of CBL genes in *Nitraria tangutorum* Bobr. and functional analysis of *NtCBL1-1* under drought and salt stress. *For. Res.* **2023**, *3*, 28. [CrossRef]
63. Chen, Y.; Li, M.; Gong, L.; Song, Y. Effects of Exogenous Signal Substances on POD, CAT Activity and ROS Content in *Cistanche deserticola* Y. C. Ma Seeds During Germination and Haustorium Formation. *Chin. Agric. Sci. Bull.* **2014**, *30*, 128–132.
64. Li, Y.; Zhou, Q.; Li, F.; Liu, X.; Luo, Y. Effects of tetrabromobisphenol A as an emerging pollutant on wheat (*Triticum aestivum*) at biochemical levels. *Chemosphere* **2008**, *74*, 119–124. [CrossRef] [PubMed]
65. Ge, H.; Zhang, F. Effects of Tetrabromobisphenol a Stress on Growth and Physiological Characteristics of Soybean Seedling. *Bull. Environ. Contam. Toxicol.* **2017**, *98*, 141–146. [CrossRef] [PubMed]
66. Zhang, Y.; Chen, Y.; Guo, Y.; Ma, Y.; Yang, M.; Fu, R.; Sun, Y. Elevated CO_2 delayed yellowing by maintaining chlorophyll biosynthesis and inhibiting chlorophyll degradation and carotenoid accumulation of postharvest broccoli. *Postharvest Biol. Technol.* **2022**, *194*, 112089. [CrossRef]
67. Steer, B.T.; Walker, D.A. Inhibition of Chlorophyll Synthesis by High Concentrations of Carbon Dioxide. *Plant Physiol.* **1965**, *40*, 577–581. [CrossRef] [PubMed]
68. Li, Y.L.; Jin, Z.X.; Li, J.M. Interactive effects of copper stress and arbuscular mycorrhizal fungi on photosynthetic characteristics and chlorophyll fluorescence parameters of elsholtzia splendens. *Pak. J. Bot.* **2017**, *49*, 1531–1540.
69. Laisk, A.; Oja, V.; Rasulov, B.; Eichelmann, H.; Sumberg, A. Quantum Yields and Rate Constants of Photochemical and Nonphotochemical Excitation Quenching (Experiment and Model). *Plant Physiol.* **1997**, *115*, 803–815. [CrossRef] [PubMed]
70. Dahal, K.; Vanlerberghe, G.C. Growth at Elevated CO_2 Requires Acclimation of the Respiratory Chain to Support Photosynthesis. *Plant Physiol.* **2018**, *178*, 82–100. [CrossRef]
71. Gandin, A.; Duffes, C.; Day, D.A.; Cousins, A.B. The Absence of Alternative Oxidase AOX1A Results in Altered Response of Photosynthetic Carbon Assimilation to Increasing CO_2 in Arabidopsis thaliana. *Plant Cell Physiol.* **2012**, *53*, 1627–1637. [CrossRef]
72. Hedrich, R.; Neimanis, S.; Savchenko, G.; Felle, H.H.; Kaiser, W.M.; Heber, U. Changes in apoplastic pH and membrane potential in leaves in relation to stomatal responses to CO_2, malate, abscisic acid or interruption of water supply. *Planta* **2001**, *213*, 594–601. [CrossRef] [PubMed]
73. Engineer, C.B.; Hashimoto-Sugimoto, M.; Negi, J.; Israelsson-Nordström, M.; Azoulay-Shemer, T.; Rappel, W.J.; Iba, K.; Schroeder, J.I. CO_2 Sensing and CO_2 peculation of Stomatal Conductance: Advances and Open Questions. *Trends Plant Sci.* **2016**, *21*, 16–30. [CrossRef] [PubMed]
74. Mao, Z.J.; Wang, Y.J.; Wang, X.W.; Voronin, P.Y. Effect of doubled CO_2 on morphology: Inhibition of stomata development in growing birch *Betula platyphylla* Suk. leaves. *Russ. J. Plant Physiol.* **2005**, *52*, 171–175. [CrossRef]
75. Ma, X.N.; Bai, L. Elevated CO_2 and Reactive Oxygen Species in Stomatal Closure. *Plants* **2021**, *10*, 410. [CrossRef] [PubMed]
76. Wang, Z.; Li, L.; Khan, D.; Chen, Y.; Pu, X.; Wang, X.; Guan, M.; Rengel, Z.; Chen, Q. Nitric oxide acts downstream of reactive oxygen species in phytomelatonin receptor 1 (PMTR1)-mediated stomatal closure in Arabidopsis. *J. Plant Physiol.* **2023**, *282*, 153917. [CrossRef] [PubMed]

77. Correa Rojo, A.; Heylen, D.; Aerts, J.; Thas, O.; Hooyberghs, J.; Ertaylan, G.; Valkenborg, D. Towards Building a Quantitative Proteomics Toolbox in Precision Medicine: A Mini-Review. *Front. Physiol.* **2021**, *12*, 723510. [CrossRef]
78. Wang, L.; Wang, F.; Zhang, Y.; Ma, Y.; Guo, Y.; Zhang, X. Enhancing the ascorbate–glutathione cycle reduced fermentation by increasing NAD+ levels during broccoli head storage under controlled atmosphere. *Postharvest Biol. Technol.* **2020**, *165*, 111169. [CrossRef]
79. Sicher, R.C.; Hatch, A.L.; Stumpf, D.K.; Jensen, R.G. Ribulose 1,5-Bisphosphate and Activation of the Carboxylase in the Chloroplast. *Plant Physiol.* **1981**, *68*, 252–255. [CrossRef]
80. Fish, L.E.; Bogorad, L. Identification and analysis of the maize P700 chlorophyll a apoproteins PSI-A1 and PSI-A2 by high pressure liquid chromatography analysis and partial sequence determination. *J. Biol. Chem.* **1986**, *261*, 8134–8139. [CrossRef]
81. Fernandez-Velasco, J.G.; Jamshidi, A.; Gong, X.S.; Zhou, J.; Ueng, R.Y. Photosynthetic electron transfer through the cytochrome b6f complex can bypass cytochrome f. *J. Biol. Chem.* **2001**, *276*, 30598–30607. [CrossRef]
82. Ustynyuk, L.Y.; Tikhonov, A.N. Plastoquinol Oxidation: Rate-Limiting Stage in the Electron Transport Chain of Chloroplasts. *Biochemistry* **2022**, *87*, 1084–1097. [CrossRef] [PubMed]
83. de Weerd, F.L.; van Stokkum, I.H.M.; van Amerongen, H.; Dekker, J.P.; van Grondelle, R. Pathways for energy transfer in the core light-harvesting complexes CP43 and CP47 of photosystem II. *Biophys. J.* **2002**, *82*, 1586–1597. [CrossRef]
84. Bricker, T.M.; Frankel, L.K. The structure and function of CP47 and CP43 in Photosystem II. *Photosynth. Res.* **2002**, *72*, 131–146. [CrossRef] [PubMed]
85. Karapetyan, N.V. Organization and role of the long-wave chlorophylls in the photosystem I of the Cyanobacterium spirulina. *Membr. Cell Biol.* **1998**, *12*, 571–584. [PubMed]
86. Ishikita, H.; Loll, B.; Biesiadka, J.; Saenger, W.; Knapp, E.W. Redox potentials of chlorophylls in the photosystem II reaction center. *Biochemistry* **2005**, *44*, 4118–4124. [CrossRef]
87. Xu, Y.H.; Liu, R.; Yan, L.; Liu, Z.Q.; Jiang, S.C.; Shen, Y.Y.; Wang, X.F.; Zhang, D.P. Light-harvesting chlorophyll-binding proteins are required for stomatal response to abscisic acid in *Arabidopsis*. *J. Exp. Bot.* **2012**, *63*, 1095–1106. [CrossRef] [PubMed]
88. Brettel, K.; Leibl, W. Electron transfer in photosystem I. *Biochim. Biophys. Acta* **2001**, *1507*, 100–114. [CrossRef] [PubMed]
89. Sunde, R.A.; Hoekstra, W.G. Structure, Synthesis and Function of Glutathione Peroxidase. *Nutr. Rev.* **1980**, *38*, 265–273. [CrossRef]
90. Babich, H.; Liebling, E.J.; Burger, R.F.; Zuckerbraun, H.L.; Schuck, A.G. Choice of DMEM, formulated with or without pyruvate, plays an important role in assessing the in vitro cytotoxicity of oxidants and prooxidant nutraceuticals. *Vitr. Cell. Dev. Biol. -Anim.* **2009**, *45*, 226–233. [CrossRef]
91. Zhang, D.; Li, S.; Wang, G.; Guo, D.; Xing, K.; Zhang, S. Biochemical responses of the copepod *Centropages tenuiremis* to CO_2-driven acidified seawater. *Water Sci. Technol.* **2012**, *65*, 30–37. [CrossRef]
92. Liu, Q.; Wang, S.W.; Du, Y.L.; Yin, K.D. Improved drought tolerance in soybean by protein elicitor AMEP412 induced ROS accumulation and scavenging. *Biotechnol. Biotechnol. Equip.* **2022**, *36*, 401–412. [CrossRef]
93. Calatayud, A.; San Bautista, A.; Pascual, B.; Maroto, J.V.; Lopez-Galarza, S. Use of chlorophyll fluorescence imaging as diagnostic technique to predict compatibility in melon graft. *Sci. Hortic.* **2013**, *149*, 13–18. [CrossRef]
94. Xu, L.; Hu, Y.; Jin, G.; Lei, P.; Sang, L.; Luo, Q.; Liu, Z.; Guan, F.; Meng, F.; Zhao, X. Physiological and Proteomic Responses to Drought in Leaves of *Amygdalus mira* (*Koehne*) Yü et Lu. *Front. Plant Sci.* **2021**, *12*, 620499. [CrossRef]
95. Perez-Riverol, Y.; Bai, J.W.; Bandla, C.; García-Seisdedos, D.; Hewapathirana, S.; Kamatchinathan, S.; Kundu, D.J.; Prakash, A.; Frericks-Zipper, A.; Eisenacher, M.; et al. The PRIDE database resources in 2022: A hub for mass spectrometry-based proteomics evidences. *Nucleic Acids Res.* **2022**, *50*, D543–D552. [CrossRef]

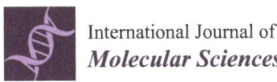

International Journal of
Molecular Sciences

Article

Evolution of the *WRKY* Family in Angiosperms and Functional Diversity under Environmental Stress

Weihuang Wu [1] , Jinchang Yang [1], Niu Yu [1], Rongsheng Li [1] , Zaixiang Yuan [1], Jisen Shi [2],* and Jinhui Chen [2],*

[1] State Key Laboratory of Tree Genetics and Breeding, Research Institute of Tropical Forestry, Chinese Academy of Forestry, Guangzhou 510520, China; wh879966@163.com (W.W.); jcyang@caf.ac.cn (J.Y.); niuyu@caf.ac.cn (N.Y.); fjlrs@tom.com (R.L.); yzx0090@163.com (Z.Y.)
[2] State Key Laboratory of Tree Genetics and Breeding, Nanjing Forestry University, Nanjing 210037, China
* Correspondence: jshi@njfu.edu.cn (J.S.); chenjh@njfu.edu.cn (J.C.)

Abstract: The transcription factor is an essential factor for regulating the responses of plants to external stimuli. The WRKY protein is a superfamily of plant transcription factors involved in response to various stresses (e.g., cold, heat, salt, drought, ions, pathogens, and insects). During angiosperm evolution, the number and function of WRKY transcription factors constantly change. After suffering from long-term environmental battering, plants of different evolutionary statuses ultimately retained different numbers of *WRKY* family members. The WRKY family of proteins is generally divided into three large categories of angiosperms, owing to their conserved domain and three-dimensional structures. The WRKY transcription factors mediate plant adaptation to various environments via participating in various biological pathways, such as ROS (reactive oxygen species) and hormone signaling pathways, further regulating plant enzyme systems, stomatal closure, and leaf shrinkage physiological responses. This article analyzed the evolution of the *WRKY* family in angiosperms and its functions in responding to various external environments, especially the function and evolution in Magnoliaceae plants. It helps to gain a deeper understanding of the evolution and functional diversity of the *WRKY* family and provides theoretical and experimental references for studying the molecular mechanisms of environmental stress.

Keywords: WRKY transcription factors; angiosperm; evolution; environmental stress

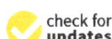

Citation: Wu, W.; Yang, J.; Yu, N.; Li, R.; Yuan, Z.; Shi, J.; Chen, J. Evolution of the *WRKY* Family in Angiosperms and Functional Diversity under Environmental Stress. *Int. J. Mol. Sci.* **2024**, *25*, 3551. https://doi.org/10.3390/ijms25063551

Academic Editor: Mateusz Labudda

Received: 31 January 2024
Revised: 12 March 2024
Accepted: 15 March 2024
Published: 21 March 2024

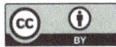

1. Introduction

The transcription factor (TF), also known as the trans-acting factor, regulates gene expression by binding cis-acting elements in the upstream region of its target gene; the expression of many abiotic stress-related genes in plants is mainly regulated in this way [1–5]. Transcription factors can be divided into two categories according to their expression patterns: constitutive and inducible transcription factors [5–8]. Constitutive transcription factors are genes that can be expressed without environmental impact, while inducible transcription factors are genes that need specific environmental conditions to be expressed. There are various types of transcription factors in plants [2,4,8]. At present, hundreds of transcription factors have been reported in plants, and they are involved in various abiotic and biological stresses, such as high salt, drought, low temperature, hormones, and pathogenic bacteria, as well as involvement in the regulation of plant growth and development [3,4,7,9,10]. Transcription factors include ARF (auxin response factor), bHLH (basic helix-loop-helix), bZIP (basic leucine zipper), CSD (cold shock domain), HSF (heat shock transcription factor), LFY (floral meristem identity genes, LEAFY), MADS (MCM1/AG/DEF/SRF), MYB (v-myb avian myeloblastosis viral oncogene homolog), NAC (NAM/ATAF/CUC), SBP (SQUAMOSA promoter binding protein), TAZ (transcriptional coactivator with PDZ binding), TiFY (TIF[F/Y]XG), and WRKY (WRKYGQK) [2,3,9].

Plant transcription factors mainly activate or inhibit the expression of downstream genes by binding the upstream regulatory sequence of target genes and interacting with other proteins or TFs to form polymers [1–3,11]. Transcription factors are mainly composed of DNA-binding regions and transcriptional regulatory regions. The former determines its specific binding with the cis-acting elements of target genes, and the latter determines its regulatory role on downstream genes [5,10,11]. Transcription factors play an important role in plant stress resistance, which can regulate the expression of signal-related genes in plants that are sensitive to high temperature, low temperature, drought, high salt, and so on [1,3,7,10]. Plant transcription factors are also key regulators of plant growth, development, and morphogenesis [3,5,12]. For example, the WRKY transcription factors are mainly involved in plant stress responses, including abiotic stresses, such as high temperature, drought, low temperature, high salt, ions, and biological stresses, such as pathogens and insects [1,3,7].

The evolution of plants gradually transitioned from aquatic to terrestrial, transitioning from algae, mosses, ferns, and gymnosperms to angiosperms. Angiosperms are further divided into basal angiosperms, magnolias, monocotyledonous plants, and dicotyledonous plants [1–3,5,7]. Magnolia plants are relatively unique, with commonly *Cinnamomum kanehirae*, *Liriodendron chinense*, and *Liriodendron tulipifera* currently available. Existing reports on the evolution of angiosperms have hardly systematically studied the evolution of magnolia plants. This study analyzes the grouping, structure, origin, evolution, functional differentiation, environmental selection pressure, whole genome duplication events, growth, development, biotic stress, and abiotic stress of the *WRKY* family in angiosperms from the perspective of the overall evolution of angiosperms. This study can better and more comprehensively explain the evolution of the *WRKY* gene family in angiosperms and the functional diversity in response to external stress, providing more theoretical and experimental references for deeper research into the biological functions of *WRKY* genes and plant environmental adaptability.

2. Results

2.1. Grouping Characteristics of the WRKY Family

To analyze the evolution of the *WRKY* family from the perspective of the overall evolution of angiosperms, the *WRKY* family protein sequences of two basal angiosperms, three magnolia plants, six monocotyledonous plants, and thirteen dicotyledonous plants were selected from the "Phytozome" website to construct a phylogenetic tree of twenty-four species of angiosperms. A total of 2274 genes were classified into three major groups and seven subgroups. The second largest group, Group II, was divided into five subgroups (Figure 1). A total of 24 angiosperm species were identified, including two basal angiosperms: *Amborella trichopoda* and *Nymphaea colorata*. Three magnolias were identified: *Cinnamomum kanehirae*, *Liriodendron chinense* and *Liriodendron tulipifera*. Six monocotyledons were also identified: *Brachypodium distachyon*, *Brachypodium arbuscula*, *Oryza sativa*, *Sorghum bicolor*, *Zea mays*, *Zostera marina*. Thirteen dicotyledonous plants were studied, including *Arabidopsis thaliana*, *Carya illinoinensis*, *Coffea arabica*, *Corymbia citriodora*, *Gossypium hirsutum*, *Malus pumila*, *Cirus trifoliata*, *Populus trichocarpa*, *Portulaca amilis*, *Sinapis alba*, *Theobroma cacao*, *Vigna unguiculata* and *Vitis vinifera*.

Although the number of members of the *WRKY* family varied among the species of different evolutionary statuses, they were all divided into three major groups and seven subgroups (Table 1). The minimum number of members of the group I subgroup was seven, namely *Amborella trichopoda*, *Liriodectron chinense*, *Zostela marina*, *Oryza sativa*, and the largest, *Sinapis alba*. The subgroups II-A, II-B, II-C, II-D, and II-E of *Amborella trichopoda* had the fewest members, with two, five, six, six, and three, respectively. In contrast, *Gossypium hirsutum* had the highest number of members in the same five subgroups. The number of group II-A in *Zostela marina* was also at least two, while the number of group II-B in *Portulaca amilis* and *Brachypodium distachyon* was also at least five. The lowest number of subgroups in group III was only five in *Nymphaea colorata*, and the highest number was fifty-one in *Sinapis alba*. This result indicates that the number of subgroups in different species varied wildly, suggesting that they may have undergone environmental screening during the evolutionary process, ultimately retaining the current number of families.

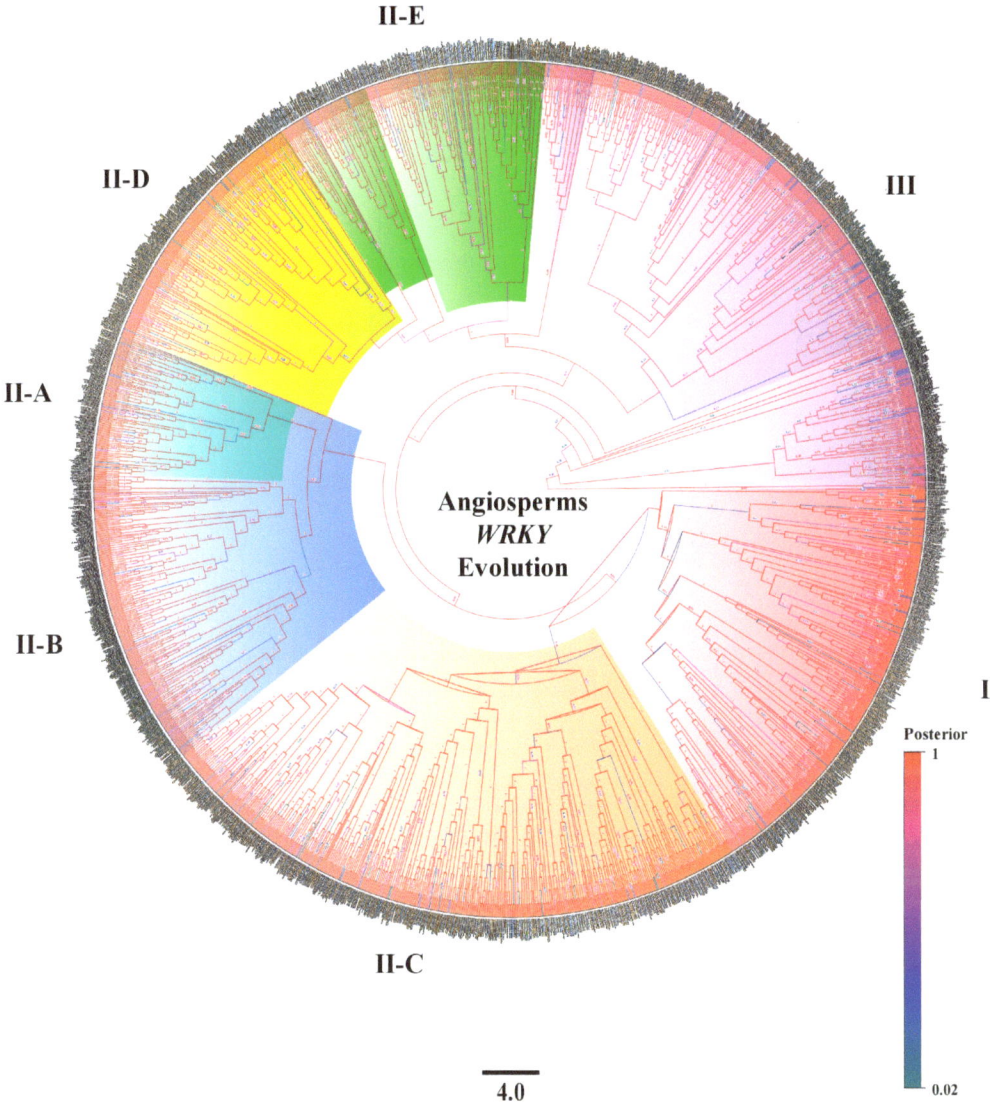

Figure 1. Twenty-four species of angiosperms from the WRKY evolutionary tree. A total of 2274 WRKY genes are divided into three major groups and seven subgroups, I, II-A II-E, and III, with the different colors representing different subgroup branches. The bottom 4.0 represents the branch length scale, and the posterior represents the Bayesian posterior value of the branch.

2.2. The Structural Characteristics and Grouping of the WRKY Family

The WRKY transcription factors are mainly a family composed of one or two WRKY domains. In recent years, with the release of various plant genome data, the *WRKY* gene family has been identified within the genome, and the expression patterns of the *WRKY* genes in different plants in response to abiotic stress have been explored using qRT-PCR and RNA-seq. The verification of their functions combined with traditional molecular experimental methods has become a hotspot in botany research.

Table 1. Number of members in different subgroups of 24 species of angiosperms.

Species	Group I	Group II-A	Group II-B	Group II-C	Group II-D	Group II-E	Group III
Amborella trichopoda	7	2	5	6	3	3	8
Nymphaea colorata	18	6	9	10	7	10	5
Cinnamomum kanehirae	15	6	8	12	9	12	11
Liriodendron chinense	7	3	6	8	4	7	9
Liriodendron tulipifera	9	6	7	13	6	7	10
Brachypodium arbuscula	13	4	8	23	7	10	26
Brachypodium distachyon	17	5	5	16	10	10	26
Oryza sativa	7	4	8	19	6	11	51
Sorghum bicolor	9	5	8	20	7	11	36
Zea mays	15	7	12	30	12	17	44
Zostera marina	7	2	8	10	6	6	7
Arabidopsis thaliana	12	3	8	18	7	7	28
Carya illinoinensis	17	6	13	24	9	10	12
Cirus trifoliata	10	3	8	13	5	7	9
Coffea arabica	23	5	15	28	13	11	32
Corymbia citriodora	16	6	11	18	5	8	15
Gossypium hirsutum	36	16	31	69	28	26	32
Malus pumila	23	6	15	25	14	13	28
Populus trichocarpa	23	5	9	24	13	12	14
Portulaca amilis	12	5	5	14	10	8	21
Sinapis alba	41	8	26	64	24	19	51
Theobroma cacao	10	3	8	14	6	6	18
Vigna unguiculata	15	6	15	22	7	11	22
Vitis vinifera	14	3	8	15	9	6	12

Note: The different background colors represent different classifications of plants; from top to bottom, they were basal angiosperms, Magnolia, Monocotyledonous, and Dicotyledonous. The table is arranged in order based on the first character of the plant Latin scientific names and different colored backgrounds represent different evolutionary branch plant categories.

The main structure of the WRKY transcription factor is composed of four bata folds and zinc finger structures, with approximately 60 amino acids. Its motif is CX4-5CX22-23HXH (C2H2) or CX7CX23HXH (C2H2). It is highly conserved in the WRKYGQK heptapeptide region, so it is called the WRKY domain. In most WRKY domains, there are two intron insertion sites, PR and VQR. Different variants in the WRKY domain, WRRY, WSKY, WKRY, WVKY, or WKKY, replace the WRKY amino acid sequence. The zinc finger structure at the end of the folded sheet is mainly formed by the highly conservative Cys/His residues, and the N-terminal is connected via Gly to form hydrogen bonds, and then forms the β chain β folding sheet.

The WRKY family is mainly divided into three types according to the number of N-terminal conservative domains and the type of C-terminal zinc finger. The first type is the zinc finger structure containing two WRKY domains and one C2H2. The second type contains only one WRKY domain and one C2H2 zinc finger structure. The second group is further divided into five subgroups according to different amino acid sequences, namely II (a), II (b), II (c), II (d), and II (e); The third category contains only one WRKY domain, which is the same as the second category. The difference is that its zinc finger structure is C2HC, which is different from the previous two types of zinc finger structures.

Through the previous evolutionary tree analysis and species tree analysis, it was found that the evolution of the WRKY family is conserved (Figure 2). Therefore, through multiple alignment analysis, it was found that the domain sequence of the WRKY family is also very conservative, mainly including the WRKYGQK signature sequence (Figure 2A) and β fold (Figure 2B). The WRKY domain has approximately 60 amino acids, with the sequence WRKYGQK13-14-CX4-5CX22-23HXH (C2H2) or WRKYGQKX13-14-CX7CX23HXH (C2H2), and WRKYGQK typically becomes a signature sequence (Figure 2A). Group I contains two WRKY domains, with the second WRKY domain containing a PR intron insertion fragment located between the C2 and H2 sequences. Group II contains a WRKY domain with two intron insertion fragments, namely the PR intron and VQR intron. Group III contains a WRKY domain, as well as the PR intron and VQR intron insertion fragments, but the domain C-terminus contains the -HXC sequence, which is different from the other two sets of sequences.

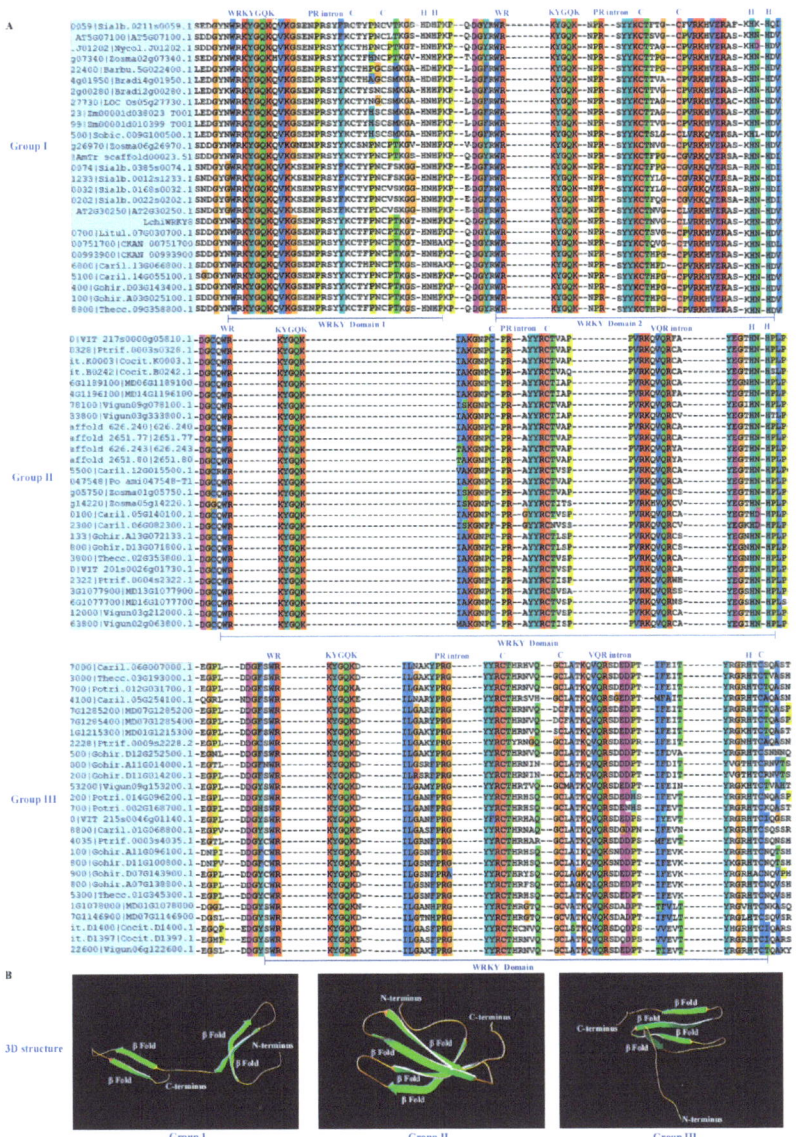

Figure 2. Domain sequence conservation and 3D structure of the WRKY family. (**A**) The sequences of the three subgroups of WRKY all contain WRKYGQK signature sequences, with two types of PR intron and VQR intron insertions. Group I contains two WRKY domains, while the other subgroups only contain one WRKY domain. Different colored backgrounds represent different base conservatism. (**B**) The three-dimensional spatial connectivity domains of the three subgroups all contain four β folds.

The 3D structural analysis of the WRKY family shows that all three subgroups contain four β folds and distribute evenly from the N-terminus to the C-terminus (Figure 2B). The sequence and spatial structure of the WRKY family indicate that they are highly conserved among 24 species of angiosperms, with plants from different evolutionary positions sharing the same WRKY domain and β folding; therefore, it is necessary to further explore the biological functions of the *WRKY* family.

2.3. Origin and Evolution of the WRKY Family

The *WRKY* family is one of the largest transcription factor families in plants. The first *WRKY* gene was cloned from sweet potato, and then it was continuously cloned from other species, such as wild oats (*Avena fatua* L.), parsley (*Petroselenium crispum* L.), and *Arabidopsis thaliana* [1,2,4]. As for the origin of the WRKY gene, the research results show that it originated from eukaryotic organisms approximately 1.5 to 2 billion years ago, but it has not appeared in fungi and animals so far. Therefore, it is speculated that the *WRKY* gene exists exclusively in plants [2,6,7]. Compared with non-flowering plants, the WRKY transcription factor plays a more important role in flowering plants. In particular, the third subfamily *WRKY* gene, which is the fastest evolving *WRKY* gene with the best adaptability, is mainly formed after the differentiation of monocots and dicots; the number of *WRKY* families also changes with the evolution of plants [4,7].

We selected 24 species of angiosperms, including basal angiosperms, monocotyledonous, and dicotyledonous plants, for species evolution analyses, and the results of reconstructing the phylogenetic tree indicate that the evolution of the *WRKY* family is consistent with the evolutionary status of the species genome. Among them, the basal angiosperms include *Amborella trichopoda* and *Nymphaea colorata*, the magnolias include *Cinnamomum kanehirae*, *Liriodendron chinense*, and *Liriodendron tulipifera*, as well as six monocotyledonous plants and thirteen dicotyledonous plants.

The number of gene families is also related to the evolutionary status of a species. Overall, the lower the evolutionary status, the smaller the number of family members in a species. If a whole genome replication event occurs in a species, the number of gene family members would also increase. From the perspective of the evolutionary status of the species, the whole genome duplication (WGD) event is also related to the evolutionary status [13]. The higher the plant, the more genome replication events may occur. In the long-term process of species evolution, plants continuously adapt to the environment and evolve many functions. Many genes lose their function or only retain some functions after the occurrence of whole genome doubling events, resulting in different numbers of genes retained in plants and ultimately forming different numbers of genes.

Among the 24 species of angiosperms, the total number of *WRKY* families in *Amborella trichopoda* is at least 34 (Table 2). Only four plants experienced two WGD events, *Cinnamomum kanehirae* from Magnoliaceae [14], *Carya illinoinensis*, *Sinapis alba*, and *Vitis vinifera* from Dicotyledonous, among others, all experienced a WGD event. The frequency of genome duplication in dicotyledonous plants is higher than that in magnolia, monocotyledonous, and basal angiosperms, and the total number of *WRKY* families in most dicotyledonous plants is also higher than in other angiosperms. For example, the most members of the dicotyledonous plant family are *Gossypium hirsutum* with 238 genes, the least is *Cirus trifoliata* with 55 genes, the most members of the monocotyledonous plant family is *Zea mays* with 137 genes, the least is *Zostela marina* with 46 genes, the most members of the magnolia family is *Cinnamomum kanehirae* with 73 genes, the least are *Lirioderon chinense* with 44 genes, and the most members of the basal angiosperm family are *Nymphaea corata* with 65 genes. The minimum number is *Amborella trichopoda*, with 34 genes.

Int. J. Mol. Sci. **2024**, *25*, 3551

Table 2. Total number of *WRKY* families and whole genome replication events in 24 species of angiosperms.

Species	Family	Taxonomy	WGD	Total Number
Amborella trichopoda	Amborellaceae	ANITA Basal angiosperms	1	34
Nymphaea colorata	Nymphaeaceae	ANITA Basal angiosperms	1	65
Liriodendron chinense	Magnoliaceae	Magnoliids	1	44
Liriodendron tulipifera	Magnoliaceae	Magnoliids	1	58
Cinnamomum kanehirae	Lauraceae	Magnoliids	2	73
Zostera marina	Zosteraceae	Monocotyledonous	1	46
Brachypodium distachyon	Poaceae	Monocotyledonous	1	89
Brachypodium arbuscula	Poaceae	Monocotyledonous	1	91
Sorghum bicolor	Poaceae	Monocotyledonous	1	96
Oryza sativa	Poaceae	Monocotyledonous	1	106
Zea mays	Poaceae	Monocotyledonous	1	137
Cirus trifoliata	Rutaceae	Dicotyledonous	1	55
Theobroma cacao	Malvaceae	Dicotyledonous	1	65
Vitis vinifera	Vitaceae	Dicotyledonous	2	67
Portulaca amilis	Portulacaceae	Dicotyledonous	1	75
Corymbia citriodora	Myrtaceae	Dicotyledonous	1	79
Arabidopsis thaliana	Brassicaceae	Dicotyledonous	1	83
Carya illinoinensis	Juglandaceae	Dicotyledonous	2	91
Vigna unguiculata	Fabaceae	Dicotyledonous	1	98
Populus trichocarpa	Salicaceae	Dicotyledonous	1	100
Malus pumila	Rosaceae	Dicotyledonous	1	124
Coffea arabica	Rubiaceae	Dicotyledonous	1	127
Sinapis alba	Brassicaceae	Dicotyledonous	2	233
Gossypium hirsutum	Malvaceae	Dicotyledonous	1	238

Note: WGD stands for whole genome duplication event, and the total number represents the total number of *WRKY* family members per species. The table is arranged in ascending order based on the total number of plants in different classifications and different colored backgrounds represent different evolutionary branch plant categories.

The total number of *WRKY* families in the 24 species of angiosperms and the results of the WGD events indicate that the genetic functional diversity of dicotyledonous plants may be more abundant than monocotyledonous, magnolia, and basal angiosperms, and may also be more adaptable to environmental changes. Therefore, further exploration of the functional differentiation of basal angiosperms, magnolias, monocots, and dicots can help to better understand the functional differences of the *WRKY* family.

To explore the relationship with the *WRKY* family of different species during the evolutionary process, 24 species of angiosperms were analyzed using the "timetree" website (http://www.timetree.org/, accessed on 19 March 2024). The results showed that there are significant differences in the differentiation time of species with different evolutionary positions (Figure 3). The functional differentiation of gymnosperms and angiosperms began around 196 MYA, while basal angiosperms and magnolia plants underwent functional differentiation around 175 MYA. By 170 MYA, magnolia and monocotyledonous plants became more capable of differentiation, gradually forming independent evolutionary clades. After relatively brief evolution, monocots and dicots further underwent functional differentiation at 160 MYA, forming two independent branching species. Through continuous evolution, different species in each branch also underwent functional differentiation at different evolutionary time points, forming a variety of species today.

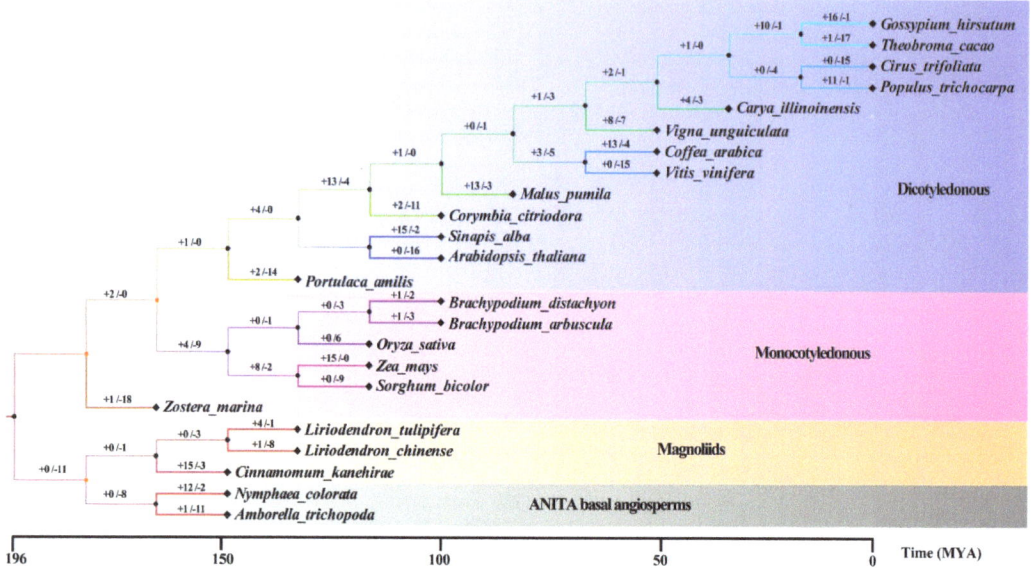

Figure 3. The evolutionary statuses and functional divergence times of 24 species of angiosperms. The numerical values on the branch represent the number of expansions and contractions, + represents expansion, - represents contraction, and the bottom coordinates represent the species divergence time, and different colored backgrounds represent different evolutionary branch plant categories.

Through the analysis of the expansion and contraction of the *WRKY* family, it is concluded that the number of expansions and contractions of plants with different evolutionary statuses was different, and the number of plants with the same evolutionary status was also different. For example, the basal angiosperm plant *Amborella trichopoda* had more shrinkage gene numbers than the expansion ones, and conversely, *Nymphaea colorata* had much more expansion gene numbers than the contraction ones. *Liriodendron tulipifera* and *Cinnamomum kanehirae* had a greater number of expansions than the shrinkage number, and *Liriodendron chinense* had fewer expansion numbers than the shrinkage ones.

2.4. The Environmental Selection Pressure of the WRKY Family

By conducting an environmental selection pressure analysis on the *WRKY* family genes, the results showed that most of them undergo positive selection during environmental changes, and as long as a small number of genes undergo negative selection, they may gradually lose their function in subsequent evolution, which may also affect the number of members of the gene family [2–5]. By combining these results with the previous analysis, it can be concluded that angiosperms undergo more whole genome replication events, more genes undergo positive selection during environmental changes, and ultimately obtain more family members [4–6].

After analyzing the *WRKY* family Ka/Ks value of the 24 species of angiosperms, it was found that the plants with different evolutionary statuses suffer from different environmental selection pressures [5,7], and the ratio of positive and negative selection is also different. As shown in Table 3, three plants showed positive selection, the other fourteen plants showed negative selection, and seven plants did not undergo synonymous or nonsynonymous substitution.

Table 3. Analysis of environmental selection pressures in the *WRKY* family.

Species	Taxonomy	Gene Pairs	Ka/Ks < 1	Ka/Ks > 1	Selection Pressure	Singe Copy
Amborella trichopoda	ANITA Basal angiosperms	0	0	0	\	6
Nymphaea colorata	ANITA Basal angiosperms	18	12	6	Negative	10
Cinnamomum kanehirae	Magnoliids	0	0	0	\	9
Liriodendron chinense	Magnoliids	5	3	2	Negative	7
Liriodendron tulipifera	Magnoliids	6	2	4	Positive	7
Brachypodium arbuscula	Monocotyledonou	105	57	48	Negative	14
Brachypodium distachyon	Monocotyledonou	0	0	0	\	15
Oryza sativa	Monocotyledonou	229	140	89	Negative	13
Sorghum bicolor	Monocotyledonou	157	67	90	Positive	11
Zea mays	Monocotyledonou	366	201	165	Negative	19
Zostera marina	Monocotyledonou	7	5	2	Negative	7
Arabidopsis thaliana	Dicotyledonous	18	5	13	Positive	11
Carya illinoinensis	Dicotyledonous	0	0	0	\	15
Cirus trifoliata	Dicotyledonous	7	3	4	Positive	8
Coffea arabica	Dicotyledonous	0	0	0	\	21
Corymbia citriodora	Dicotyledonous	0	0	0	\	12
Gossypium hirsutum	Dicotyledonous	115	71	44	Negative	32
Malus pumila	Dicotyledonous	27	21	6	Negative	17
Populus trichocarpa	Dicotyledonous	18	8	10	Positive	18
Portulaca amilis	Dicotyledonous	0	0	0	\	13
Sinapis alba	Dicotyledonous	55	30	25	Negative	33
Theobroma cacao	Dicotyledonous	7	4	3	Negative	9
Vigna unguiculata	Dicotyledonous	15	9	6	Negative	13
Vitis vinifera	Dicotyledonous	9	8	1	Negative	11

Note: Gene pairs represent the number of genes that underwent base substitutions, and the number 0 indicates that the sequences without genes in the species underwent substitutions. The table is arranged in order of the first character of the plant Latin scientific names and different colored backgrounds represent different evolutionary branch plant categories.

For basic angiosperms, eighteen genes undergo replacement in water lilies, but under environmental selection conditions, only six genes are positively selected, indicating that the environment would eliminate unfavorable genes and retain favorable ones. No base substitution occurred in the genes of *Amborella trichopoda*, indicating that the *WRKY* gene sequence was stable and conserved during evolution, and no mutations occurred. The selection pressure of magnolia plants is different from that of basal angiosperms. The *WRKY* gene of the camphor tree did not undergo base substitution, indicating a relatively stable evolutionary process. *Liriodendron chinense* and *Liriodendron tulipifera* are different species of magnolia plants, but they exhibit completely different adaptations in environmental selection. Five genes of *Liriodendron chinense* undergo base substitution, while six genes of *Liriodendron tulipifera* undergo base substitution. However, *Liriodendron chinense* undergoes purification selection from the environment, while *Liriodendron tulipifera* undergoes positive selection from the environment. This indicates that during the evolutionary process, species of the same evolutionary status, due to differences in their living environment, experience differences in the evolution of the *WRKY* family, ultimately affecting the number of members of the *WRKY* family.

The environmental selection pressure of the *WRKY* gene varied more among different species of dicots, most of which were purified selection; only a few were positive selection, and some plants did not undergo base substitution. For example, no gene substitution occurred for *Corymbia citriodora*, *Carya illinoinensis*, *Coffea arabica*, and *Portulaca amilis*. *Arabidopsis thaliana*, *Cirus trifoliata*, and *Populus trichocarpa* all suffered positive selection, and the other plant *WRYK* genes all suffered from environmental purification selection. The *WRKY* gene of the monocots and dicots was subjected to a similar pattern of environmental selection pressure, and most plants were subjected to environmental purification selection; only a few of them had positive selection or no base substitution. For example, *Sorghum bicolor* suffered from positive selection, *Brachypodium distachyon* did not undergo base substitution, and plants such as *Oryza sativa* and *Zea mays* suffered from purification selection.

The above results showed that the base substitution of the *WRKY* gene in most plants was mainly subjected to the purification selection of the environment and the elimination of unfavorable genes, and only a few plants had a positive selection of the environment for base substitution. In some plants, the *WRKY* gene was relatively stable and did not undergo base substitution. Therefore, plants with different evolutionary positions also have genes that undergo base substitution in the process of adapting to the environment and eliminate unfavorable genes after environmental selection to achieve better evolution.

The number of single-copy genes varied among the species of different evolutionary statuses. The gene tree analysis of single-copy genes in the *WRKY* family showed that single-copy genes were also relatively conserved (Figure S1 and Table 3). Overall, there were a total of 331 single-copy genes in the 24 species of angiosperms, with *Amborella trichopoda* having only six genes and *Sinapis alba* having thirty-three genes. Compared with the evolutionary tree grouping of the *WRKY* family genes, group I had the highest number of single-copy genes, while the other subgroups had little or almost no single-copy genes.

2.5. Development Function of WRKY Transcription Factor

The diversity of this gene family in plants is related to the life cycle of plants and their response to environmental stress. At present, the research on the *WRKY* gene has mainly focused on the growth and development of plants, and the response to resistance, such as seed germination, and the response to abiotic stresses, such as drought and low temperature. Studies have shown that the *WRKY* gene can regulate plant resistance through over-expression or gene knockout, which is also conducive to revealing the signal pathway mediated by the *WRKY* gene.

The WRKY transcription factor mainly regulates the expression of specific target genes and is subject to environmental factors and biological stress (such as bacteria, fungi, viruses, and other pathogens) or abiotic stress (such as exogenous hormones, high temperature, low temperature, high salt, mechanical injury, etc.), and the expression is specific in different tissues. The signal transduction pathways involved in WRKY regulation include plant hormone salicylic acid (SA), abscisic acid (ABA), jasmonic acid (JA), and the enzyme calmodulin (CaM).

The *WRKY* gene also regulates the growth, development, and reproductive senescence of plants, such as seed development, dormancy, germination, flowering, and the senescence of plants, and further regulates the growth, development, and metabolism of plants. In terms of biosynthesis, the 42 *GmWRKY* genes of *Gentiana macrophylla* can participate in secoiridoid biosynthesis, promoting the accumulation of secondary metabolites [15]. The *Lagerstroemia indica* L. contains 61 *LiWRKY* genes involved in regulating anthocyanin biosynthesis [16]. Among the 72 *JsWRKY* genes of *Jasminum sambac*, the overexpression of *JsWRKY51* can enhance the accumulation of β-ocimene, which regulates the synthesis of aromatic hydrocarbon components [8]. In tomatoes, *SlWRKY75* can maintain auxin homeostasis and promote plant resistance [17]. In rose petals, *RhWRKY30* can promote the expression of the *RhCAD* gene and enhance the biosynthesis content of lignin [18]. The transcriptome of *Melastoma dodecandrum* revealed that the *MedWRKY* gene is involved in growth and development and is highly expressed in roots and mature fruits [19].

The senescence process at the end of the plant life cycle is inevitable, and the *WRKY* gene plays a regulatory role in petal senescence. In terms of senescence, the transcription factor TgWRKY75 of the tulip activates the biosynthesis of ABA and SA, accelerating the petal senescence process of the tulip [20]. This indicates that the WRKY transcription factor can not only positively regulate the aging process, but also participate in this process as a negative regulatory factor. In general, it is particularly important to study the function of the *WRKY* gene in the whole process of plant growth, development, metabolism, and senescence.

2.6. Functions of the WRKY Family in Biotic Stress

Plants grow in the natural environment and adapt to the changing environment through their defense mechanisms. Systemic acquired resistance and induced systemic resistance are two important ways for plants to resist pathogens. When plants are invaded by pathogens, they will resist the invasion of pathogens through a series of physiological reactions, such as the waxy layer of their leaves and the secretion of their body surface. The plant resistance pathway is regulated by salicylic acid and jasmonic acid, which activate or inhibit the expression of disease resistance genes through signal transduction [11].

In tomatoes, the overexpression of *SlWRKY75* can reduce the content of IAA, reduce the expansion of auxin proteins, upregulate the expression of the PRs and NPR1 genes, and enhance potato resistance to the *Pseudomonas syringae* pv. *Tomato* (*Pst*) DC3000 pathogen [17]. The full-length transcriptome and RNA-seq analyses of sesame revealed that the *WRKY* gene is highly expressed in response to *Corynespora casicola* stress and is a hub gene in the coexpression regulatory network [21]. The domain of *Arabidopsis AtWRKY45* is susceptible to two pathogens, *Pseudomonas syringae* pv. *Pisi* and *Ralstonia pseudosolanacearum*, which specifically recognize anchoring, thereby inhibiting the pathogen immune response in Arabidopsis [22]. The *Cicer arietinum* L. *WRKY* gene responds to *Ascomycta rabiei* infection and exhibits differential expression trends with other transcription factors during the response process [23]. Recent research has proposed a new method to capture the binding transcription factors of the *SERRATE(SE)* genes through CRISPR-dCas9 (CASPA dCas9). The results showed that the transcription factors AtWRKY19 and AtPAR2 jointly promote the expression of the *SE* genes and enhance the pathogen resistance of *Arabidopsis* [24].

Insects or pathogens in the environment can cause damage to plant growth. Therefore, increasing the biological resistance of plants helps them better adapt to environmental growth. Whether it is crops, horticultural plants, or woody plants, these are all plants that are beneficial for human survival and development, and in-depth research on their molecular mechanisms is of great significance.

2.7. Functions of the WRKY Family in Abiotic Stress

Under abiotic stress, to resist the influence of an adverse environment through a series of physiological regulation and metabolic processes [25–27], plants can normally grow, forming a complex gene regulation network in which the WRKY transcription factor plays a very important role [28]. With the continuous development of biotechnology, the expression pattern of the *WRKY* family in response to abiotic stress was verified via RNA-seq, real-time quantitative PCR, and other technologies, and the regulation mechanism of the *WRKY* family was expounded [26].

The WRKY transcription factor regulates the response of plants to abiotic stress. For example, in wheat, TaWRKY transcription factors are involved in regulating the response to aluminum and manganese ion stress [29]. The transcriptome of low-phosphorus-stressed wheat revealed that *TaWRKY74s* is the major gene involved, which may regulate plant adaptation to low-phosphorus stress through ABA and auxin signaling [30]. In *Pyrus betulifolia*, the *PbWRKY* gene responds to both high temperature and drought stress and exhibits a high expression trend [31]. The transcriptome of *Gossypium anomalum* seedlings revealed that the *GaWRKY* gene is involved in salt stress response, and was validated via qRT-PCR to be consistent with RNA-seq data [32].

The 145 *TrWRKY* genes of the white clone respond to cold stress, and most genes are upregulated in the early stages of cold stress [33]. The 64 *DhWRKY* genes of *Dendrobium huoshanense* respond to hormone and low temperature stress. *DhWRKY42* significantly responds to jasmonic acid stress [34]. The *WRKY* family of *Liriodendron chinense* also participates in the abiotic stress response, and *LchiWRKY18* and *36* are involved in high temperature and drought stress responses, with high expression levels [35]. *StWRKY016*, *StWRKY045*, and *StWRKY055* in potatoes specifically respond to high-temperature stress in leaf tissues [7].

The *WRKY* gene family is involved in both biological and abiotic stress functions, regulating plant adaptation to different environments (Figure 4). Biological stress mainly includes insect stress, pathogen stress, and microbial stress. Abiotic stress mainly includes temperature, ion, and osmotic stress. In the long-term evolutionary process, the *WRKY* family exhibits diverse functions in adapting to environmental changes, and there are also differences in the biological functions of different subgroups. For example, most genes respond to abiotic stress, but have little response to the third group of *WRKY* members. In some species, the third group of *WRKY* members almost do not respond to abiotic stress but respond to biological stress. The *LchiWRKY18* and *36* genes of *Liriodendron chinense* are both members of the second group and participate in the response to high temperature and drought abiotic stress [35]. Combined with the promoters of downstream target genes *LchiHSPs* and *LchiMED26*, the expression of these target genes promotes plant response to abiotic stress environments.

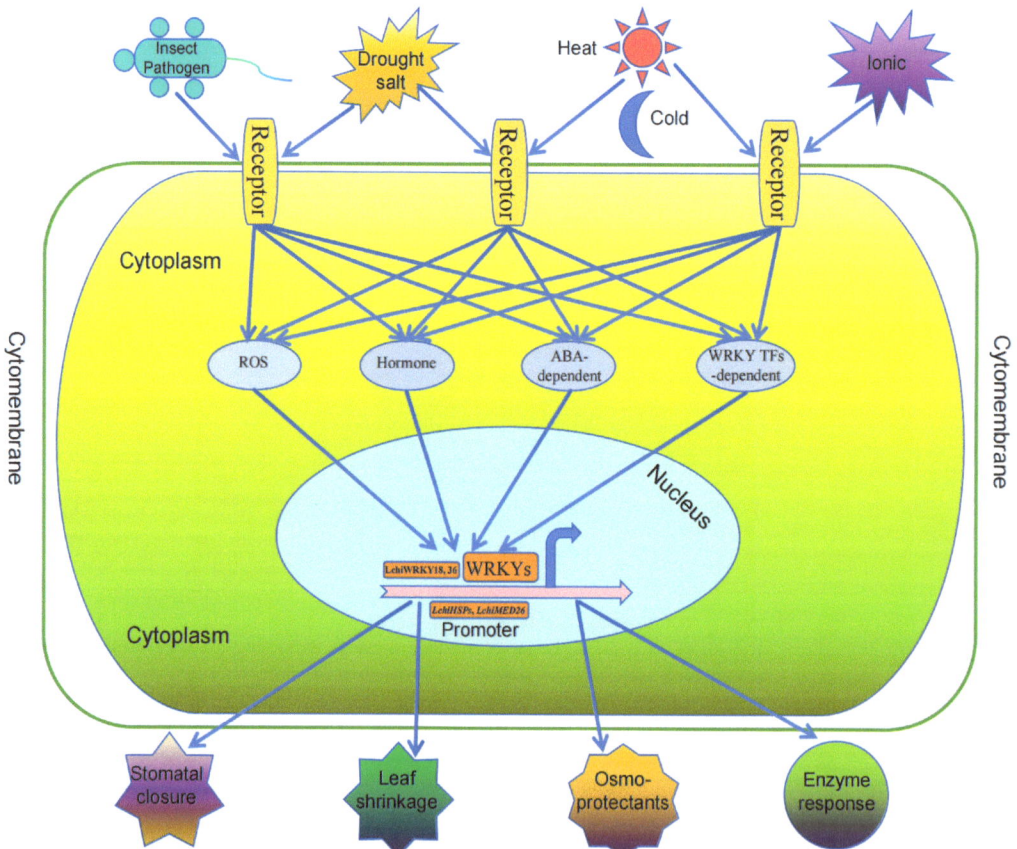

Figure 4. *WRKY* functional diversity summary chart. The different shapes in the upper part represent different external environmental stress conditions, the middle part represents the overall cell, and the bottom represents the different responses after stress.

Environmental stress includes many factors, including temperature, osmotic stress, and ion stress, which mainly affect plant growth [26,27]. Insect and pathogen stress is mainly biological stress that occurs during a certain stage of plant growth and changes in the external environment (Figure 4). In the living environment of angiosperms, stimulated by environmental factors, cells in the body begin to respond to these environmental stresses. The receptors on the cell membrane perceive environmental stimuli and transmit signals to various signaling pathways within the cell, such as ROS, hormones, ABA-dependent substances, and WRKY transcription factors. These substances then feed the signals back to various WRKY transcription factors in the nucleus for a response. These transcription factors further bind to the promoter sequences of downstream target genes, activating the expression of various downstream target genes. After the expression of these target genes, various response mechanisms are activated, such as stomatal closure, leaf shrinkage, the production of osmotic protective substances, and the activation of enzyme system responses, promoting plant adaptation to environmental changes.

3. Discussion

3.1. The Evolution of the WRKY Family in Higher Plants Is Relatively Conservative

Plants also undergo whole genome duplication events during their evolutionary process, and the number of occurrences varies among plants of different evolutionary statuses [28,36,37]. Overall, there are more plants with dicotyledonous leaves that experience WGD twice than other plants, while monocotyledonous plants and basal angiosperms rarely experience WGD events twice [36,37]. Magnolia plants only have camphor trees experiencing WGD events twice [14]. Most plants undergo a WGD event and retain the replicated genes to form the current total number of *WRKY* families.

WRKY also undergoes multiple functional differentiation during the purification process, with functional differentiation occurring in gymnosperms and angiosperms around 196 MYA. By 175 MYA, the basal angiosperms had undergone functional differentiation with magnolia and monocotyledonous plants, forming three branches of plant evolution. After a long period of evolution, around 160 MYA, monocotyledonous and dicotyledonous plants underwent functional differentiation, forming new plant branches.

Compared to the evolutionary statuses and functional differentiation times of plant genomes, the functional differentiation time of basal angiosperms and magnolias *WRKY* family is earlier and slower than that of the genome (Figure S2). The evolutionary status of the *WRKY* family in magnolias and basal angiosperms is the same, which may be due to differences in the evolutionary process between the genomes and individual families.

3.2. The Environment Selection Preserves the Existing WRKY Number of Family Members and Different Expansion–Contraction Ratios

Environmental selection eliminates unfavorable genes in plants and preserves favorable genes, so the analysis of environmental selection can better understand the replacement of gene bases in plants during the process of adapting to environmental changes, and thus understand the stability of plant genes [38,39]. Most genes in plants undergo environmental selection during their evolutionary process. The *WRKY* selection pressure analysis from basal angiosperms to monocotyledonous plants shows that most genes undergoing base substitution are subjected to environmental purification selection. Only some plant genes undergo positive selection, and dicotyledonous plants have more positive selection than monocotyledonous plants.

The expansion and contraction of gene families are also key factors affecting the number of families. Further analysis of the expansion and contraction of the *WRKY* family in angiosperms shows that most plants experience more expansion than contraction, while some plants experience less expansion than contraction. Many species of monocotyledonous plants may experience contraction, and only *Zea mays* has a greater expansion than contraction. Magnolia plants are relatively unique, with only the number of contracted of *Liriodendron chinense* greater than the number of expanded ones. Combined with the total number analysis of the *WRKY* family, the number of *Liriodendron chinense* is less than the other two species. These results indicate that the total number of *WRKY* family members is not only related to the number of WGD events but also the degree of environmental selection and expansion–contraction, ultimately determining the total number of family members.

3.3. The Conservatism of Domain and 3D Structure of the WRKY Family

The WRKY domain is mainly specifically bound to the cis-regulating element W-box (T) (T) TGAC (C/T) sequence of the target gene promoter to regulate the expression of the downstream target gene. The core conserved sequence of this cis-regulating element is TGAC, which is also the key sequence that the WRKY protein can specifically bind to [1,4,9]. Through the bioinformatics and functional analysis of the promoter, it is concluded that in the stress-related promoter sequence, the W-box, is generally combined into the promoter via clustering [40]. Among the genes related to disease resistance and aging, the W-box mainly starts the expression of these genes, and the WRKY transcription factor is mainly involved in the response of these processes in the response of plants to environmental stress [3–5]. In addition, some experiments have shown that the WRKY transcription factor also has a regulatory effect on plant growth and development. Some WRKY proteins may participate in seed development and ABA-mediated growth inhibition after germination, regulating the formation of leaf hair and the senescence process.

The three-dimensional structure of a protein determines its function. The WRKY family consists of four main components, which are β-fold proteins. Its main characteristic sequence is WRKYGQK, which also contains two types of intron insertion sequences, the PR intron and VQR intron. The former is mainly inserted after the WRKYGQK sequence, while the latter is mainly inserted after the second C base of C-C. According to the analysis of multiple sequences in the *WRKY* family of basal angiosperms, magnolias, and monocotyledonous plants, it can be concluded that *WRKY* is relatively conserved in family evolution.

The first subgroup of the WRKY family in THE 24 species of angiosperms contains two WRKY domains, and PR intron insertion mainly occurs in the second WRKY domain sequence. The second and third subgroups both contain a WRKY domain, and both intron insertion sequences, the PR intron and VQR intron, appear in these two subgroups. The three-dimensional structure of *WRKY* is also very conservative, with four north tower folds in the three-dimensional structures of different subgroups across the 24 species of angiosperms. The above results indicate that the *WRKY* family has a very stable grouping quantity and sequence structure during the evolutionary process, and plants of different evolutionary positions have the same function.

3.4. Functional Diversity of the WRKY Family in Angiosperms

The *WRKY* gene family is involved in many biological processes in plants, including biotic stress and abiotic stress [3,4,41]. Biological stress mainly refers to insect, pathogen, and microbial stress, while abiotic stress mainly includes temperature, osmotic, and ion stress [3,41,42]. When plants adapt to different environments, the receptors on the cell membrane first sense the external stimuli, stimulate changes in various physiological indicators of the cytoplasm, stimulate the expression of transcription factors in the nucleus, and then combine with downstream target gene promoters to induce the expression of target genes, promoting plant adaptation to various environments [4,12,41].

The overexpression of the splicing variant *AtrWRKY42-2* in *Amaranthus Paniculatus* enhances the expression of the *AtrCYP76AD1* gene and increases the biosynthesis of betaine [43]. In tulips, the overexpression of *TgWRKY75* enhances the expression of the *TgNCED3* gene, increases ABA and SA biosynthesis, and jointly promotes the leaf senescence process [20]. Under calcium ion stress, the *SlWRKY* gene in potatoes participates in both the positive and negative regulation of the stress response, promoting crop adaptation to heavy metal environments [44]. In wheat, silencing the *TaWRKY31* gene leads to poor plant growth status and poorer resistance to drought stress. The overexpression of the *TaWRKY31* gene in *Arabidopsis thaliana* can enhance its drought resistance, reduce water loss rate, and reduce stomatal opening [45]. The overexpression of the maize *ZmB12D* gene in *Arabidopsis thaliana* enhances its waterlogging tolerance. Enzymatic hybridization experiments have shown that *ZmB12D* interacts with *ZmWRKY70*, regulating maize waterlogging resistance [46]. The *PmWRKY70* gene was cloned from the *Prunus mume* cultivar "Guhong zhusha", and the overexpression of *PmWRKY57* enhanced the cold stress resistance of *Arabidopsis thaliana* plants [47].

The *WRKY* family is involved in plant regulation with group specificity, with the majority of abiotic stresses being mainly mediated by the second group. The first and third groups are primarily involved in biological stress or other tissue growth and development processes. For example, in magnolia plants, the *WRKY* family of *Liriodendron chinense* is mainly the group II involved in high temperature and drought stress, and *LchiWRKY18* (II-e) and *LchiWRKY36* (II-d) reach their expression peaks at the 24-h and 72-h time points of stress [35]. The group IIc GhWRKY transcription factor in cotton enhances plant resistance to *Fusarium oxysporum* stress by mediating *GhMKK2* flavonoid synthesis [48].

In summary, the *WRKY* family is relatively conservative in terms of grouping and 3D structure in the evolution of angiosperms. However, in plants of different evolutionary positions, due to the different environmental adaptability of plants, different evolutionary processes, such as WGD events, environmental selection pressures, and family expansions and contractions ultimately result in differences in the number of *WRKY* family members among different plants, leading to various differential characteristics in adapting to the environment. This may be the underlying mechanism of plant diversity, and with the continuous development of science and technology and in-depth research, more functions of the *WRKY* family will continue to be explored.

4. Materials and Methods

Twenty-four WRKY family protein sequences from the plant genome website Phytozome(V13) (https://phytozome-next.jgi.doe.gov/, accessed on 19 March 2024) were used [49]. We found and downloaded the *WRKY* keyword in the search box, checked for no duplicate sequences, and then used OrthoFinder2 software to analyze the species evolution status of the *WRKY* family [50,51]. We organized the *WRKY* sequences of each species into a "Fasta" format file, and then placed the "Fasta" files of 24 species in the same folder. Then, we ran the command line "orthofinder2 -f folder" to obtain the results. We used the default parameter "Fasttree" in the program to construct the species tree. For all the other parameters, we used the default parameters in the software [50,51]. The time of species functional differentiation was analyzed on the "time tree" website (http://www.timetree.org/, accessed on 19 March 2024) and was displayed at the bottom of the evolutionary tree [52].

The construction of the phylogenetic tree was first carried out using ClustalX (v2.1) software to perform the multiple sequence alignments and save them into the "Fasta" format. Then, the evolutionary tree was constructed using BEAST (v2.6.6) software. The "Fasta" format files were converted into XML files using the BEAUTi (v2.6.6) program and the site model was set to Dayoff. Then, the BEAST (v2.6.6) program was imported for 10,000,000 MCMC sampling to construct a Bayesian evolutionary tree [53]. Finally, the parameter burning percentage was selected to 90 through the TreeAnnotator (v2.6.6) program and the posterior probability limit was set to 1 [53]. Then, we checked for low memory, annotated the evolutionary tree, and used Figtree (v1.4.3) to obtain the evolutionary tree and the posterior values of all the branches, which were displayed with two decimal places on the evolutionary tree.

The 3D structural analysis was conducted through the online website NCBI (https://www.ncbi.nlm.nih.gov/Structure/CN3D/cn3d.shtml, accessed on 19 March 2024), which imported the protein sequences from the *WRKY* family to obtain the PDB files. Then, a 3D browsing program Cn3D (v4.3.1) was downloaded from the website to visualize the

Int. J. Mol. Sci. **2024**, 25, 3551

spatial structure and obtain the 3D structural maps. The domain sequence conservatism of the *WRKY* family was obtained through multiple sequence alignment analysis using ClustalX (v2.1). The conservatism of the WRKY domain was then segmented and visualized by integrating the conservatism of different sequence fragments. The Ka and Ks values were calculated using KaKs_Calculator_3.0 (V3.0), and the select pressure was measured according to the Ka/ks value [54–56].

5. Conclusions

During the process of adapting to the environment, plants undergo changes in their genes, enzyme systems, and biological pathways to better adapt to the environment. WRKY transcription factors are involved in the various life activities of plants. Although the number varies among different angiosperms, they are generally divided into three major groups and seven subgroups. In terms of evolution, WRKY's domain is relatively conservative and contains WRKYQGK signature sequences. The tertiary structure of the WRKY protein is highly conserved across different subgroups, each containing four β-folds. Due to the varying number of replication events throughout the entire genome and the different environmental choices experienced during evolution, different plants ultimately retain different numbers of *WRKY* family members. According to the evolutionary results of the *WRKY* family in basal angiosperms, magnolia plants, and monocotyledonous and dicotyledonous plants, the higher the evolutionary status, the relatively more members of the *WRKY* family, and the better their potential for adapting to environmental changes.

The human living environment is deteriorating, and global warming and rising temperatures are constantly breaking new records. Plants constantly adapt to new high temperature and drought environments, and the expression and response of WRKY transcription factors in the body are crucial for plants to survive in high temperature and drought environments. There are also various other environmental factors, such as phosphorus stress, low temperature stress, and salt stress, which can limit plant growth. Therefore, studying the *WRKY* gene family is crucial for revealing the biological mechanisms of plant adaptation to the environment.

With the rapid development of science and technology and the maturity of biotechnology, such as genetic manipulation, more and more research will continue to emerge. The molecular mechanisms of plant environmental stress will become more in-depth, and the functional diversity of the *WRKY* gene family will become clearer with the deepening of scientific research.

Supplementary Materials: The following supporting information can be downloaded at: https://www.mdpi.com/article/10.3390/ijms25063551/s1.

Author Contributions: W.W. performed the analysis of the data and wrote the manuscript. J.Y., N.Y., R.L., Z.Y., J.S. and J.C. revised the manuscript. All authors have read and agreed to the published version of the manuscript.

Funding: This research was funded by the Sub project of the Guangdong Province Key Field Research and Development Program "Research on Targeted Cultivation of *Mytilaria laosensis* New Strain" (Grant number 2020B020215002). The funding bodies had no role in the design of the study and collection, analysis, and interpretation of data and in writing the manuscript.

Institutional Review Board Statement: Not applicable.

Informed Consent Statement: Not applicable.

Data Availability Statement: The data in this article has been publicly published and can be downloaded from the website and the Supplementary Data (data S1–S6) provided in the article.

Acknowledgments: We greatly appreciate the support of the Guangzhou Collaborative Innovation Center on Science Tech of ecology and Landscape project (Grant number 202206010058). We are especially grateful to Sheng Zhu from the College of Life Science of Nanjing Forestry University for helping with the bioinformatics analysis. We greatly appreciate the valuable suggestions provided by the editors and reviewers.

Conflicts of Interest: The authors declare no conflicts of interest. The funders had no role in the design of the study; in the collection, analyses, or interpretation of data; in the writing of the manuscript; or in the decision to publish the results.

References

1. Javed, T.; Gao, S. WRKY transcription factors in plant defense. *Trends Genet.* **2023**, *39*, 787–801. [CrossRef] [PubMed]
2. Goyal, P.; Devi, R.; Verma, B.; Hussain, S.; Arora, P.; Tabassum, R.; Gupta, S. WRKY transcription factors: Evolution, regulation, and functional diversity in plants. *Protoplasma* **2023**, *260*, 331–348. [CrossRef] [PubMed]
3. Rai, G.K.; Mishra, S.; Chouhan, R.; Mushtaq, M.; Chowdhary, A.A.; Rai, P.K.; Kumar, R.R.; Kumar, P.; Perez-Alfocea, F.; Colla, G.; et al. Plant salinity stress, sensing, and its mitigation through WRKY. *Front. Plant Sci.* **2023**, *14*, 1238507. [CrossRef] [PubMed]
4. Khoso, M.A.; Hussain, A.; Ritonga, F.N.; Ali, Q.; Channa, M.M.; Alshegaihi, R.M.; Meng, Q.; Ali, M.; Zaman, W.; Brohi, R.D.; et al. WRKY transcription factors (TFs): Molecular switches to regulate drought, temperature, and salinity stresses in plants. *Front. Plant Sci.* **2022**, *13*, 1039329. [CrossRef] [PubMed]
5. Hsin, K.T.; Hsieh, M.-C.; Lee, Y.-H.; Lin, K.-C.; Cheng, Y.-S. Insight into the Phylogeny and Binding Ability of WRKY Transcription Factors. *Int. J. Mol. Sci.* **2022**, *23*, 2895. [CrossRef] [PubMed]
6. Wani, S.H.; Anand, S.; Singh, B.; Bohra, A.; Joshi, R. WRKY transcription factors and plant defense responses: Latest discoveries and future prospects. *Plant Cell Rep.* **2021**, *40*, 1071–1085. [CrossRef] [PubMed]
7. Cheng, Z.; Luan, Y.; Meng, J.; Sun, J.; Tao, J.; Zhao, D. WRKY Transcription Factor Response to High-Temperature Stress. *Plants* **2021**, *10*, 2211. [CrossRef] [PubMed]
8. Lu, Z.; Wang, X.; Mostafa, S.; Noor, I.; Lin, X.; Ren, S.; Cui, J.; Jin, B. WRKY Transcription Factors in *Jasminum sambac*: An Insight into the Regulation of Aroma Synthesis. *Biomolecules* **2023**, *13*, 1679. [CrossRef]
9. Guo, X.; Ullah, A.; Siuta, D.; Kukfisz, B.; Iqbal, S. Role of WRKY Transcription Factors in Regulation of Abiotic Stress Responses in Cotton. *Life* **2022**, *12*, 1410. [CrossRef]
10. Zhang, J.; Zhao, H.; Chen, L.; Lin, J.; Wang, Z.; Pan, J.; Yang, F.; Ni, X.; Wang, Y.; Wang, Y.; et al. Multifaceted roles of WRKY transcription factors in abiotic stress and flavonoid biosynthesis. *Front. Plant Sci.* **2023**, *14*, 1303667. [CrossRef]
11. Wang, H.; Cheng, X.; Yin, D.; Chen, D.; Luo, C.; Liu, H.; Huang, C. Advances in the Research on Plant WRKY Transcription Factors Responsive to External Stresses. *Curr. Issues Mol. Biol.* **2023**, *45*, 2861–2880. [CrossRef] [PubMed]
12. Dos Santos, T.B.; Ribas, A.F.; de Souza, S.G.H.; Budzinski, I.G.F.; Domingues, D.S. Physiological Responses to Drought, Salinity, and Heat Stress in Plants: A Review. *Stresses* **2022**, *2*, 113–135. [CrossRef]
13. Chen, J.; Hao, Z.; Guang, X.; Zhao, C.; Wang, P.; Xue, L.; Zhu, Q.; Yang, L.; Sheng, Y.; Zhou, Y.; et al. Liriodendron genome sheds light on angiosperm phylogeny and species-pair differentiation. *Nat. Plants* **2019**, *5*, 18–25. [CrossRef] [PubMed]
14. Chaw, S.M.; Liu, Y.-C.; Wu, Y.-W.; Wang, H.-Y.; Lin, C.-Y.I.; Wu, C.-S.; Ke, H.-M.; Chang, L.-Y.; Hsu, C.-Y.; Yang, H.-T.; et al. Stout camphor tree genome fills gaps in understanding of flowering plant genome evolution. *Nat. Plants* **2019**, *5*, 63–73. [CrossRef] [PubMed]
15. Yin, Y.; Fu, H.; Mi, F.; Yang, Y.; Wang, Y.; Li, Z.; He, Y.; Yue, Z. Genomic characterization of WRKY transcription factors related to secoiridoid biosynthesis in *Gentiana macrophylla*. *BMC Plant Biol.* **2024**, *24*, 66. [CrossRef] [PubMed]
16. Gu, C.; Hong, S.; Wang, J.; Shang, L.; Zhang, G.; Zhao, Y.; Ma, Q.; Ma, D. Identification and expression analysis of the bZIP and WRKY gene families during anthocyanins biosynthesis in *Lagerstroemia indica* L. *Hortic. Environ. Biotechnol.* **2024**, *65*, 169–180. [CrossRef]
17. Yang, M.; Wang, Y.; Chen, C.; Xin, X.; Dai, S.; Meng, C.; Ma, N. Transcription factor WRKY75 maintains auxin homeostasis to promote tomato defense against *Pseudomonas syringae*. *Plant Physiol.* **2024**, kiae025. [CrossRef]
18. Li, D.; Li, X.; Wang, Z.; Wang, H.; Gao, J.; Liu, X.; Zhang, Z. Transcription factors RhbZIP17 and RhWRKY30 enhance resistance to *Botrytis cinerea* by increasing lignin content in rose petals. *J. Exp. Bot.* **2024**, *75*, 1633–1646. [CrossRef]
19. Tang, R.; Zhu, Y.; Yang, S.; Wang, F.; Chen, G.; Chen, J.; Zhao, K.; Liu, Z.; Peng, D. Genome-Wide Identification and Analysis of WRKY Gene Family in *Melastoma dodecandrum*. *Int. J. Mol. Sci.* **2023**, *24*, 14904. [CrossRef]
20. Meng, L.; Yang, H.; Yang, J.; Ye, T.; Xiang, L.; Chan, Z.; Wang, Y. Tulip transcription factor TgWRKY75 activates salicylic acid and abscisic acid biosynthesis to synergistically promote petal senescence. *J. Exp. Bot.* **2024**, erae021. [CrossRef]
21. Jia, M.; Ni, Y.; Zhao, H.; Liu, X.; Yan, W.; Zhao, X.; Wang, J.; He, B.; Liu, H. Full-length transcriptome and RNA-Seq analyses reveal the resistance mechanism of sesame in response to *Corynespora cassiicola*. *BMC Plant Biol.* **2024**, *24*, 64. [CrossRef] [PubMed]
22. Kim, H.; Kim, J.; Choi, D.S.; Kim, M.-S.; Deslandes, L.; Jayaraman, J.; Sohn, K.H. Molecular basis for the interference of the Arabidopsis WRKY54-mediated immune response by two sequence-unrelated bacterial effectors. *Plant J. Cell Mol. Biol.* **2024**. [CrossRef]
23. Deokar, A.A.; Sagi, M.; Tar'an, B. Genetic Analysis of Partially Resistant and Susceptible Chickpea Cultivars in Response to *Ascochyta rabiei* Infection. *Int. J. Mol. Sci.* **2024**, *25*, 1360. [CrossRef] [PubMed]
24. Chen, W.; Wang, J.; Wang, Z.; Zhu, T.; Zheng, Y.; Hawar, A.; Chang, Y.; Wang, X.; Li, D.; Wang, G.; et al. Capture of regulatory factors via CRISPR-dCas9 for mechanistic analysis of fine-tuned SERRATE expression in *Arabidopsis*. *Nat. Plants* **2024**, *10*, 86–99. [CrossRef] [PubMed]
25. Czarnocka, W.; Karpiński, S. Friend or foe? Reactive oxygen species production, scavenging, and signaling in plant response to environmental stresses. *Free Radic. Biol. Med.* **2018**, *122*, 4–20. [CrossRef] [PubMed]

26. Ahanger, M.A.; Akram, N.A.; Ashraf, M.; Alyemeni, M.N.; Wijaya, L.; Ahmad, P. Plant responses to environmental stresses—From gene to biotechnology. *AoB Plants* **2017**, *9*, plx025. [CrossRef] [PubMed]
27. Xie, X.; He, Z.; Chen, N.; Tang, Z.; Wang, Q.; Cai, Y. The Roles of Environmental Factors in Regulation of Oxidative Stress in Plant. *BioMed Res. Int.* **2019**, *2019*, 9732325. [CrossRef]
28. Doebley, J.; Lukens, L. Transcriptional regulators and the evolution of plant form. *Plant Cell* **1998**, *10*, 1075–1082. [CrossRef]
29. Luo, D.; Xian, C.; Zhang, W.; Qin, Y.; Li, Q.; Usman, M.; Sun, S.; Xing, Y.; Dong, D. Physiological and Transcriptomic Analyses Reveal Commonalities and Specificities in Wheat in Response to Aluminum and Manganese. *Curr. Issues Mol. Biol.* **2024**, *46*, 367–397. [CrossRef]
30. Li, X.Z.; Zhang, X.-T.; Bie, X.-M.; Zhang, J.; Jiang, D.-J.; Tang, H.; Wang, F. Transcriptome analysis of axillary buds in low phosphorus stress and functional analysis of TaWRKY74s in wheat. *BMC Plant Biol.* **2024**, *24*, 1. [CrossRef]
31. Ma, P.; Guo, G.; Xu, X.; Luo, T.; Sun, Y.; Tang, X.; Heng, W.; Jia, B.; Liu, L. Transcriptome Analysis Reveals Key Genes Involved in the Response of *Pyrus betuleafolia* to Drought and High-Temperature Stress. *Plants* **2024**, *13*, 309. [CrossRef] [PubMed]
32. Yu, H.; Guo, Q.; Ji, W.; Wang, H.; Tao, J.; Xu, P.; Chen, X.; Ali, W.; Wu, X.; Shen, X.; et al. Transcriptome Expression Profiling Reveals the Molecular Response to Salt Stress in *Gossipium anomalum* Seedlings. *Plants* **2024**, *13*, 312. [CrossRef] [PubMed]
33. Li, M.; Zhang, X.; Zhang, T.; Bai, Y.; Chen, C.; Guo, D.; Guo, C.; Shu, Y. Genome-wide analysis of the WRKY genes and their important roles during cold stress in white clover. *PeerJ* **2023**, *11*, e15610. [CrossRef] [PubMed]
34. Zhang, Y.; Zhang, W.; Manzoor, M.A.; Sabir, I.A.; Zhang, P.; Cao, Y.; Song, C. Differential involvement of WRKY genes in abiotic stress tolerance of *Dendrobium huoshanense*. *Ind. Crops Prod.* **2023**, *204*, 117295. [CrossRef]
35. Wu, W.; Zhu, S.; Xu, L.; Zhu, L.; Wang, D.; Liu, Y.; Liu, S.; Hao, Z.; Lu, Y.; Yang, L.; et al. Genome-wide identification of the Liriodendron chinense WRKY gene family and its diverse roles in response to multiple abiotic stress. *BMC Plant Biol.* **2022**, *22*, 25. [CrossRef] [PubMed]
36. Soltis, D.E.; Bell, C.D.; Kim, S.; Soltis, P.S. Origin and early evolution of angiosperms. *Ann. N. Y. Acad. Sci.* **2008**, *1133*, 3–25. [CrossRef] [PubMed]
37. Wikstrom, N.; Savolainen, V.; Chase, M.W. Evolution of the angiosperms: Calibrating the family tree. *Proc. Biol. Sci.* **2001**, *268*, 2211–2220. [CrossRef]
38. Chen, M.; Li, M.; Zhao, L.; Song, H. Deciphering evolutionary dynamics of WRKY genes in Arachis species. *BMC Genom.* **2023**, *24*, 48. [CrossRef]
39. Tang, W.; Wang, F.; Chu, H.; You, M.; Lv, Q.; Ji, W.; Deng, X.; Zhou, B.; Peng, D. WRKY transcription factors regulate phosphate uptake in plants. *Environ. Exp. Bot.* **2023**, *208*, 105241. [CrossRef]
40. An, X.; Liu, Q.; Jiang, H.; Dong, G.; Tian, D.; Luo, X.; Chen, C.; Li, W.; Liu, T.; Zou, L.; et al. Bioinformatics Analysis of WRKY Family Genes in Flax (*Linum usitatissimum*). *Life* **2023**, *13*, 1258. [CrossRef]
41. Li, W.; Pang, S.; Lu, Z.; Jin, B. Function and Mechanism of WRKY Transcription Factors in Abiotic Stress Responses of Plants. *Plants* **2020**, *9*, 1515. [CrossRef] [PubMed]
42. Mohanta, T.K.; Park, Y.; Bae, H. Novel Genomic and Evolutionary Insight of WRKY Transcription Factors in Plant Lineage. *Sci. Rep.* **2016**, *6*, 37309. [CrossRef] [PubMed]
43. Yang, R.; Huang, T.; Song, W.; An, Z.; Lai, Z.; Liu, S. Identification of WRKY gene family members in amaranth based on a transcriptome database and functional analysis of AtrWRKY42-2 in betalain metabolism. *Front. Plant Sci.* **2023**, *14*, 1300522. [CrossRef] [PubMed]
44. Khan, I.; Asaf, S.; Jan, R.; Bilal, S.; Lubna; Khan, A.L.; Kim, K.-M.; Al-Harrasi, A. Genome-wide annotation and expression analysis of WRKY and bHLH transcriptional factor families reveal their involvement under cadmium stress in tomato (*Solanum lycopersicum* L.). *Front. Plant Sci.* **2023**, *14*, 1100895. [CrossRef] [PubMed]
45. Ge, M.; Tang, Y.; Guan, Y.; Lv, M.; Zhou, C.; Ma, H.; Lv, J. TaWRKY31, a novel WRKY transcription factor in wheat, participates in regulation of plant drought stress tolerance. *BMC Plant Biol.* **2024**, *24*, 27. [CrossRef] [PubMed]
46. Gu, L.; Hou, Y.; Sun, Y.; Chen, X.; Wang, H.; Zhu, B.; Du, X. ZmB12D, a target of transcription factor ZmWRKY70, enhances the tolerance of Arabidopsis to submergence. *Plant Physiol. Biochem.* **2024**, *206*, 108322. [CrossRef] [PubMed]
47. Wang, Y.; Dong, B.; Wang, N.; Zheng, Z.; Yang, L.; Zhong, S.; Fang, Q.; Xiao, Z.; Zhao, H. A WRKY Transcription Factor PmWRKY57 from *Prunus mume* Improves Cold Tolerance in *Arabidopsis thaliana*. *Mol. Biotechnol.* **2023**, *65*, 1359–1368. [CrossRef]
48. Wang, L.; Guo, D.; Zhao, G.; Wang, J.; Zhang, S.; Wang, C.; Guo, X. Group IIc WRKY transcription factors regulate cotton resistance to *Fusarium oxysporum* by promoting GhMKK2-mediated flavonoid biosynthesis. *New Phytol.* **2022**, *236*, 249–265. [CrossRef]
49. Goodstein, D.M.; Shu, S.; Howson, R.; Neupane, R.; Hayes, R.D.; Fazo, J.; Mitros, T.; Dirks, W.; Hellsten, U.; Putnam, N.; et al. Phytozome: A comparative platform for green plant genomics. *Nucleic Acids Res.* **2012**, *40*, D1178–D1186. [CrossRef]
50. Emms, D.M.; Kelly, S. OrthoFinder: Phylogenetic orthology inference for comparative genomics. *Genome Biol.* **2019**, *20*, 238. [CrossRef]
51. Emms, D.M.; Kelly, S. OrthoFinder: Solving fundamental biases in whole genome comparisons dramatically improves orthogroup inference accuracy. *Genome Biol.* **2015**, *16*, 157. [CrossRef]
52. Kumar, S.; Suleski, M.; Craig, J.M.; Kasprowicz, A.E.; Sanderford, M.; Li, M.; Stecher, G.; Hedges, S.B. TimeTree 5: An Expanded Resource for Species Divergence Times. *Mol. Biol. Evol.* **2022**, *39*, msac174. [CrossRef]

53. Barido-Sottani, J.; Morlon, H. The ClaDS rate-heterogeneous birth-death prior for full phylogenetic inference in BEAST2. *Syst. Biol.* **2023**, *72*, 1180–1187. [CrossRef]

54. Li, J.; Zhang, Z.; Vang, S.; Yu, J.; Wong, G.K.-S.; Wang, J. Correlation between Ka/Ks and Ks is related to substitution model and evolutionary lineage. *J. Mol. Evol.* **2009**, *68*, 414–423. [CrossRef]

55. Peterson, G.I.; Masel, J. Quantitative prediction of molecular clock and ka/ks at short timescales. *Mol. Biol. Evol.* **2009**, *26*, 2595–2603. [CrossRef]

56. Hurst, L.D. The Ka/Ks ratio: Diagnosing the form of sequence evolution. *Trends Genet.* **2002**, *18*, 486. [CrossRef] [PubMed]

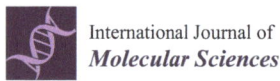

International Journal of
Molecular Sciences

MDPI

Review

NO and H₂S Contribute to Crop Resilience against Atmospheric Stressors

Francisco J. Corpas

Group of Antioxidants, Free Radicals and Nitric Oxide in Biotechnology, Food and Agriculture, Department of Stress, Development and Signaling in Plants, Estación Experimental del Zaidín, Spanish National Research Council (CSIC), Profesor Albareda 1, E-18008 Granada, Spain; javier.corpas@eez.csic.es

Abstract: Atmospheric stressors include a variety of pollutant gases such as CO_2, nitrous oxide (NOx), and sulfurous compounds which could have a natural origin or be generated by uncontrolled human activity. Nevertheless, other atmospheric elements including high and low temperatures, ozone (O_3), UV-B radiation, or acid rain among others can affect, at different levels, a large number of plant species, particularly those of agronomic interest. Paradoxically, both nitric oxide (NO) and hydrogen sulfide (H_2S), until recently were considered toxic since they are part of the polluting gases; however, at present, these molecules are part of the mechanism of response to multiple stresses since they exert signaling functions which usually have an associated stimulation of the enzymatic and non-enzymatic antioxidant systems. At present, these gasotransmitters are considered essential components of the defense against a wide range of environmental stresses including atmospheric ones. This review aims to provide an updated vision of the endogenous metabolism of NO and H_2S in plant cells and to deepen how the exogenous application of these compounds can contribute to crop resilience, particularly, against atmospheric stressors stimulating antioxidant systems.

Keywords: acid rain; abiotic stress; gasotransmitters; oxidative stress; ozone; persulfidation; posttranslational modifications; *S*-nitrosation

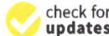

check for updates

Citation: Corpas, F.J. NO and H₂S Contribute to Crop Resilience against Atmospheric Stressors. *Int. J. Mol. Sci.* **2024**, *25*, 3509. https://doi.org/10.3390/ijms25063509

Academic Editors: Philippe Jeandet and Mateusz Labudda

Received: 10 March 2024
Revised: 16 March 2024
Accepted: 18 March 2024
Published: 20 March 2024

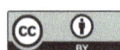
1. Introduction

Higher plants, as sessile organisms, are recurrently subjected to environmental changes throughout their life cycle. Among the different atmospheric stressors, it can be mentioned that high and low temperatures, hailstorms, absence of rain (drought), extreme rain (waterlogging), ozone, ultraviolet (UV-B) radiation, CO_2, methane, or nitrogen oxide (NOx) among others which effects on plants can be increased under the current climate change pattern [1–3]. The majority of them have a natural origin, but the negative effects of some of them could be increased by human activity. Furthermore, these atmospheric pollutants can affect extensive areas, but others can affect more restricted areas due to local phenomena, for example, the emissions of polluting gases by volcanoes or certain industries. However, the degree of pollution effects on a specific plant will depend on its intensity and the distance from the emission source.

Nitric oxide ($^\bullet NO$) is a free radical that is part of the nitrogen cycle and in the atmosphere, in the presence of oxygen, it quickly transforms into nitrogen dioxide ($^\bullet NO_2$), and both constitute nitrogen oxide (NOx). Figure 1a,b illustrates how atmospheric $^\bullet NO$, as a pollutant, participates in the formation of acid rain as well as in the destruction of the ozone layer [4,5]. For many plant species, the negative effects triggered by nitrogen oxides (NOx) have been estimated when the level of NOx is around 30 μg/m³. However, there is experimental evidence suggesting that moderate concentrations of NOx may have both positive and negative plant growth responses [6,7].

On the other hand, atmospheric hydrogen sulfide (H_2S) comes from different sources such as volcanoes, geothermal vents, or wetlands where it is generated by bacteria during the anaerobic decay of organic sulfur compounds [8–10]. In the atmosphere, H_2S is oxidized to sulfur dioxide (SO_2), which then can be converted to sulfuric acid (H_2SO_4) and participates in acid rain (Figure 1a).

(a) Acid rain

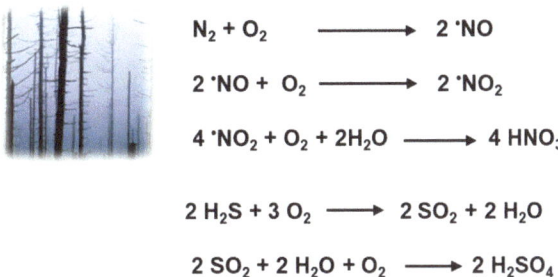

$$N_2 + O_2 \longrightarrow 2\ ^\bullet NO$$

$$2\ ^\bullet NO + O_2 \longrightarrow 2\ ^\bullet NO_2$$

$$4\ ^\bullet NO_2 + O_2 + 2H_2O \longrightarrow 4\ HNO_3$$

$$2\ H_2S + 3\ O_2 \longrightarrow 2\ SO_2 + 2\ H_2O$$

$$2\ SO_2 + 2\ H_2O + O_2 \longrightarrow 2\ H_2SO_4$$

(b) Ozone layer destruction

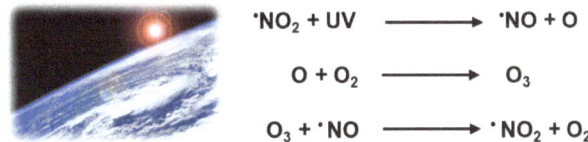

$$^\bullet NO_2 + UV \longrightarrow\ ^\bullet NO + O$$

$$O + O_2 \longrightarrow O_3$$

$$O_3 +\ ^\bullet NO \longrightarrow\ ^\bullet NO_2 + O_2$$

Figure 1. Nitric oxide ($^\bullet NO$) and hydrogen sulfide (H_2S) participate in atmospheric pollution such as acid rain and the destruction of the ozone layer. (**a**) Nitrogen (N_2) has a greater presence in the atmosphere but in the occurrence of atmospheric oxygen, it quickly transforms into nitrogen dioxide ($^\bullet NO_2$). Nitrogen oxides are acidic, and they can form nitric acid (HNO_3) which can be dissolved in water, giving rise to acid rain. Similarly, H_2S can also react with O_2 to generate sulfur dioxide (SO_2) which reacts with water droplets in clouds to create sulfuric acid (H_2SO_4). (**b**) $^\bullet NO_2$ due to ultraviolet (UV) radiation generates $^\bullet NO$ and atomic oxygen, which together with O_2 generates ozone, which reacts with $^\bullet NO$, generating $^\bullet NO_2$ and oxygen, which constitutes the photolytic cycle of the destruction of the O_3 layer.

From the time when $^\bullet NO$ and H_2S were identified and characterized in the 18th century, these molecules have been considered toxic molecules that exert negative effects on all organisms. At the end of the 20th century, it was found that $^\bullet NO$ and H_2S can be generated endogenously in both animal and plant cells [11–14]. As a result, the concept of "toxic" molecules changed, and to date, they have been shown to both exert regulatory and signaling functions in many plant processes such as seed germination, root development, plant growth, stomatal movement, senescence, fruit development and ripening as well as response mechanisms to both abiotic and biotic stresses [15–17]. Thus, both $^\bullet NO$ and H_2S have paradoxical effects as atmospheric pollutants but also as signaling molecules that are endogenously generated in cells. Likewise, there are numerous examples that their exogenous application, individually or in combination, exerts beneficial effects against atmospheric stress.

This review aims to provide an updated vision of the endogenous metabolism of $^\bullet NO$ and H_2S in plant cells and to deepen how the exogenous application of these compounds can contribute to crop resilience against some representative atmospheric stressors such as extreme temperature, O_3, UV-B radiation, and acid rain.

2. $^\bullet NO$ and H_2S Metabolism in Higher Plants

Our knowledge about $^\bullet NO$ and H_2S metabolism has increased significantly during the last decade considering that these two molecules were considered toxic until they were found to be endogenously generated in animal cells [13,14].

The enzymatic generation of $^\bullet$NO in higher plants has been very controversial since its generation was discovered. Currently, two main enzymatic pathways have been generally accepted, the reductive and the oxidative pathways [18–20]. The reductive pathway is the one that uses nitrate and nitrite as substrates using NADH as an electron donor, being linked to the nitrate reductase (NR) and nitrite reductase (NiR) activities [21–24]. On the other hand, there is the oxidative pathway, which is considered similar to the nitric oxide synthase (NOS) of animal cells, since it starts with L-arginine using NADPH as the electron donor and FAD, FMN, calcium, calmodulin, and tetrabiopterin as cofactors, so it is called L-Arg-dependent NOS-like activity because the gene similar to that of animal organisms that encodes it has not been identified [25–27]. In addition, there is another possible route that, from polyamines or oximes, seems to be involved in the generation of $^\bullet$NO [28–30]. However, we must not rule out other possible enzymatic or non-enzymatic sources that should be involved in the generation of $^\bullet$NO.

The generation of H_2S in plants is part of the sulfate assimilation pathway and the cysteine biosynthesis pathway. Currently, there are several enzymes located in different subcellular compartments involved in the generation of H_2S [31,32]. Figure 2a,b shows the main enzymatic source involved in the generation of $^\bullet$NO and H_2S in higher plants.

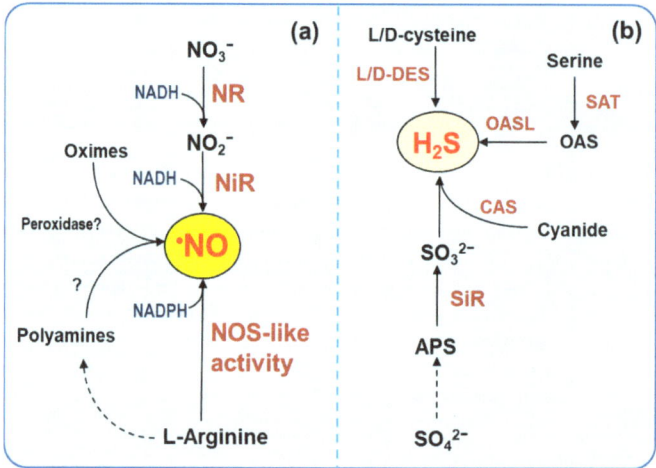

Figure 2. Main enzymatic source of $^\bullet$NO and H_2S in higher plant cells. (**a**) Nitrate reductase (NR), nitrite reductase (NiR), and L-arginine-dependent nitric oxide synthase (NOS)-like activity are the recognized major candidates for enzymatic $^\bullet$NO sources in the different subcellular compartments of higher plants. (**b**) The biosynthesis of H_2S in plants is part of sulfur and cysteine metabolism which primarily involves several enzymes located in the cytosol, plastids, and mitochondria including L/D-cysteine desulfhydrase (L/D-DES), cyanoalanine synthase (CAS), serine acetyltransferase (SAT), sulfite reductase (SiR), and O-acetyl-l-serine(thiol)lyase (OASL), also named cysteine synthase. APS, adenosine 5′-phosphosulfate. Dashed line, indicates different stages. ?, unidentified.

3. $^\bullet$NO- and H_2S-Derived Posttranslational Modifications (PTMs) as Tools to Regulate Plant Metabolism

$^\bullet$NO and derived molecules called reactive nitrogen species (RNS) can affect the function of different macromolecules through their specific interactions. Among the RNS, it is worth highlighting peroxynitrite ($ONOO^-$) which is the result of the chemical reaction between $^\bullet$NO and superoxide radical ($O_2^{\bullet-}$) [33] or S-nitrosoglutathione (GSNO), which results from the interaction of $^\bullet$NO with reduced glutathione (GSH) [34,35]. RNS can mediate several post-translational modifications (PTMs) that affect different macromolecules including peptides, proteins, fatty acids, and nucleotides. Thus, RNS interacts with thiol groups present in Cys residues to generate the corresponding S-nitrosated protein, with tyrosine residues to generate tyrosine nitration or bind to metals present in certain proteins in a process designed as metal nitrosylation [36–39]. $^\bullet$NO can also interact with other biomolecules including unsaturated fatty acids (FAs) to form the corresponding nitro-FAs [40] and nucleic acids through guanine or guanosine to generate 8-nitroguanine or 8-nitroguanosine, respectively [41,42].

H$_2$S mediates another PTM named persulfidation which involves its interaction with the thiol group (-SH) of susceptible Cys residues. Similar to *S*-nitrosation, persulfidation is a reversible covalent interaction but, in this case, the thiol group is converted into a persulfide (-SSH) group which can affect positively or negatively the function of the target proteins [43,44]. Figure 3 illustrates the main PTMs mediated by $^\bullet$NO and H$_2$S. However, in a cellular context, it should be considered that the thiol groups of Cys residues are susceptible to being targets of other thiol-based oxidative posttranslational modifications (OxiPTMs) mediated by glutathione (*S*-glutathionylation), H$_2$O$_2$ (*S*-sulfenylation), fatty acids (*S*-acylation) or cyanide (*S*-cyanylation) that can compete with each other depending on their cellular concentrations and the subcellular location of the target protein [45–49]. However, in conditions of oxidative stress resulting from environmental stress, some of them may have a greater preponderance, such as an increase in H$_2$O$_2$.

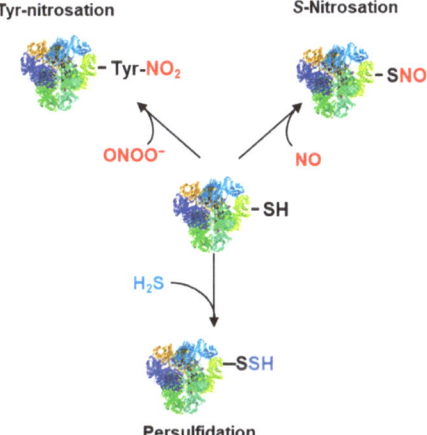

Figure 3. Protein postranslational modifications (PTMs) mediated by either $^\bullet$NO (*S*-nitrosation and tyrosine nitration) or H$_2$S (persulfidation). ONOO$^-$, peroxynitrite.

4. Stomata Movement, a Process Regulated by $^\bullet$NO and H$_2$S

Stomata are specialized cells that regulate gas exchange in the leaves and stomatal closure is one of the response mechanisms against atmospheric stress [50–52]. It is interesting to mention that both $^\bullet$NO and H$_2$S are molecules that, although they may be polluting molecules, are also generated endogenously by regulating stomatal closure through PTMs including tyrosine nitration, *S*-nitrosation, and persulfidation. Thus, $^\bullet$NO and H$_2$S are part of the crosstalk with other signal molecules such as abscisic acid (ABA), Ca^{2+}, H$_2$O$_2$, and ethylene among others participate in the regulation of stomatal movement [53–58]. Figure 4 shows a simple model of the main signals involved in the stomata closure where it highlights the main effect of $^\bullet$NO and H$_2$S. Thus, $^\bullet$NO seems to be generated either via NR or a NOS-like activity whereas H$_2$S is generated by an L-cysteine desulfhydrase (LCD) activity. NR can be inhibited by tyrosine nitration (NO$_2$-Tyr) [24]. On the other hand, H$_2$O$_2$ is produced by a respiratory burst oxidase homolog (RBOH) type D/F. H$_2$S triggers the generation of H$_2$O$_2$ by persulfidation of RBOH [59] whereas it can be inhibited by *S*-nitrosation. $^\bullet$NO can inactivate the ABA receptor PYR/PYL/RCAR by a process of tyrosine nitration (NO$_2$-Tyr), but $^\bullet$NO can also negatively regulate the open stomata 1 (OST1)/sucrose nonfermenting 1 (SNF1)-related protein kinase 2.6 (SnRK2.6) complex by *S*-nitrosation (Cys-NO). But SnRK2.6 can be activated by persulfidation [60,61]. On the other hand, ethylene induces H_2S production in guard cells and this H_2S can then inhibit the synthesis of ethylene by the inhibition of 1-aminocyclopropane-1-carboxylic acid oxidase (ACO) activity by persulfidation (Cys-SSH) at Cys60 [62].

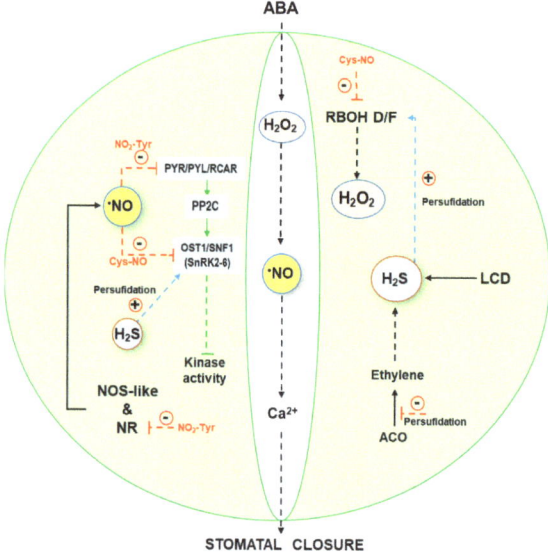

Figure 4. Simple model of the signaling cascade mediated by abscisic acid (ABA), H_2O_2, ethylene and Ca^{2+} where $^\bullet NO$ and H_2S participate in the stomatal closure in response to atmospheric stresses. PP2C, protein phosphatase 2C; PYR/PYL/RCAR, pyrabactin resistance1/PYR1-like/regulatory components of ABA receptor. Red dashed lines indicate inhibitory effects. Blue dashed arrows indicate positive effects. Green dashed line, indicates blocking of activity.

Thus, it is well established that stomata movement as it has happened with photosynthesis activity can be affected by numerous atmospheric pollutants [63–68].

5. Atmospheric Pollutants and Higher Plant Response—What Happens to $^\bullet NO$ and H_2S When It Is Applied Exogenously?

At present, it is known that plants can emit $^\bullet NO$ [11,69–71] and H_2S [12,72,73] to their surrounding atmosphere; however, plants could also release other gases such as CO_2, nitrous oxide (N_2O) [74,75] and methane (CH_4) [76,77] which are part of the greenhouse gases that contribute to global warming. At the same time, it is important to note that atmospheric $^\bullet NO$/NOx and H_2S may be adsorbed at the leaf's surface through the stomata [65,78–80], and depending on their concentration, these gases can have either negative or beneficial effects on higher plants. For example, it has been pointed out that $^\bullet NO$ seems to be a key signaling molecule in the mechanism of response against higher levels of atmospheric gases including CO_2, N_2O, CH_4, or O_3 which usually provoke stress in plants that have associated oxidative stress because they trigger an uncontrolled increase in the generation of ROS and RNS associated with a lower antioxidant capacity [81]. Thus, the harmful or beneficial effects of the gas exchanges between plants and the surrounding atmosphere will depend on their final concentration inside the cells.

On the other hand, $^\bullet NO$ and H_2S as signaling molecules that are involved in numerous biological processes in higher plants, have started to be applied exogenously as alternative biotechnology tools since it has been proven that they can exert benefit effects to palliate the negative effects caused by different atmospheric factors such as high and low temperatures, O_3, UV-B radiation or acid rain among others.

5.1. High and Low Temperature

Higher plants, during their development, are exposed to seasonal changes in temperature; consequently, they have developed the corresponding strategic adaptations that have allowed them to survive in a specific ecosystem [82–84]. However, plants can also undergo unusual extreme temperatures provoking undesirable effects. For example, *Arabidopsis thaliana* exposed to heat stress (38 °C) experiences an increase in the H_2O_2 content in chloroplasts which triggers the *S*-sulfenylation of the 2-phosphoglycolate phosphatase 1 at Cys86 producing its inhibition and, consequently, provoking the accumulation of 2-phosphoglycolate which has toxic effects because it inhibits the enzymes triose-phosphate isomerase and phosphofructokinase which are required for CO_2 assimilation [85]. In these cases, plants have to trigger a different mechanism of responses in which ${}^\bullet$NO and H_2S, along with other regulatory molecules, participate to react and alleviate possible damages caused by extreme temperatures [86–91].

Tables 1 and 2 show some examples of how ${}^\bullet$NO and H_2S applied exogenously can contribute to reducing the damage associated with high and low temperatures and how antioxidant systems are stimulated to alleviate oxidative damages associated with extreme temperatures. It should be mentioned that in the majority of studies in plants, the most widely used donors are sodium nitroprusside (SNP) for ${}^\bullet$NO and sodium hydrosulfide (NaHS) for H_2S. The main reason is that both donors have a low economic cost compared to other ${}^\bullet$NO donors such as GSNO or NONOates or H_2S donors such as GYY4137 or sulfobiotic-H_2S donors 5a, 8ℓ, and 8o. SNP and NaHS donors are usually applied either by spraying the aerial part of the plant or by adding it to the nutrient solution.

5.2. Ozone (O_3)

According to the predictions of Wang et al. [92], the increase in atmospheric O_3 has been estimated to be 20–25% by 2050 and it has already been proven that a high content of O_3 can negatively affect plant metabolism and growth [93–95] which usually triggers an increase in ROS metabolism [96,97]. For example, in tobacco plants exposed to O_3, an accumulation of ${}^\bullet$NO and H_2O_2 was found [98]. In the case of *Phaseolus vulgaris*, O_3 reduces the chlorophyll content and increases the content of ROS [99]. Tables 1 and 2 show some representative examples of how ${}^\bullet$NO and H_2S applied exogenously to plants can contribute to providing metabolic adaptations to high levels of atmospheric O_3.

5.3. UV-B Radiation

UV radiation is a non-ionizing radiation that is produced by the sun and three categories of UV radiation can be distinguished according to the wavelength: 315–400 nm corresponds to UV-A, 280–315 nm to UV-B, and 100–280 nm to UV-C. UV-B radiation is the most studied in plants due to its increase on the earth's surface as a consequence of the depletion of the stratospheric O_3 layer since the atmosphere intercepts around 77% UV radiation. In this sense, plants under UV-B radiation trigger nonspecific responses such as DNA damage and an increase in ROS production as well as specific ones that involve photomorphogenic signals affecting the gene expression of *UV-resistance locus 8* (*UVR8*) and *constitutive photomorphogenesis 1* (*COP1*) accompanied by the transcription factor elongated hypocotyl 5 (HY5) [100–104].

Accumulating data indicate that in plants under UV-B radiation, the metabolism of ${}^\bullet$NO and H_2S is exacerbated and contributes to palliating the damaged symptoms [105–110]. For example, in leaves of kidney beans (*Phaseolus vulgaris*) exposed to UV-B stress it was found that ${}^\bullet$NO generation was associated with a NOS-like activity being mediated by H_2O_2 [106]. Additionally, the exogenous application of ${}^\bullet$NO and H_2S has been shown to contribute at different levels to diminishing the negative impact of UV-B radiation mainly by stimulating at gene and protein levels the different antioxidant systems. Tables 1 and 2 display representative examples of how exogenous ${}^\bullet$NO and H_2S applied can palliate the negative impact of UV-B radiation in plants.

5.4. Acid Rain

As mentioned above, acid rain is the consequence of the presence of NOx and/or SO_2 in the air during precipitation (Figure 1a). Acid rain damages plant growth since it affects photosynthesis and, in general, triggers a response of the antioxidant systems to palliate the oxidative stress [5,111,112]. Some examples show that the exogenous application of several compounds such as glutathione, melatonin, or silicon could help to palliate the harmful effect on plants [113]. In the model plant, *Arabidopsis thaliana* exposed to acid rain has been found to have an active nitrogen metabolism which has an elevated •NO production and provides a tolerance to acid rain [111]. Table 1 summarizes how the exogenous •NO application modulates the plant response to acid rain.

Table 1. Main effects of the exogenous application of •NO plants exposed to diverse atmospheric stressors.

•NO Donor	Plant Species	Effects	Ref.
		Low temperature	
0.1 mM SNP	Jujube (*Ziziphus jujube*) fruit	Exogenous NO inhibits the development of chilling injury by maintaining cellular redox homeostasis through the presence of *S*-nitrosation of superoxide dismutase and catalase.	[114]
0.2 mM SNP	Cowpea (*Vigna unguiculata*)	Diminish the production of ROS and the content of MDA. Delay the degradation of photosynthetic pigments, increase the content of proline, and the activity of antioxidant enzymes such as SOD, catalase, and component of the ascorbate-glutathione cycle.	[115]
50 µM GSNO	Chinese Cabbage (*Brassica rapa*)	Simultaneous •NO treatment with brassinosteroids increases the leaf area, stem diameter, chlorophyll content, dry and fresh weight, and proline content. Decrease the MDA content.	[116]
		High temperature	
50 µM SNP	Wheat (*Triticum aestivum* L.)	Improve growth and photosynthetic parameters. Mitigate the oxidative stress. Increase membrane stability index.	[117,118]
100 µM SNP	Rice (*Oryza sativa* L.)	•NO interacts with ethylene and H_2S metabolism. Activation of the antioxidant system such as components of the ascorbate–glutathione cycle, accumulation of osmolytes with the concomitant increase in thermos tolerance.	[119,120]
		Ozone (O_3)	
50 µM SNP	*Arabidopsis thaliana*	•NO enhances O_3-induced cell death, possibly by altering the NO–ROS balance. Decrease salicylic acid and increase jasmonic acid concentrations.	[121]
200 µM SNP	Wheat (*Triticum aestivum* L.)	NO is involved in ozone tolerance. It enhances the net photosynthetic rate while reducing H_2O_2, membrane peroxidation, and electrolyte leakage. Increase SOD and POD activities.	[122]
		UV-B radiation	
SNP	Bean (*Phaseolus vulgaris*) leaves	Decrease chlorophyll contents and oxidative damage to the thylakoid membrane. Increase activities of SOD, APX, and catalase.	[123]
100 µM SNP	Maize (*Zea mays* L.) leaves	Induce the accumulation of flavonoids and anthocyanin that absorb UV-B radiation.	[124]
0.8 mM SNP	Soybean leaves (*Glycine max* L.)	Up-regulate the gene expression and activity of antioxidant enzymes	[125]

Table 1. *Cont.*

•NO Donor	Plant Species	Effects	Ref.
		Acid rain	
0.5 mM SNP	Longan (*Dimocarpus longana*) seedlings	Under acid rain (pH 3.0), exogenous •NO provokes an increase in total chlorophyll, soluble protein, and soluble sugar as well as the activity of antioxidant enzymes (SOD, POD and CAT) whereas it decreases the MDA content.	[126]
0.1 mM SNP	*Arabidopsis thaliana*	•NO treatment decreases the leaf necrosis whereas it increases the fresh weight.	[111]
0.25 mM SNP	*Vigna radiata* seedlings	Under simulated acid rain (pH 2), exogenous •NO triggers an increase in antioxidant activities (SOD, POD, and APX), NR activiy and NO content whereas it decreases MDA content.	[7]

APX, ascorbate peroxidase. CAT, catalase. GSNO, S-nitrosoglutathione. MDA, malondialdehyde. NR, nitrtate reductase. POD, peroxidase. SNP, sodium nitroprusside. SOD, superoxide dismutase.

Table 2. Main effects of the exogenous application of H2S plants exposed to diverse environmental stressors.

H$_2$S Donor	Plant Species	Effects	Ref.
		Low Temperature	
50 µM NaHS	Cucumber (*Cucumis sativus* L.)	Increase the content of GSH' and cucurbitacin C. H$_2$O$_2$ as a downstream signal of IAA mediates H$_2$S-induced chilling tolerance.	[127,128]
0.5 mM NaHS	Pepper (*Capsicum annuum* L.)	Increase the content of endogenous H$_2$S and the integrity of the membrane system. Enhance the photosynthetic rate, stomatal conductance, transpiration rate, and photosynthesis. Reduce the intercellular CO$_2$ concentration. Increase antioxidant activities (SOD, catalase, and ascorbate-glutathione cycle).	[129]
0.5 mM NaHS	Blueberry (*Vaccinium corymbosum*) leaves	Promote the electron transfer from Q A to Q B on the PSII acceptor side and alleviate the degradation of chlorophyll and carotenoids. Increase proline content.	[130]
0.5 mM NaHS	Alfalfa (*Medicago truncatula*)	Improve the height, number of leaves, and fresh and dry shoot weights. Increase tolerance by regulating the antioxidant defense system and enhancing photosynthetic capacity.	[131]
		High temperature	
100 µM NaHS	Strawberry (*Fragaria* × *ananassa* cv. 'Camarosa')	Induction of gene expression of antioxidant enzymes (cAPX, CAT, MnSOD, GR), heat shock proteins (HSP70, HSP80, HSP90) and aquaporins (PIP).	[132]
500 µM NaHS	Maize (*Zea mays* L.)	Improve seed germination and increase antioxidant enzymes. Accumulation of proline.	[133]
50 µM NaHS or 10 µM GYY4137	Poplar (*Populus trichocarpa*)	Increase GSNOR activity and reduce HT-induced damage to the photosynthetic system.	[134]
100 µM NaHS or 10 µM GYY4137	*Arabidopsis thaliana*	Enhance seed germination rate under HT. Increase gene expression of *ABI5* (ABA-INSENSITIVE 5).	[135]
		UV B radiation	
125 µM NaHS	Borage (*Borago officinalis* L.)	Decrease the MDA carbonyl groups, and H$_2$O$_2$ content. Increase the activities of APX and guaiacol peroxidase.	[136]

ABA, abscisic acid. APX, ascorbate peroxidase. CAT, catalase. GSH, reduced glutathione. IAA, indole-3-acetic acid. MDA, malondialdehyde. NaHS, sodium hydrosulfide. SOD, superoxide dismutase.

6. Conclusions and Future Perspectives

•NO and H$_2$S have become paradoxical molecules in plant biology since they have gone from being hazardous molecules to becoming essential molecules in cellular metabolism, regulating physiological processes from seed germination, root development, photosynthesis, senescence, stomatal closure, formation of flowers and fruit ripening, in addition to participating in the response mechanisms against challenging environments. Paradoxically, the available information demonstrates that the exogenous application of these molecules can be biotechnological tools that allow for promoting crop resilience [137,138]. In most cases, these gasotransmitters stimulate enzymatic and non-enzymatic antioxidant systems, for example, the APX activity is upregulated by S-nitrosation and persulfidation [139,140] which makes it possible to alleviate oxidative damage associated with atmospheric stressors, protecting the functionality of cells, and maintaining photosynthetic activity (Figure 5). Although we are still in the basic studies to understand the intimate molecular mechanisms exerted by $^{\bullet}$NO and H_2S, it would be of great interest to establish protocols on how the exogenous application of these molecules can allow us to combat atmospheric stressors or other types of abiotic or biotic stresses, allowing us to connect the basic knowledge and its application to the agricultural productive sector [141,142].

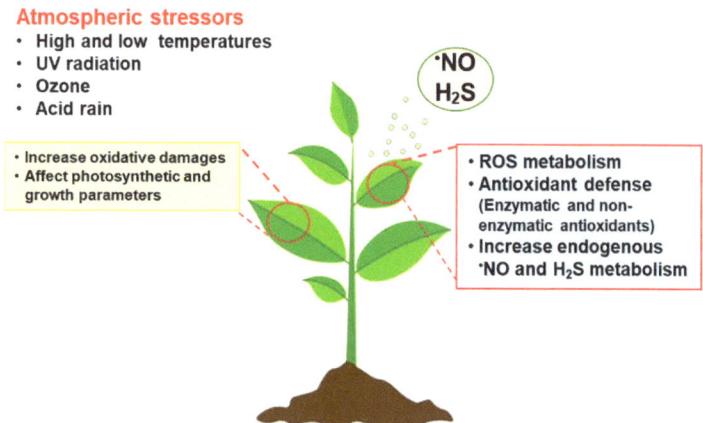

Figure 5. Working model of the main effects of the exogenous application of $^{\bullet}$NO or H_2S under several atmospheric stressors which trigger an active ROS metabolism with the induction of antioxidant systems.

Funding: F.J.C. research is supported by European Regional Development Fund co-financed grants from the Ministry of Science and Innovation (PID2019-103924GB-I00), the AEI (10.13039/501100011033), and Junta de Andalucía (P18-FR-1359), Spain.

Conflicts of Interest: Author has no conflict of interest to declare.

References

1. Bal, S.K.; Minhas, P.S. Atmospheric Stressors: Challenges and Coping Strategies. In *Abiotic Stress Management for Resilient Agriculture*; Minhas, P., Rane, J., Pasala, R., Eds.; Springer: Singapore, 2017. [CrossRef]
2. Bornman, J.F.; Barnes, P.W.; Robson, T.M.; Robinson, S.A.; Jansen, M.A.K.; Ballaré, C.L.; Flint, S.D. Linkages between stratospheric ozone, UV radiation and climate change and their implications for terrestrial ecosystems. *Photochem. Photobiol. Sci.* **2019**, *18*, 681–716. [CrossRef]
3. Roy, S.; Kapoor, R.; Mathur, P. Revisiting Changes in Growth, Physiology and Stress Responses of Plants under the Effect of Enhanced CO_2 and Temperature. *Plant Cell Physiol.* **2024**, *65*, 4–19. [CrossRef] [PubMed]
4. Ravishankara, A.R.; Daniel, J.S.; Portmann, R.W. Nitrous oxide (N_2O): The dominant ozone-depleting substance emitted in the 21st century. *Science* **2009**, *326*, 123–125. [CrossRef]
5. Shi, Z.; Zhang, J.; Xiao, Z.; Lu, T.; Ren, X.; Wei, H. Effects of acid rain on plant growth: A meta-analysis. *J. Environ. Manage* **2021**, *297*, 113213. [CrossRef] [PubMed]
6. Chaparro-Suarez, I.G.; Meixner, F.X.; Kesselmeier, J. Nitrogen dioxide (NO_2) uptake by vegetation controlled by atmospheric concentrations and plant stomatal aperture. *Atmos. Environ.* **2011**, *45*, 5742–5750. [CrossRef]
7. Jiao, R.; Zhang, M.; Wei, Z.; Xu, J.; Zhang, H. Alleviative effects of nitric oxide on *Vigna radiata* seedlings under acidic rain stress. *Mol. Biol. Rep.* **2021**, *48*, 2243–2251. [CrossRef]

8. Williams-Jones, G.; Rymer, H. Hazards of volcanic gases. In *The Encyclopedia of Volcanoes*; Academic Press: Cambridge, MA, USA, 2015; pp. 985–992.
9. Lloyd, D. Hydrogen sulfide: Clandestine microbial messenger? *Trends Microbiol.* **2006**, *14*, 456–462. [CrossRef]
10. Fuentes-Lara, L.O.; Medrano-Macías, J.; Pérez-Labrada, F.; Rivas-Martínez, E.N.; García-Enciso, E.L.; González-Morales, S.; Juárez-Maldonado, A.; Rincón-Sánchez, F.; Benavides-Mendoza, A. From Elemental Sulfur to Hydrogen Sulfide in Agricultural Soils and Plants. *Molecules* **2019**, *24*, 2282. [CrossRef] [PubMed]
11. Klepper, L. Nitric oxide (NO) and nitrogen dioxide (NO$_2$) emissions from herbicide-treated soybean plants. *Atmos. Environ.* **1979**, *13*, 537–542. [CrossRef]
12. Sekiya, J.; Schmidt, A.; Wilson, L.G.; Filner, P. Emission of Hydrogen Sulfide by Leaf Tissue in Response to L-Cysteine. *Plant Physiol.* **1982**, *70*, 430–436. [CrossRef]
13. Palmer, R.M.; Ferrige, A.G.; Moncada, S. Nitric oxide release accounts for the biological activity of endothelium-derived relaxing factor. *Nature* **1987**, *327*, 524–526. [CrossRef]
14. Abe, K.; Kimura, H. The possible role of hydrogen sulfide as an endogenous neuromodulator. *J. Neurosci.* **1996**, *6*, 1066–1071. [CrossRef] [PubMed]
15. Yamasaki, H.; Cohen, M.F. Biological consilience of hydrogen sulfide and nitric oxide in plants: Gases of primordial earth linking plant, microbial and animal physiologies. *Nitric Oxide* **2016**, *55–56*, 91–100. [CrossRef] [PubMed]
16. Mishra, V.; Singh, P.; Tripathi, D.K.; Corpas, F.J.; Singh, V.P. Nitric oxide and hydrogen sulfide: An indispensable combination for plant functioning. *Trends Plant Sci.* **2021**, *26*, 1270–1285. [CrossRef] [PubMed]
17. Sharma, G.; Sharma, N.; Ohri, P. Harmonizing hydrogen sulfide and nitric oxide: A duo defending plants against salinity stress. *Nitric Oxide* **2024**, *144*, 1–10. [CrossRef] [PubMed]
18. Astier, J.; Gross, I.; Durner, J. Nitric oxide production in plants: An update. *J. Exp. Bot.* **2018**, *69*, 3401–3411. [CrossRef] [PubMed]
19. Kolbert, Z.; Barroso, J.B.; Brouquisse, R.; Corpas, F.J.; Gupta, K.J.; Lindermayr, C.; Loake, G.J.; Palma, J.M.; Petřivalský, M.; Wendehenne, D.; et al. A forty year journey: The generation and roles of NO in plants. *Nitric Oxide* **2019**, *93*, 53–70. [CrossRef] [PubMed]
20. Corpas, F.J.; González-Gordo, S.; Palma, J.M. NO source in higher plants: Present and future of an unresolved question. *Trends Plant Sci.* **2022**, *27*, 116–119. [CrossRef] [PubMed]
21. Yamasaki, H.; Sakihama, Y.; Takahashi, S. An alternative pathway for nitric oxide production in plants: New features of an old enzyme. *Trends Plant Sci.* **1999**, *4*, 128–129. [CrossRef]
22. Rockel, P.; Strube, F.; Rockel, A.; Wildt, J.; Kaiser, W.M. Regulation of nitric oxide (NO) production by plant nitrate reductase in vivo and in vitro. *J. Exp. Bot.* **2002**, *53*, 103–110. [CrossRef]
23. Mohn, M.A.; Thaqi, B.; Fischer-Schrader, K. Isoform-Specific NO Synthesis by *Arabidopsis thaliana* Nitrate Reductase. *Plants* **2019**, *8*, 67. [CrossRef]
24. Costa-Broseta, Á.; Castillo, M.; León, J. Post-translational modifications of nitrate reductases autoregulates nitric oxide biosynthesis in Arabidopsis. *Int. J. Mol. Sci.* **2021**, *22*, 549. [CrossRef]
25. Ribeiro, E.A., Jr.; Cunha, F.Q.; Tamashiro, W.M.; Martins, I.S. Growth phase-dependent subcellular localization of nitric oxide synthase in maize cells. *FEBS Lett.* **1999**, *445*, 283–286. [CrossRef] [PubMed]
26. Corpas, F.J.; Barroso, J.B. Peroxisomal plant nitric oxide synthase (NOS) protein is imported by peroxisomal targeting signal type 2 (PTS2) in a process that depends on the cytosolic receptor PEX7 and calmodulin. *FEBS Lett.* **2014**, *588*, 2049–2054. [CrossRef] [PubMed]
27. Astier, J.; Jeandroz, S.; Wendehenne, D. Nitric oxide synthase in plants: The surprise from algae. *Plant Sci.* **2018**, *268*, 64–66. [CrossRef] [PubMed]
28. Tun, N.N.; Santa-Catarina, C.; Begum, T.; Silveira, V.; Handro, W.; Floh, E.I.; Scherer, G.F. Polyamines induce rapid biosynthesis of nitric oxide (NO) in *Arabidopsis thaliana* seedlings. *Plant Cell Physiol.* **2006**, *47*, 346–354. [CrossRef] [PubMed]
29. Yamasaki, H.; Cohen, M.F. NO signal at the crossroads: Polyamine-induced nitric oxide synthesis in plants? *Trends Plant Sci.* **2006**, *11*, 522–524. [CrossRef] [PubMed]
30. López-Gómez, P.; Buezo, J.; Urra, M.; Cornejo, A.; Esteban, R.; Fernández de Los Reyes, J.; Urarte, E.; Rodríguez-Dobreva, E.; Chamizo-Ampudia, A.; Eguaras, A.; et al. A new oxidative pathway of nitric oxide production from oximes in plants. *Mol. Plant* **2024**, *17*, 178–198. [CrossRef] [PubMed]
31. Gotor, C.; Laureano-Marín, A.M.; Moreno, I.; Aroca, Á.; García, I.; Romero, L.C. Signaling in the plant cytosol: Cysteine or sulfide? *Amino Acids* **2015**, *47*, 2155–2164. [CrossRef]
32. González-Gordo, S.; Palma, J.M.; Corpas, F.J. Appraisal of H$_2$S metabolism in *Arabidopsis thaliana*: In silico analysis at the subcellular level. *Plant Physiol. Biochem.* **2020**, *155*, 579–588. [CrossRef]
33. Radi, R. Oxygen radicals, nitric oxide, and peroxynitrite: Redox pathways in molecular medicine. *Proc. Natl. Acad. Sci. USA* **2018**, *115*, 5839–5848. [CrossRef]
34. Corpas, F.J.; Alché, J.D.; Barroso, J.B. Current overview of S-nitrosoglutathione (GSNO) in higher plants. *Front. Plant Sci.* **2013**, *4*, 126. [CrossRef] [PubMed]
35. Broniowska, K.A.; Diers, A.R.; Hogg, N. S-nitrosoglutathione. *Biochim. Biophys. Acta* **2013**, *1830*, 3173–3181. [CrossRef]
36. Perazzolli, M.; Dominici, P.; Romero-Puertas, M.C.; Zago, E.; Zeier, J.; Sonoda, M.; Lamb, C.; Delledonne, M. Arabidopsis nonsymbiotic hemoglobin AHb1 modulates nitric oxide bioactivity. *Plant Cell.* **2004**, *16*, 2785–2794. [CrossRef] [PubMed]

37. Corpas, F.J.; González-Gordo, S.; Palma, J.M. Protein nitration: A connecting bridge between nitric oxide (NO) and plant stress. *Plant Stress.* **2021**, *2*, 100026. [CrossRef]
38. Claudiane da Veiga, J.; Silveira, N.M.; Seabra, A.B.; Bron, I.U. Exploring the power of nitric oxide and nanotechnology for prolonging postharvest shelf-life and enhancing fruit quality. *Nitric Oxide* **2024**, *142*, 26–37. [CrossRef]
39. Mata-Pérez, C.; Sánchez-Vicente, I.; Arteaga, N.; Gómez-Jiménez, S.; Fuentes-Terrón, A.; Oulebsir, C.S.; Calvo-Polanco, M.; Oliver, C.; Lorenzo, Ó. Functions of nitric oxide-mediated post-translational modifications under abiotic stress. *Front. Plant Sci.* **2023**, *14*, 1158184. [CrossRef] [PubMed]
40. Mata-Pérez, C.; Sánchez-Calvo, B.; Padilla, M.N.; Begara-Morales, J.C.; Luque, F.; Melguizo, M.; Jiménez-Ruiz, J.; Fierro-Risco, J.; Peñas-Sanjuán, A.; Valderrama, R.; et al. Nitro-Fatty Acids in Plant Signaling: Nitro-Linolenic Acid Induces the Molecular Chaperone Network in Arabidopsis. *Plant Physiol.* **2016**, *170*, 686–701. [CrossRef] [PubMed]
41. Izbiańska, K.; Floryszak-Wieczorek, J.; Gajewska, J.; Meller, B.; Kuźnicki, D.; Arasimowicz-Jelonek, M. RNA and mRNA Nitration as a Novel Metabolic Link in Potato Immune Response to *Phytophthora infestans*. *Front. Plant Sci.* **2018**, *9*, 672. [CrossRef]
42. Petřivalský, M.; Luhová, L. Nitrated Nucleotides: New Players in Signaling Pathways of Reactive Nitrogen and Oxygen Species in Plants. *Front. Plant Sci.* **2020**, *11*, 598. [CrossRef]
43. Aroca, A.; Zhang, J.; Xie, Y.; Romero, L.C.; Gotor, C. Hydrogen sulfide signaling in plant adaptations to adverse conditions: Molecular mechanisms. *J. Exp. Bot.* **2021**, *72*, 5893–5904. [CrossRef]
44. Corpas, F.J.; González-Gordo, S.; Muñoz-Vargas, M.A.; Rodríguez-Ruiz, M.; Palma, J.M. The *Modus Operandi* of Hydrogen Sulfide(H$_2$S)-Dependent Protein Persulfidation in Higher Plants. *Antioxidants* **2021**, *10*, 1686. [CrossRef]
45. Dixon, D.P.; Skipsey, M.; Grundy, N.M.; Edwards, R. Stress-induced protein S-glutathionylation in Arabidopsis. *Plant Physiol.* **2005**, *138*, 2233–2344. [CrossRef]
46. García, I.; Arenas-Alfonseca, L.; Moreno, I.; Gotor, C.; Romero, L.C. HCN Regulates Cellular Processes through Posttranslational Modification of Proteins by S-cyanylation. *Plant Physiol.* **2019**, *179*, 107–123. [CrossRef]
47. Huang, J.; Willems, P.; Wei, B.; Tian, C.; Ferreira, R.B.; Bodra, N.; Martínez Gache, S.A.; Wahni, K.; Liu, K.; Vertommen, D.; et al. Mining for protein S-sulfenylation in *Arabidopsis* uncovers redox-sensitive sites. *Proc. Natl. Acad. Sci. USA* **2019**, *116*, 21256–21261. [CrossRef]
48. Kumar, M.; Carr, P.; Turner, S.R. An atlas of Arabidopsis protein S-acylation reveals its widespread role in plant cell organization and function. *Nat. Plants* **2022**, *8*, 670–681. [CrossRef]
49. Corpas, F.J.; González-Gordo, S.; Rodríguez-Ruiz, M.; Muñoz-Vargas, M.A.; Palma, J.M. Thiol-based Oxidative Posttranslational Modifications (OxiPTMs) of Plant Proteins. *Plant Cell Physiol.* **2022**, *63*, 889–900. [CrossRef] [PubMed]
50. McAinsh, M.R.; Evans, N.H.; Montgomery, L.T.; North, K.A. Calcium signalling in stomatal responses to pollutants. *New Phytol.* **2002**, *153*, 441–447. [CrossRef] [PubMed]
51. Neill, S.; Barros, R.; Bright, J.; Desikan, R.; Hancock, J.; Harrison, J.; Morris, P.; Ribeiro, D.; Wilson, I. Nitric oxide, stomatal closure, and abiotic stress. *J. Exp. Bot.* **2008**, *59*, 165–176. [CrossRef]
52. Li, Y.; Gao, Z.; Lu, J.; Wei, X.; Qi, M.; Yin, Z.; Li, T. SlSnRK2.3 interacts with SlSUI1 to modulate high temperature tolerance via Abscisic acid (ABA) controlling stomatal movement in tomato. *Plant Sci.* **2022**, *321*, 111305. [CrossRef] [PubMed]
53. Bright, J.; Desikan, R.; Hancock, J.T.; Weir, I.S.; Neill, S.J. ABA-induced NO generation and stomatal closure in Arabidopsis are dependent on H$_2$O$_2$ synthesis. *Plant J.* **2006**, *45*, 113–122. [CrossRef] [PubMed]
54. García-Mata, C.; Lamattina, L. Gasotransmitters are emerging as new guard cell signaling molecules and regulators of leaf gas exchange. *Plant Sci.* **2013**, *201–202*, 66–73. [CrossRef] [PubMed]
55. Scuffi, D.; Álvarez, C.; Laspina, N.; Gotor, C.; Lamattina, L.; García-Mata, C. Hydrogen sulfide generated by L-cysteine desulfhydrase acts upstream of nitric oxide to modulate abscisic acid-dependent stomatal closure. *Plant Physiol.* **2014**, *166*, 2065–2076. [CrossRef] [PubMed]
56. Pantaleno, R.; Scuffi, D.; García-Mata, C. Hydrogen sulphide as a guard cell network regulator. *New Phytol.* **2021**, *230*, 451–456. [CrossRef] [PubMed]
57. Shimizu, T.; Kanno, Y.; Suzuki, H.; Watanabe, S.; Seo, M. Arabidopsis NPF4.6 and NPF5.1 control leaf stomatal aperture by regulating abscisic acid transport. *Genes* **2021**, *12*, 885. [CrossRef]
58. Hasan, M.M.; Liu, X.D.; Yao, G.Q.; Liu, J.; Fang, X.W. Ethylene-mediated stomatal responses to dehydration and rehydration in seed plants. *J. Exp. Bot.* **2024**, *17*, erae060. [CrossRef]
59. Shen, J.; Zhang, J.; Zhou, M.; Zhou, H.; Cui, B.; Gotor, C.; Romero, L.C.; Fu, L.; Yang, J.; Foyer, C.H.; et al. Persulfidation-based Modification of Cysteine Desulfhydrase and the NADPH Oxidase RBOHD Controls Guard Cell Abscisic Acid Signaling. *Plant Cell* **2020**, *32*, 1000–1017. [CrossRef]
60. Chen, S.; Wang, X.; Jia, H.; Li, F.; Ma, Y.; Liesche, J.; Liao, M.; Ding, X.; Liu, C.; Chen, Y.; et al. Persulfidation-induced structural change in SnRK2.6 establishes intramolecular interaction between phosphorylation and persulfidation. *Mol. Plant* **2021**, *14*, 1814–1830. [CrossRef]
61. Chen, S.; Jia, H.; Wang, X.; Shi, C.; Wang, X.; Ma, P.; Wang, J.; Ren, M.; Li, J. Hydrogen sulfide positively regulates abscisic acid signaling through persulfidation of SnRK2.6 in guard cells. *Mol. Plant* **2020**, *13*, 732–744. [CrossRef]
62. Jia, H.; Chen, S.; Liu, D.; Liesche, J.; Shi, C.; Wang, J.; Ren, M.; Wang, X.; Yang, J.; Shi, W.; et al. Ethylene-Induced Hydrogen Sulfide Negatively Regulates Ethylene Biosynthesis by Persulfidation of ACO in Tomato Under Osmotic Stress. *Front. Plant Sci.* **2018**, *9*, 1517. [CrossRef]

63. Coyne, P.I.; Bingham, G.E. Photosynthesis and Stomatal Light Responses in Snap Beans Exposed to Hydrogen Sulfide and Ozone. *J. Air Pollut. Control. Assoc.* **1978**, *28*, 1119–1123. [CrossRef]

64. Zhang, L.; Vet, R.; Brook, J.R.; Legge, A.H. Factors affecting stomatal uptake of ozone by different canopies and a comparison between dose and exposure. *Sci. Total Environ.* **2006**, *370*, 117–132. [CrossRef]

65. Ren, Z.; Wang, R.Y.; Huang, X.Y.; Wang, Y. Sulfur Compounds in Regulation of Stomatal Movement. *Front. Plant Sci.* **2022**, *13*, 846518. [CrossRef]

66. Cheng, C.; Wu, Q.; Wang, M.; Chen, D.; Li, J.; Shen, J.; Hou, S.; Zhang, P.; Qin, L.; Acharya, B.R.; et al. Maize Mitogen-Activated Protein Kinase 20 mediates high-temperature-regulated stomatal movement. *Plant Physiol.* **2023**, *193*, 2788–2805. [CrossRef]

67. Merilo, E.; Laanemets, K.; Hu, H.; Xue, S.; Jakobson, L.; Tulva, I.; Gonzalez-Guzman, M.; Rodriguez, P.L.; Schroeder, J.I.; Broschè, M.; et al. PYR/RCAR receptors contribute to ozone-, reduced air humidity-, darkness-, and CO_2-induced stomatal regulation. *Plant Physiol.* **2013**, *162*, 1652–1668. [CrossRef] [PubMed]

68. Ač, A.; Jansen, M.A.K.; Grace, J.; Urban, O. Unravelling the neglected role of ultraviolet radiation on stomata: A meta-analysis with implications for modelling ecosystem-climate interactions. *Plant Cell Environ.* **2024**. [CrossRef]

69. Dean, J.V.; Harper, J.E. Nitric oxide and nitrous oxide production by soybean and winged bean during the in vivo nitrate reductase assay. *Plant Physiol.* **1986**, *82*, 718–723. [CrossRef] [PubMed]

70. Liu, B.; Rennenberg, H.; Kreuzwieser, J. Hypoxia induces stem and leaf nitric oxide (NO) emission from poplar seedlings. *Planta* **2015**, *241*, 579–589. [CrossRef]

71. Welle, M.; Niether, W.; Stöhr, C. The underestimated role of plant root nitric oxide emission under low-oxygen stress. *Front. Plant Sci.* **2024**, *15*, 1290700. [CrossRef]

72. Rennenberg, H.; Filner, P. Stimulation of H_2S emission from pumpkin leaves by inhibition of glutathione synthesis. *Plant Physiol.* **1982**, *69*, 766–770. [CrossRef]

73. Rennenberg, H. Role of O-acetylserine in hydrogen sulfide emission from pumpkin leaves in response to sulfate. *Plant Physiol.* **1983**, *73*, 560–565. [CrossRef] [PubMed]

74. Lenhart, K.; Behrendt, T.; Greiner, S.; Steinkamp, J.; Well, R.; Giesemann, A.; Keppler, F. Nitrous oxide effluxes from plants as a potentially important source to the atmosphere. *New Phytol.* **2019**, *221*, 1398–1408. [CrossRef] [PubMed]

75. Qin, S.; Pang, Y.; Hu, H.; Liu, T.; Yuan, D.; Clough, T.; Wrage-Mönnig, N.; Luo, J.; Zhou, S.; Ma, L.; et al. Foliar N_2O emissions constitute a significant source to atmosphere. *Glob. Change Biol.* **2024**, *30*, e17181. [CrossRef] [PubMed]

76. Barba, J.; Bradford, M.A.; Brewer, P.E.; Bruhn, D.; Covey, K.; van Haren, J.; Megonigal, J.P.; Mikkelsen, T.N.; Pangala, S.R.; Pihlatie, M.; et al. Methane emissions from tree stems: A new frontier in the global carbon cycle. *New Phytol.* **2019**, *222*, 18–28. [CrossRef] [PubMed]

77. Barba, J.; Brewer, P.E.; Pangala, S.R.; Machacova, K. Methane emissions from tree stems—Current knowledge and challenges: An introduction to a Virtual Issue. *New Phytol.* **2024**, *241*, 1377–1380. [CrossRef] [PubMed]

78. Aghajanzadeh, T.; Kopriva, S.; Hawkesford, M.J.; Koprivova, A.; De Kok, L.J. Atmospheric H_2S and SO_2 as sulfur source for *Brassica juncea* and *Brassica rapa*: Impact on the glucosinolate composition. *Front. Plant Sci.* **2015**, *6*, 924. [CrossRef]

79. Homyak, P.M.; Blankinship, J.C.; Marchus, K.; Lucero, D.M.; Sickman, J.O.; Schimel, J.P. Aridity and plant uptake interact to make dryland soils hotspots for nitric oxide (NO) emissions. *Proc. Natl. Acad. Sci. USA* **2016**, *113*, E2608–E2616. [CrossRef]

80. Ausma, T.; De Kok, L.J. Atmospheric H_2S: Impact on Plant Functioning. *Front. Plant Sci.* **2019**, *10*, 743. [CrossRef]

81. Kabange, N.R.; Mun, B.G.; Lee, S.M.; Kwon, Y.; Lee, D.; Lee, G.M.; Yun, B.W.; Lee, J.H. Nitric oxide: A core signaling molecule under elevated GHGs (CO_2, CH_4, N_2O, O_3)-mediated abiotic stress in plants. *Front. Plant Sci.* **2022**, *13*, 994149. [CrossRef] [PubMed]

82. Hatfield, J.L.; Prueger, J.H. Temperature extremes: Effect on plant growth and development. *Weather. Clim. Extrem.* **2015**, *10*, 4–10. [CrossRef]

83. Alamri, S.A.; Siddiqui, M.H.; Al-Khaishany, M.Y.; Khan, M.N.; Ali, H.M.; Alakeel, K.A. Nitric oxide-mediated cross-talk of proline and heat shock proteins induce thermotolerance in *Vicia faba* L. *Environ. Exp. Bot.* **2019**, *161*, 290–302. [CrossRef]

84. De Leone, M.J.; Yanovsky, M.J. The Circadian Clock and Thermal Regulation in Plants: Novel Findings on the Role of Positive Circadian Clock-Regulators in Temperature Responses. *J. Exp. Bot.* **2024**, erae045. [CrossRef]

85. Fu, Z.W.; Ding, F.; Zhang, B.L.; Liu, W.C.; Huang, Z.H.; Fan, S.H.; Feng, Y.R.; Lu, Y.T.; Hua, W. Hydrogen peroxide sulfenylates and inhibits the photorespiratory enzyme PGLP1 to modulate plant thermotolerance. *Plant Commun.* **2024**, 100852. [CrossRef]

86. Chaki, M.; Valderrama, R.; Fernández-Ocaña, A.M.; Carreras, A.; Gómez-Rodríguez, M.V.; López-Jaramillo, J.; Begara-Morales, J.C.; Sánchez-Calvo, B.; Luque, F.; Leterrier, M.; et al. High temperature triggers the metabolism of S-nitrosothiols in sunflower mediating a process of nitrosative stress which provokes the inhibition of ferredoxin-NADP reductase by tyrosine nitration. *Plant Cell Environ.* **2011**, *34*, 1803–1818. [CrossRef]

87. Sun, Y.Y.; Wang, J.Q.; Xiang, R.H.; Li, Z.G. Key role of reactive oxygen species-scavenging system in nitric oxide and hydrogen sulfide crosstalk-evoked thermotolerance in maize seedlings. *Front. Plant Sci.* **2022**, *13*, 967968. [CrossRef]

88. Corpas, F.J. Hydrogen Sulfide: A New Warrior against Abiotic Stress. *Trends Plant Sci.* **2019**, *24*, 983–988. [CrossRef]

89. Chae, H.B.; Bae, S.B.; Paeng, S.K.; Wi, S.D.; Thi Phan, K.A.; Lee, S.Y. S-nitrosylation switches the Arabidopsis redox sensor protein, QSOX1, from an oxidoreductase to a molecular chaperone under heat stress. *Plant Physiol. Biochem.* **2024**, *206*, 108219. [CrossRef] [PubMed]

90. Mishra, S.; Chowdhary, A.A.; Bhau, B.S.; Srivastava, V. Hydrogen sulphide-mediated alleviation and its interplay with other signalling molecules during temperature stress. *Plant Biol.* **2022**, *24*, 569–575. [CrossRef] [PubMed]
91. Kolupaev, Y.E.; Yemets, A.I.; Yastreb, T.O.; Blume, Y.B. The role of nitric oxide and hydrogen sulfide in regulation of redox homeostasis at extreme temperatures in plants. *Front. Plant Sci.* **2023**, *14*, 1128439. [CrossRef]
92. Wagg, S.; Mills, G.; Hayes, F.; Wilkinson, S.; Cooper, D.; Davies, W.J. Reduced soil water availability did not protect two competing grassland species from the negative effects of increasing background ozone. *Environ. Pollut.* **2012**, *165*, 91–99. [CrossRef] [PubMed]
93. Skärby, L.; Ro-Poulsen, H.; Wellburn, F.A.; Sheppard, L.J. Impacts of ozone on forests: A European perspective. *New Phytol.* **1998**, *139*, 109–122. [CrossRef]
94. Grulke, N.E.; Heath, R.L. Ozone effects on plants in natural ecosystems. *Plant Biol.* **2020**, *22*, 12–37. [CrossRef]
95. Jimenez-Montenegro, L.; Lopez-Fernandez, M.; Gimenez, E. Worldwide research on the ozone influence in plants. *Agronomy* **2021**, *11*, 1504. [CrossRef]
96. Singh, A.A.; Ghosh, A.; Agrawal, M.; Agrawal, S.B. Secondary metabolites responses of plants exposed to ozone: An update. *Environ. Sci. Pollut. Res. Int.* **2023**, *30*, 88281–88312. [CrossRef] [PubMed]
97. Nowroz, F.; Hasanuzzaman, M.; Siddika, A.; Parvin, K.; Caparros, P.G.; Nahar, K.; Prasad, P.V.V. Elevated tropospheric ozone and crop production: Potential negative effects and plant defense mechanisms. *Front. Plant Sci.* **2024**, *14*, 1244515. [CrossRef] [PubMed]
98. Pasqualini, S.; Meier, S.; Gehring, C.; Madeo, L.; Fornaciari, M.; Romano, B.; Ederli, L. Ozone and nitric oxide induce cGMP-dependent and -independent transcription of defence genes in tobacco. *Plant Signal. Behav.* **2009**, *181*, 860–870. [CrossRef]
99. Caregnato, F.F.; Bortolin, R.C.; Divan Junior, A.M.; Moreira, J.C. Exposure to elevated ozone levels differentially affects the antioxidant capacity and the redox homeostasis of two subtropical *Phaseolus vulgaris* L. varieties. *Chemosphere* **2013**, *93*, 320–330. [CrossRef]
100. Favory, J.J.; Stec, A.; Gruber, H.; Rizzini, L.; Oravecz, A.; Funk, M.; Albert, A.; Cloix, C.; Jenkins, G.I.; Oakeley, E.J.; et al. Interaction of COP1 and UVR8 regulates UV-B-induced photomorphogenesis and stress acclimation in Arabidopsis. *EMBO J.* **2009**, *28*, 591–601. [CrossRef]
101. Jenkins, G.I. Signal transduction in responses to UV-B radiation. *Annu. Rev. Plant Biol.* **2009**, *60*, 407–431. [CrossRef] [PubMed]
102. Shi, C.; Liu, H. How plants protect themselves from ultraviolet-B radiation stress. *Plant Physiol.* **2021**, *187*, 1096–1103. [CrossRef]
103. Fang, F.; Lin, L.; Zhang, Q.; Lu, M.; Skvortsova, M.Y.; Podolec, R.; Zhang, Q.; Pi, J.; Zhang, C.; Ulm, R.; et al. Mechanisms of UV-B light-induced photoreceptor UVR8 nuclear localization dynamics. *New Phytol.* **2022**, *236*, 1824–1837. [CrossRef] [PubMed]
104. Sharma, A.; Pridgeon, A.J.; Liu, W.; Segers, F.; Sharma, B.; Jenkins, G.I.; Franklin, K.A. *Elongated Hypocotyl5* (*HY5*) and HY5 *Homologue* (*HYH*) maintain shade avoidance suppression in UV-B. *Plant J.* **2023**, *115*, 1394–1407. [CrossRef] [PubMed]
105. A-H-Mackerness, S.; John, C.F.; Jordan, B.; Thomas, B. Early signaling components in ultraviolet-B responses: Distinct roles for different reactive oxygen species and nitric oxide. *FEBS Lett.* **2001**, *489*, 237–242. [CrossRef] [PubMed]
106. Zhang, L.; Zhao, L. Production of nitric oxide under ultraviolet-b irradiation is mediated by hydrogen peroxide through activation of nitric oxide synthase. *J. Plant Biol.* **2008**, *51*, 395–400. [CrossRef]
107. Krasylenko, Y.A.; Yemets, A.I.; Sheremet, Y.A.; Blume, Y.B. Nitric oxide as a critical factor for perception of UV-B irradiation by microtubules in Arabidopsis. *Physiol. Plant* **2012**, *145*, 505–515. [CrossRef] [PubMed]
108. Jiao, C.; Wang, P.; Yang, R.; Tian, L.; Gu, Z. IP3 Mediates Nitric Oxide-Guanosine 3′,5′-Cyclic Monophosphate (NO-cGMP)-Induced Isoflavone Accumulation in Soybean Sprouts under UV-B Radiation. *J. Agric. Food Chem.* **2016**, *64*, 8282–8288. [CrossRef] [PubMed]
109. Li, Q.; Wang, Z.; Zhao, Y.; Zhang, X.; Zhang, S.; Bo, L.; Wang, Y.; Ding, Y.; An, L. Putrescine protects hulless barley from damage due to UV-B stress via H_2S- and H_2O_2-mediated signaling pathways. *Plant Cell Rep.* **2016**, *35*, 1155–1168. [CrossRef]
110. Cassia, R.; Amenta, M.; Fernández, M.B.; Nocioni, M.; Dávila, V. The Role of Nitric Oxide in the Antioxidant Defense of Plants Exposed to UV-B Radiation. In *Reactive Oxygen, Nitrogen and Sulfur Species in Plants: Production, Metabolism, Signaling and Defense Mechanisms*; John and Wiley and Sons: Hoboken, NJ, USA, 2019; pp. 555–572.
111. Qiao, F.; Zhang, X.M.; Liu, X.; Chen, J.; Hu, W.J.; Liu, T.W.; Liu, J.Y.; Zhu, C.Q.; Ghoto, K.; Zhu, X.Y.; et al. Elevated nitrogen metabolism and nitric oxide production are involved in Arabidopsis resistance to acid rain. *Plant Physiol. Biochem.* **2018**, *127*, 238–247. [CrossRef]
112. Debnath, B.; Sikdar, A.; Islam, S.; Hasan, K.; Li, M.; Qiu, D. Physiological and Molecular Responses to Acid Rain Stress in Plants and the Impact of Melatonin, Glutathione and Silicon in the Amendment of Plant Acid Rain Stress. *Molecules* **2021**, *26*, 862. [CrossRef]
113. Debnath, B.; Irshad, M.; Mitra, S.; Li, M.; Liu, S.; Rizwan, H.M.; Pan, T.; Qiu, D. Acid rain deposition modulates photosynthesis, enzymatic and non-enzymatic antioxidant activities in tomato. *Int. J. Environ. Res.* **2018**, *12*, 203–214. [CrossRef]
114. Zhang, S.; Liu, L.; Wu, Z.; Wang, L.; Ban, Z. S-nitrosylation of superoxide dismutase and catalase involved in promotion of fruit resistance to chilling stress: A case study on *Ziziphus jujube* Mill. *Postharvest Biol. Technol.* **2023**, *197*, 112210. [CrossRef]
115. Song, X.; Xu, Z.; Zhang, J.; Liang, L.; Xiao, J.; Liang, Z.; Yu, G.; Sun, B.; Huang, Z.; Tang, Y.; et al. NO and GSH alleviate the inhibition of low-temperature stress on cowpea seedlings. *Plants* **2023**, *12*, 1317. [CrossRef]
116. Gao, X.; Ma, J.; Tie, J.; Li, Y.; Hu, L.; Yu, J. BR-Mediated Protein S-Nitrosylation alleviated low-temperature stress in mini chinese cabbage (*Brassica rapa* ssp. *pekinensis*). *Int. J. Mol. Sci.* **2022**, *23*, 10964. [CrossRef]

117. Sehar, Z.; Mir, I.R.; Khan, S.; Masood, A.; Khan, N.A. Nitric Oxide and Proline Modulate Redox Homeostasis and Photosynthetic Metabolism in Wheat Plants under High Temperature Stress Acclimation. *Plants* **2023**, *12*, 1256. [CrossRef]
118. Rasheed, F.; Mir, I.R.; Sehar, Z.; Fatma, M.; Gautam, H.; Khan, S.; Anjum, N.A.; Masood, A.; Sofo, A.; Khan, N.A. Nitric oxide and salicylic acid regulate glutathione and ethylene production to enhance heat stress acclimation in wheat involving sulfur assimilation. *Plants* **2022**, *11*, 3131. [CrossRef]
119. Gautam, H.; Sehar, Z.; Rehman, M.T.; Hussain, A.; AlAjmi, M.F.; Khan, N.A. Nitric Oxide Enhances Photosynthetic Nitrogen and Sulfur-Use Efficiency and Activity of Ascorbate-Glutathione Cycle to Reduce High Temperature Stress-Induced Oxidative Stress in Rice (*Oryza sativa* L.) Plants. *Biomolecules* **2021**, *11*, 305. [CrossRef]
120. Gautam, H.; Fatma, M.; Sehar, Z.; Mir, I.R.; Khan, N.A. Hydrogen Sulfide, Ethylene, and Nitric Oxide Regulate Redox Homeostasis and Protect Photosynthetic Metabolism under High Temperature Stress in Rice Plants. *Antioxidants* **2022**, *11*, 1478. [CrossRef]
121. Ahlfors, R.; Brosché, M.; Kollist, H.; Kangasjärvi, J. Nitric oxide modulates ozone-induced cell death, hormone biosynthesis and gene expression in Arabidopsis thaliana. *Plant J.* **2009**, *58*, 1–12. [CrossRef]
122. Li, C.; Song, Y.; Guo, L.; Gu, X.; Muminov, M.A.; Wang, T. Nitric oxide alleviates wheat yield reduction by protecting photosynthetic system from oxidation of ozone pollution. *Environ. Pollut.* **2018**, *236*, 296–303. [CrossRef]
123. Shi, S.; Wang, G.; Wang, Y.; Zhang, L.; Zhang, L. Protective effect of nitric oxide against oxidative stress under ultraviolet-B radiation. *Nitric Oxide* **2005**, *13*, 1–9. [CrossRef]
124. Kim, T.-Y.; Jo, M.-H.; Hong, J.-H. Protective effect of nitric oxide against oxidative stress under UV-B radiation in maize leaves. *J. Environ. Sci. Int.* **2010**, *19*, 1323–1334. [CrossRef]
125. Santa-Cruz, D.M.; Pacienza, N.A.; Zilli, C.G.; Tomaro, M.L.; Balestrasse, K.B.; Yannarelli, G.G. Nitric oxide induces specific isoforms of antioxidant enzymes in soybean leaves subjected to enhanced ultraviolet-B radiation. *J. Photochem. Photobiol. B* **2014**, *141*, 202–209. [CrossRef]
126. Liu, J.F.; Wang, M.Y.; Yang, C.; Zhu, A.J. Effects of exogenous nitric oxide on physiological characteristics of longan (*Dimocarpus longana*) seedlings under acid rain stress. *Ying Yong Sheng Tai Xue Bao* **2013**, *24*, 2235–2240.
127. Liu, Z.; Li, Y.; Cao, C.; Liang, S.; Ma, Y.; Liu, X.; Pei, Y. The role of H_2S in low temperature-induced cucurbitacin C increases in cucumber. *Plant Mol. Biol.* **2019**, *99*, 535–544. [CrossRef]
128. Zhang, X.; Zhang, Y.; Xu, C.; Liu, K.; Bi, H.; Ai, X. H_2O_2 Functions as a Downstream Signal of IAA to Mediate H_2S-Induced Chilling Tolerance in Cucumber. *Int. J. Mol. Sci.* **2021**, *22*, 12910. [CrossRef]
129. Song, X.; Zhu, L.; Wang, D.; Liang, L.; Xiao, J.; Tang, W.; Xie, M.; Zhao, Z.; Lai, Y.; Sun, B.; et al. Molecular Regulatory Mechanism of Exogenous Hydrogen Sulfide in Alleviating Low-Temperature Stress in Pepper Seedlings. *Int. J. Mol. Sci.* **2023**, *24*, 16337. [CrossRef]
130. Tang, X.; An, B.; Cao, D.; Xu, R.; Wang, S.; Zhang, Z.; Liu, X.; Sun, X. Improving photosynthetic capacity, alleviating photosynthetic inhibition and oxidative stress under low temperature stress with exogenous hydrogen sulfide in blueberry seedlings. *Front. Plant Sci.* **2020**, *11*, 108. [CrossRef]
131. Gao, S.; Wang, Y.; Zeng, Z.; Zhang, M.; Yi, N.; Liu, B.; Wang, R.; Long, S.; Gong, J.; Liu, T.; et al. Integrated bioinformatic and physiological analyses reveal the pivotal role of hydrogen sulfide in enhancing low-temperature tolerance in alfalfa. *Physiol. Plant.* **2023**, *175*, e13885. [CrossRef]
132. Christou, A.; Filippou, P.; Manganaris, G.A.; Fotopoulos, V. Sodium hydrosulfide induces systemic thermotolerance to strawberry plants through transcriptional regulation of heat shock proteins and aquaporin. *BMC Plant Biol.* **2014**, *14*, 42. [CrossRef]
133. Zhou, Z.H.; Wang, Y.; Ye, X.-Y.; Li, Z.-G. Signaling molecule hydrogen sulfide improves seed germination and seedling growth of maize (*Zea mays* L.) under high temperature by inducing antioxidant system and osmolyte biosynthesis. *Front. Plant Sci.* **2018**, *9*, 1288. [CrossRef]
134. Cheng, T.; Shi, J.; Dong, Y.; Ma, Y.; Peng, Y.; Hu, X.; Chen, J. Hydrogen sulfide enhances poplar tolerance to high-temperature stress by increasing S-nitrosoglutathione reductase (GSNOR) activity and reducing reactive oxygen/nitrogen damage. *Plant Growth Regul.* **2018**, *84*, 11–23. [CrossRef]
135. Chen, Z.; Huang, Y.; Yang, W.; Chang, G.; Li, P.; Wei, J.; Yuan, X.; Huang, J.; Hu, X. The hydrogen sulfide signal enhances seed germination tolerance to high temperatures by retaining nuclear COP1 for HY5 degradation. *Plant Sci.* **2019**, *285*, 34–43. [CrossRef]
136. Rostami, F.; Nasibi, F.; Kalantari, K.M. Alleviation of UV-B radiation damages by sodium hydrosulfide (H_2S donor) pre-treatment in Borage seedlings. *J. Plant Interact.* **2019**, *14*, 519–524. [CrossRef]
137. Corpas, F.J.; Muñoz-Vargas, M.A.; González-Gordo SRodríguez-Ruiz, M.; Palma, J.M. Nitric Oxide (NO) and Hydrogen Sulfide (H_2S): New Potential Biotechnological Tools for Postharvest Storage of Horticultural Crops. *J. Plant Growth Regul.* **2023**. [CrossRef]
138. Luo, S.; Liu, Z.; Wan, Z.; He, X.; Lv, J.; Yu, J.; Zhang, G. Foliar Spraying of NaHS Alleviates Cucumber Salt Stress by Maintaining N^+/K^+ Balance and Activating Salt Tolerance Signaling Pathways. *Plants* **2023**, *12*, 2450. [CrossRef]
139. Begara-Morales, J.C.; Sánchez-Calvo, B.; Chaki, M.; Valderrama, R.; Mata-Pérez, C.; López-Jaramillo, J.; Padilla, M.N.; Carreras, A.; Corpas, F.J.; Barroso, J.B. Dual regulation of cytosolic ascorbate peroxidase (APX) by tyrosine nitration and S-nitrosylation. *J. Exp. Bot.* **2014**, *65*, 527–538. [CrossRef]
140. Aroca, Á.; Serna, A.; Gotor, C.; Romero, L.C. S-sulfhydration: A cysteine posttranslational modification in plant systems. *Plant Physiol.* **2015**, *168*, 334–342. [CrossRef]

141. Cai, H.; Han, S.; Yu, M.; Ma, R.; Yu, Z. Exogenous nitric oxide fumigation promoted the emission of volatile organic compounds in peach fruit during shelf life after long-term cold storage. *Food Res. Int.* **2020**, *133*, 109135. [CrossRef]

142. Ma, T.; Xu, S.; Wang, Y.; Zhang, L.; Liu, Z.; Liu, D.; Jin, Z.; Pei, Y. Exogenous hydrogen sulphide promotes plant flowering through the Arabidopsis splicing factor AtU2AF65a. *Plant Cell Environ.* **2024**. [CrossRef]

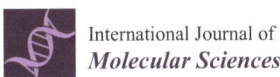

International Journal of
Molecular Sciences

Article

METACASPASE8 (MC8) Is a Crucial Protein in the LSD1-Dependent Cell Death Pathway in Response to Ultraviolet Stress

Maciej Jerzy Bernacki [1,2], Anna Rusaczonek [3], Kinga Gołębiewska [2], Agata Barbara Majewska-Fala [2], Weronika Czarnocka [3] and Stanisław Mariusz Karpiński [2,*]

1   Institute of Technology and Life Sciences—National Research Institute, Falenty, Al. Hrabska 3, 05-090 Raszyn, Poland; maciej_bernacki@sggw.edu.pl

2   Department of Plant Genetics, Breeding and Biotechnology, Institute of Biology, Warsaw University of Life Sciences, Nowoursynowska Street 159, 02-776 Warsaw, Poland; kinga_golebiewska@sggw.edu.pl (K.G.); agata.barbara.majewska@gmail.com (A.B.M.-F.)

3   Department of Botany, Institute of Biology, Warsaw University of Life Sciences, Nowoursynowska 159, 02-776 Warsaw, Poland; anna_rusaczonek@sggw.edu.pl (A.R.); weronika_czarnocka@sggw.edu.pl (W.C.)

*   Correspondence: stanislaw_karpinski@sggw.edu.pl

Abstract: LESION-SIMULATING DISEASE1 (LSD1) is one of the well-known cell death regulatory proteins in *Arabidopsis thaliana*. The *lsd1* mutant exhibits runaway cell death (RCD) in response to various biotic and abiotic stresses. The phenotype of the *lsd1* mutant strongly depends on two other proteins, ENHANCED DISEASE SUSCEPTIBILITY 1 (EDS1) and PHYTOALEXIN-DEFICIENT 4 (PAD4) as well as on the synthesis/metabolism/signaling of salicylic acid (SA) and reactive oxygen species (ROS). However, the most interesting aspect of the *lsd1* mutant is its conditional-dependent RCD phenotype, and thus, the defined role and function of LSD1 in the suppression of EDS1 and PAD4 in controlled laboratory conditions is different in comparison to a multivariable field environment. Analysis of the *lsd1* mutant transcriptome in ambient laboratory and field conditions indicated that there were some candidate genes and proteins that might be involved in the regulation of the *lsd1* conditional-dependent RCD phenotype. One of them is METACASPASE 8 (AT1G16420). This type II metacaspase was described as a cell death-positive regulator induced by UV-C irradiation and ROS accumulation. In the double *mc8*/*lsd1* mutant, we discovered reversion of the *lsd1* RCD phenotype in response to UV radiation applied in controlled laboratory conditions. This cell death deregulation observed in the *lsd1* mutant was reverted like in double mutants of *lsd1*/*eds1* and *lsd1*/*pad4*. To summarize, in this work, we demonstrated that MC8 is positively involved in EDS1 and PAD4 conditional-dependent regulation of cell death when LSD1 function is suppressed in *Arabidopsis thaliana*. Thus, we identified a new protein compound of the conditional LSD1-EDS1-PAD4 regulatory hub. We proposed a working model of MC8 involvement in the regulation of cell death and we postulated that MC8 is a crucial protein in this regulatory pathway.

Keywords: abiotic stress; *Arabidopsis thaliana*; cell death; LSD1; METACASPASES; salicylic acid; reactive oxygen species

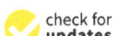

Citation: Bernacki, M.J.; Rusaczonek, A.; Gołębiewska, K.; Majewska-Fala, A.B.; Czarnocka, W.; Karpiński, S.M. METACASPASE8 (MC8) Is a Crucial Protein in the LSD1-Dependent Cell Death Pathway in Response to Ultraviolet Stress. *Int. J. Mol. Sci.* **2024**, *25*, 3195. https://doi.org/10.3390/ijms25063195

Academic Editors: Hunseung Kang and Yong-Hwan Moon

Received: 16 January 2024
Revised: 5 March 2024
Accepted: 6 March 2024
Published: 11 March 2024

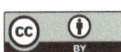
1. Introduction

Because of their sessile nature, plants cannot avoid environmental stresses by changing their place of inhabitance. Therefore, in natural environments, plants are constantly exposed to biotic and abiotic stress simultaneously, such as various pathogens, excess/deficiency of light, UV irradiation, drought, cold, heat, or salinity. Throughout the course of evolution, plants have developed many molecular and physiological mechanisms that enable them to simultaneously optimize acclimation and defense responses to variable and adverse environmental conditions [1–3]. One of the mechanisms crucial in plants response to stress is cell death (CD). CD is a molecular and physiological process that leads to the selective death of some cells, i.e., mesophyll cells, thus triggering a beneficial immune defense and acclimatory response in other cells [4,5]. In this regard, CD is a specified and highly organized process of the cells' self-elimination. It plays a crucial role in plant development [6,7], immune defense [8] and acclimatory responses [1,2]. From this point of view, CD is not only the ultimate end of the cell life cycle, but most importantly, it maintains cellular homeostasis in organs and in the whole plant during unfavorable environmental conditions.

Knowledge of the molecular, physiological and genetic mechanisms of plant CD at different levels of complexity (cellular and organismal) was facilitated by the identification of different *Arabidopsis thaliana* mutants exhibiting CD deregulation [9–11]. Some of the best-known conditional CD regulators in plants are LESION-SIMULATING DISEASE 1 protein (LSD1), ENHANCED DISEASE SUSCEPTIBILITY 1 (EDS1) and PHYTOALEXIN-DEFICIENT 4 (PAD4). The dysfunctional CD phenotype of the *lsd1* mutant has been broadly studied. This mutant exhibits a runaway cell death (RCD) phenotype which is manifested by the inability to restrict CD propagation if it has been initiated by an external stimulus [3,8,12]. It has been shown that RCD can be induced in the *lsd1* mutant by the following stress factors: high light and photorespiration [13,14], root hypoxia [1,15], drought [16,17], cold [18], UV radiation [16,19] or biotic stresses [20,21]. However, the *lsd1* RCD phenotype is dependent on growing conditions and was not observed when plants were grown in multivariable field conditions [16,22]. Based on many studies, LSD1 is considered a conditional suppressor of CD which is positively regulated by EDS1 and PAD4 and integrates various signaling pathways in response to both biotic and abiotic stresses [3].

Initially, the RCD phenotype of the *lsd1* mutant was linked to the accumulation of superoxide ions produced by plasma membrane-bound NADPH oxidase [8] and only after the other reaction oxygen species (ROS) forms were identified to be involved in RCD phenotype elicitation [13,14,18,23,24]. Since in the *lsd1* mutant the initial level of antioxidative enzyme activity is lower than in the wild type [23,25], LSD1 is regarded as a positive regulator of the enzymatic antioxidant machinery. Another CD-related molecule, which is excessively accumulated in *lsd1*, is salicylic acid (SA) [16,22,23]. It has been found that the artificial blocking of SA accumulation in the *lsd1* mutant prevents RCD induction; therefore, it was proposed that SA accumulation, controlled by LSD1, is essential in triggering CD in response to stress [19].

Dysfunctional overaccumulation of SA in the *lsd1* mutant is caused by the fact that LSD1 can physically interact with proteins involved in SA signaling. It was shown that LSD1 interacts with ENHANCED DISEASE SUSCEPTIBILITY 1 (EDS1), while EDS1 forms complexes with PHYTOALEXIN-DEFICIENT 4 (PAD4) [26,27]. Both EDS1 and PAD4 possess triacylglycerol lipase domains that were originally described as components of gene-mediated and basal disease resistance [28–31]. EDS1 and PAD4 are crucial for RCD propagation in the *lsd1* mutant, because in the eds1/lsd1 and pad4/lsd1 double mutants, the RCD was inhibited regardless of the stimulus type [21–23,32]. Therefore, LSD1 is considered a negative regulator of EDS1- and PAD4-dependent pathways that lead to RCD [3].

From a molecular perspective, an LSD1 protein contains three zinc (Zn)-finger domains that are responsible for DNA/protein binding [33]. LSD1 was proven to be a transcriptional regulator and a scaffold protein [27]. The Zn-finger motifs in LSD1 belong to the C2C2 class that is also present in GaTa1-type transcription factors containing the conserved consensus sequence CxxCRxxLMYxxGaSxVxCxxC [33,34]. Using yeast two-hybrid (Y2H) assay, additional ten putative LSD1-interacting proteins were found, from which one of them was METACASPASE1 (MC1), a positive CD regulator [35].

The METACASAPASES family is interesting in the context of cell death studies. *Arabidopsis thaliana* contains nine METACASAPASES proteins, 1 to 9, that are divided into two groups [36]. Type I metacaspases (MC1, MC2 and MC3) contain zinc-finger domains, while type II (MC4-MC9) do not [36,37]. This family contains both positive and negative CD regulators. While type I metacaspases' role is relatively well understood [35], the function of the type II subfamily is still largely unknown. In the context of the LSD1-dependent cell death regulation pathway, METACASPASE 8 (MC8) seems to be especially interesting. Its expression level is strongly up-regulated in response to UV-C [38], pathogens [39] and methyl viologen [38]. It was also shown that the recessive mutants in *MC8* exhibit higher resistance to UV-C and ROS treatment [38]. Therefore, we postulated a hypothesis that MC8 is involved in the propagation of RCD in *lsd1* plants and we decided to explore the mutual interdependence of these two proteins in CD regulation.

2. Results

2.1. MC8 Is Important in the LSD1-Dependent Cell Death Pathway

Because proteins belonging to the METACASPASE family are known to be involved in cell death regulation [35,36,40], we decided to search for MC genes within microarray data published in one of our previous articles [16]. Having compared the fold changes in *MC* genes' expression level in the *lsd1* mutant and wild-type plants, we observed that only the level of *MC4* and *MC8* were significantly up-regulated (Figure 1A). Interestingly, the expression level of *MC8* was antagonistically regulated in different growing conditions, an ambient laboratory or natural field (Figure 1A). In addition, in *eds1/lsd1* and *pad4/lsd1* double mutants, which do not exhibit the specific RCD phenotype, the *MC8* fold change was not detected (Supplementary Table S1). Data from microarray experiments were confirmed using a real-time PCR (Supplementary Figure S1). Interestingly, in double *lsd1/eds1* and *lsd1/pad4* mutants that reverted the *lsd1* RCD phenotype to the wild type, there were not any significant changes in the *MC8* transcript level (Supplementary Table S1). This finding together with the reverted cell death in the double *mc8/lsd1* mutant in response to UV irradiation (Figure 1B) and the plant phenotype (Figure 1C and Supplementary Figure S2) allowed us to conclude that MC8 was an important component in the LSD1-dependent conditional cell death regulatory hub. Moreover, we proved that in *Arabidopsis thaliana* wild-type plants, *MC8* expression was strongly up-regulated in response to a combined UV-A + UV-B irradiation episode, while in response to heat or high light stress, there were no differences compared to plants growing in controlled conditions (Supplementary Figure S3).

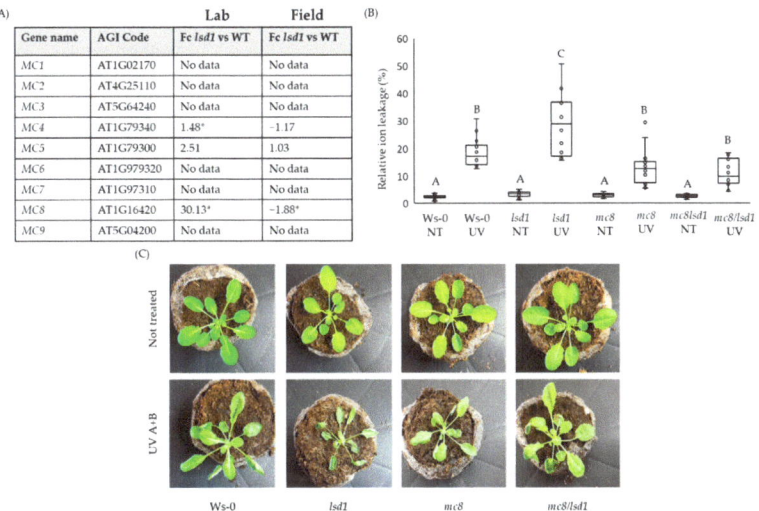

Figure 1. The role of METACASPASE 8 in conditional LSD1-dependent cell death regulation. (**A**) Analysis of transcriptomic data [16] in the context of expression changes in genes encoding METACA-CASPES family proteins, and in *lsd1* mutant grown in ambient laboratory conditions (Lab) or in natural

field conditions (Field), significant changes are marked with asterisks. FC—fold change. (**B**) Level of measured foliar ion leakage (manifesting the cell death level) for plants grown in control conditions and exposed to episode of UV-A + UV-B irradiation. Within a subgraph, values sharing the same letters are not significantly different from each other ($p > 0.001$) (n = 10–15). (**C**) Pictures of *Arabidopsis thaliana* rosettes from control conditions (upper row) and after UV-A + UV-B irradiation incidents (bottom row).

2.2. MC8 Affects LSD1-Dependent Foliar ROS and SA Levels

In control conditions, we observed a significantly lower foliar H_2O_2 level in *lsd1* and *mc8* mutants compared to wild-type plants. The concentration of foliar H_2O_2 in the double *mc8/lsd1* mutant did not differ significantly from the wild type. After the UV irradiation episode, we observed the highest foliar H_2O_2 content in the *lsd1* mutant, while in *mc8*, it was lower than in the wild-type plants. The double *mc8/lsd1* mutant did not differ from the wild type in terms of H_2O_2 content, while the *mc8* mutant demonstrated the lowest H_2O_2 content after UV stress (Figure 2A). Salicylic acid is an important cell death signaling molecule and the RCD phenotype of *lsd1* is related to high foliar SA content [19,20]. Because of this fact, we performed an analysis of SA content in foliar tissues of tested *Arabidopsis thaliana* mutants. In control conditions, the *lsd1* mutant did not differ much from the wild type, while the *mc8* plants exhibited an insignificantly lower SA content. After UV stress, foliar SA levels were strongly increased in *lsd1*, but in *mc8* and in double *lsd1/mc8* mutants, they were increased similarly like in the wild-type plants (Figure 2B).

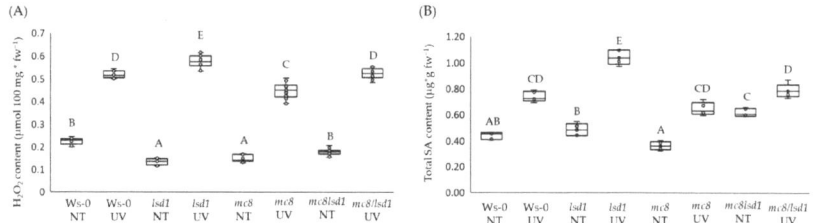

Figure 2. Foliar (**A**) H_2O_2 and (**B**) salicylic acid levels in control conditions and 24 h after UV irradiation. Within a subgraph, values sharing common letters are not significantly different from each other ($p > 0.001$) (n = 6).

2.3. High PR5 Gene Expression Level in lsd1 Is Reverted by the Mutation in MC8

PR genes' expression is strongly up-regulated in the *lsd1* mutant [19] and their expression is related to SA levels in plant tissues [41,42]. Therefore, we decided to check the expression of *PR1*, *PR2* and *PR5* in all lines being investigated in this study. In control conditions, we found similarly low expression levels of *PR1* and *PR2* in all tested genotypes. The *PR5* expression level was differentiated, and its expression was significantly higher in the *lsd1* mutant in control conditions in comparison to the wild type and other tested mutants (Figure 3A–C). After UV irradiation, *PR1* expression was higher in all tested genotypes when compared to control conditions. However, the *PR1* transcript was drastically increased in *lsd1* and *mc8/lsd1* mutants (Figure 3A). Upon UV stress, the *PR2* expression level was significantly higher in *lsd1* and *mc8/lsd1* mutants (Figure 3B). However, the expression level of *PR5* after UV stress was significantly higher only in the *lsd1* mutant when compared to the wild type (Figure 3C).

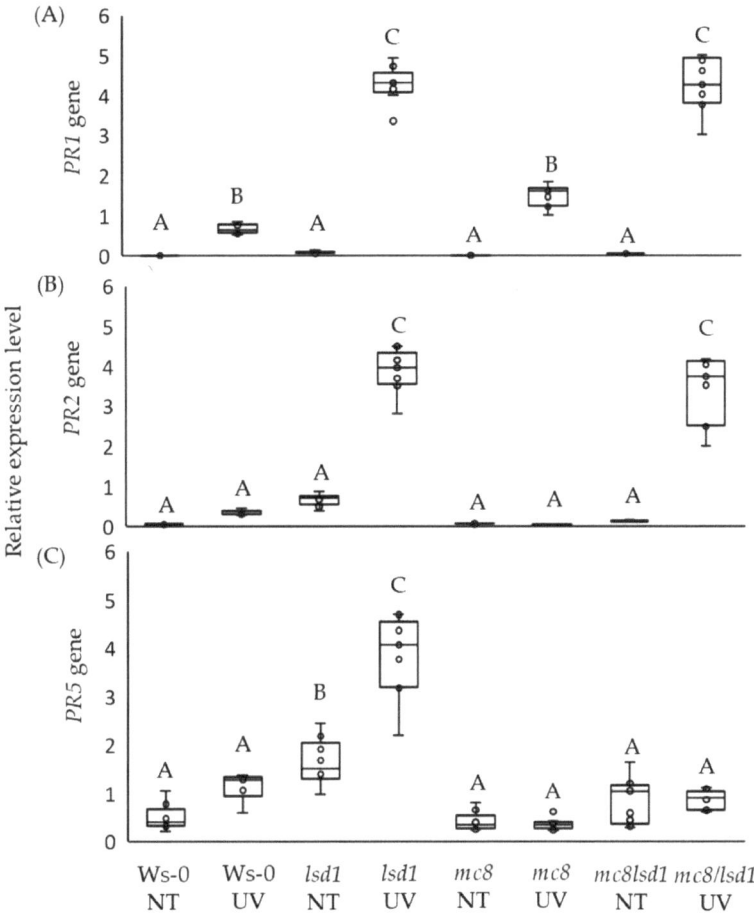

Figure 3. *PR* genes' relative expression levels in non-stress ambient laboratory conditions and in response to UV irradiation episode. (**A**) *PR1*, (**B**) *PR2* and (**C**) *PR5* expression levels in tested mutants in control conditions and 24 h after UV irradiation. Within a subgraph, values sharing common letters are not significantly different from each other ($p > 0.001$) ($n = 9$).

2.4. PR Proteins Are Degraded in Response to UV Stress

Despite the fact that we found a very strong up-regulation of *PR1* gene expression in *lsd1* and *mc8/lsd1* mutants in stress conditions (Figure 3A), we did not observe a higher PR1 protein level. In fact, the PR1 protein level was similar in wild type plants and decreased in other tested genotypes after UV stress, in comparison to control conditions (Figure 4A). Even though the expression of the *PR2* gene was strongly up-regulated in *lsd1* and *mc8/lsd1* mutants in response to UV irradiation, in *lsd1* and in mc8/*lsd1*, the level of the PR2 protein decreased (Figure 4B). The PR5 protein was present in all of the tested genotypes; however, the higher amount of this protein was found in *mc8* and *lsd1/mc8* mutants in control conditions. The level of PR5 protein decreased in response to stress in all of the tested genotypes (Figure 4C). The experiment was performed in two independent biological replicates (Supplementary Figure S4).

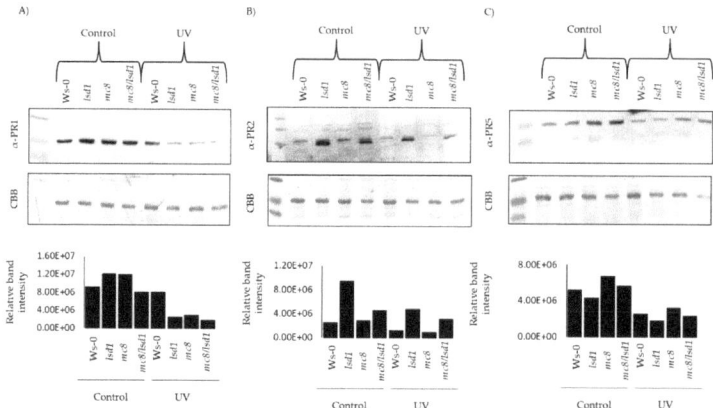

Figure 4. Level of PR proteins in response to UV irradiation. Western blot analysis of (**A**) PR1, (**B**) PR2 and (**C**) PR5 proteins in all tested genotypes in control conditions and 24 h after UV irradiation. The graphs show relative intensity of the bands (presented on gels) for each tested protein. As a loading control, CBB staining was used.

2.5. Prediction of MC8 Interaction

The protein–protein interaction of LSD1 is well known, and there is no information about any LSD1-MC8 interaction [27]. There is no prediction of the potential interaction of MC8 with LSD1, EDS1 and PAD4 nor of any other proteins which were previously described as LSD1, EDS1 and PAD4 interactors. This indicates the lack of protein–protein interaction with the above-mentioned CD-regulating proteins. Moreover, it shows that the analyzed pathway is dependent on hormones and ROS, which are regulated by LSD1/EDS1/PAD4 proteins (Supplementary Figure S5 and Supplementary Table S2).

3. Discussion

Plants are constantly exposed to various types of environmental stresses and because of that, they have developed many mechanisms and pathways to mitigate the effects of unfavorable conditions. One of the mechanisms activated during plant response to stress is programed cell death (PCD), a very old evolutionary mechanism present in all multicellular living organisms [43–45]. The role of PCD in plant response to stresses is basically the elimination of affected and/or older cells in order to induce higher tolerance and better acclimation in the other cells and maintenance of cellular homeostasis within an organism [46,47]. It is well known that this process is under conditional control of the LSD1 protein as well as EDS1 and PAD4, which are negative and positive cell death regulators, respectively [16,22,23,26,48]. Reversal of the *lsd1* RCD phenotype is nothing new. This effect was obtained by mutation in *EDS1* or *PAD4* genes in the *lsd1* mutant background, because these proteins physically interact with each other, forming a trimmer [26,27]. When there is no LSD1 protein present (*lsd1* mutant) or it is at a lower level (in field conditions), the EDS1 and PAD4 proteins are active, and when there is only EDS1 (*lsd1/pad4* mutant) present, it cannot induce a PR pathway alone [21–23,49]. Another way to revert the *lsd1* phenotype is to disable the chloroplast signal recognition particle cpSRP 43 protein (encoded by the *CAO* gene) [32]. CAO is involved in the regulation of light-harvesting antenna size and non-photochemical quenching of absorbed energy in excess by photosystem II [50]. In the *lsd1/cao* double mutant, there is a reversion of the RCD phenotype due to its reduced ability to absorb light energy [3,32]. Thus, LSD1 is a negative regulator of PCD and photorespiration and a positive regulator of the antioxidant system [3]. Another piece of evidence to support chloroplast retrograde signaling mediated by cytoplasmic LSD1/EDS1/PAD4 proteins is presented in the *lsd1/ex1* mutant which did not exhibit the RCD phenotype [51]. EXECUTER1 (EX1) is involved in singlet oxygen chloroplast retrograde signaling. ROS do not act alone in plant cells and the relation between SA and ROS in plant stress response is well known [22]. Because of this, deregulation in SA synthesis/metabolism also leads to reversion of the *lsd1* phenotype in mutants such as *lsd1/sid2* or in transgenic plants like *lsd1/NahG* [19,20]. Ours results and those of previous studies strongly suggest that a unified genetic and molecular system for the regulation of biotic and abiotic stress responses and cross-tolerance has evolved in plants [52]. Ethylene is also involved in conditional regulation by LSD1/EDS1/PAD4 PCD signaling, since impairment of this signaling pathway in the *ein2/lsd1* double mutant also leads to reversion of the RCD *lsd1* phenotype [2]. Interestingly, the *lsd1* mutant, when grown in field conditions, did not differ from the wild type in size, visually or in seed yield [16,22]. In ambient laboratory conditions, *lsd1* mutant plants are much smaller and produce much fewer seeds (fourfold lower seed yield) than the wild-type or double *eds1/lsd1* and *pad4/lsd1* plants. While all currently known ways to revert the *lsd1* RCD phenotype are related to changes in ROS, SA or ethylene signaling pathways or to LSD1-interactor proteins, in this study, we found a new protein, MC8, which, according to the current knowledge [38,53] and bioinformatic prediction (Supplementary Figure S4 and Supplementary Table S2), does not interact with LSD1 and is not involved in SA, ROS and ET synthesis/metabolism, which suggests its functions as a signal receiver (ROS/hormonal) and as the final enforcer of LSD1-dependent cell death. During the analysis of our previously performed microarray [16], in the context of genes from the METACASPASE family, we found a significant positive fold change in *MC8* in laboratory growing conditions (inducing RCD) and a significant negative fold change in field conditions (not inducing RCD). Moreover, in double *lsd1/eds1* and *lsd1/pad4* mutants with well-known reversion of the *lsd1* RCD phenotype [22,23], there was a non-positive fold change in *MC8*, which indicates that MC8 acts upstream of the LSD1/EDS1/PAD4 trimer. These results were confirmed by studies on the *mc8/lsd1* mutant. A double mutant exhibited a completely reverted RCD phenotype. This is probably caused by the fact that MC8 transcription is ROS-dependent, which was experimentally demonstrated by exogenous H_2O_2 treatment and by the induction ROS synthesis by of UV-C stress [22,38]. In conclusion, we can assume that MC8 is an important protein in the conditional LSD1/EDS1/PAD4-dependent cell death regulatory pathway. MC8 most probably is not related to SA and ROS synthesis or metabolism since in the *lsd1/mc8* double mutant, we found lower or similar foliar levels of SA and H_2O_2 to those observed in wild-type plants. It is probably involved in the very early stage of metacaspases cascades of PCD and/or the inhibition of the second burst of the ROS/SA [44,54] wave from cell organelles undergoing PCD, which was observed in the RCD of the *lsd1* mutant [23] or generally while PCD progressed in wild-type plants [44,55]. Inhibition of gene expression from the *PR* family was previously proposed as one of the reasons for the inhibition of RCD in *lsd1/eds1*, *pad4/lsd1*, *sid2/lsd1*, etc. [19,49]. However, in the *lsd1/mc8* mutant, EDS1 and PAD4 were not inhibited by LSD1. This led to the induction of *PR1* and *PR2* expression in *lsd1/mc8* on a similar level as in the *lsd1* mutant. The exception is *PR5* and its higher expression, which was observed only in the *lsd1* mutant but not in *lsd1/mc8*. It could be caused by the fact that SA and ROS levels were slightly, but statistically significantly higher in *lsd1* compared to *lsd1/mc8*. There are some alternatives to the SA-related signaling pathway [56] and there is a reverse correlation between H_2O_2 steady-state concentration and *PR5* gene expression [57]. However, the number of PR proteins appear to be different to the *PR* genes' transcription level. In general, in all of the mutants and in the wild-type plants, 24 h after UV-A + B stress, we found lower levels of PR1, PR2 and PR5. This is opposite to biotic stress, where the number of PR proteins were higher after pathogen inoculation [58]. This indicates that in response to abiotic stress (UV stress), a *PR* gene family is regulated differently on transcription and translation levels. However, this requires further research. Based on the current knowledge and on our results, we propose a model of LSD1 and MC8 interdependence in plant PCD regulation in response to UV-A + B irradiation (Figure 5). The UV episode is comprehended mostly by chloroplasts and provokes changes in the quantum-redox status of the photosynthetic electron transport chain components [3,59–62]. It leads to ROS overproduction [63], which consequently leads to increased synthesis of SA [3]. Both ROS and phytohormones act as a signal for LSD1 inhibition, which leads to EDS1 and PAD4 increasing in activity and then to the induction of cell death. Nevertheless, in other cells, LSD1 is induced, thus inhibiting EDS1 and PAD4 and preventing PCD spreading. Meanwhile, in the *lsd1* mutant, there is no LSD1, thus EDS1 and PAD4 are hyperactive and act as inhibitors of the antioxidant system [3] and are important in SA synthesis [64,65]. This altogether leads to RCD induction [66]. However, in *lsd1/mc8*, all ROS/SA/ET signaling is still deregulated because of the lack of functional LSD1 and the lack of LSD1/EDS1/PAD4 trimers, thus EDS1 and PAD4 should induce the RCD phenotype, but such phenotype in *lsd1/mc8* is not observed after UV stress. This is probably because MC8 is a receiver of the above-mentioned signals and MC8 acts upstream of all of the above-described proteins and thus is the ultimate executor of the run-away cell death process.

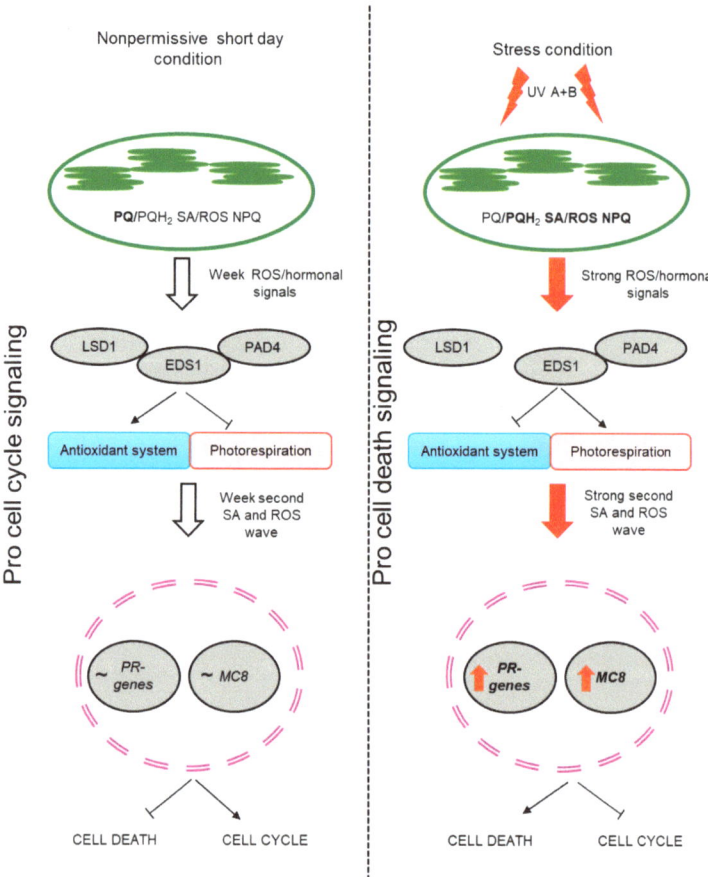

Figure 5. Proposed/hypothetical model of LSD1 and MC8 interdependence in plant cell death regulation in response to UV-A + B irradiation. We propose that MC8 is more important in the cell death pathway dependent on LSD1 than the proposed EDS1 and PAD4 proteins (there are more details in the last paragraph of the discussion). The arrow is the inducing action; The blunt-headed arrow is braking; The red arrow next to the gene names is increased expression; The tilde sign is an expression without change.

4. Materials and Methods

4.1. Plant Material

In this study, *Arabidopsis thaliana* mutants, *lsd1*, *mc8* and *mc8/lsd1*, and wild-type plants (Ws-0) were used. All used mutants were of Wassilewskija (Ws-0) background. Wild-type and *lsd1* seeds were already available in our lab, while *mc8* seeds were provided by Dr. Patrick Gallois (Faculty of Biology, Medicine and Health, University of Manchester, Manchester, UK). In order to obtain a double mutant, we crossed *lsd1* and *mc8*. A double mutant was obtained via selection in T3 generation. Correctness of the crossing was checked by PCR (Figure S6) and by RT-PCR (Figure S1). All primers used in the study are attached in the Supplementary Material (Table S3).

4.2. Growing Conditions

For all experiments described in this study, plants were grown in a walk-in-type growing chamber (Siemens, München, Germany) under the following conditions: 8/16 h photoperiod, photosynthetic photon flux density of 80 μmol photons m$^{-2}\cdot$s^{-1}, air humidity of 50% and day/night temperature of 20/18 °C.

4.3. Stress Induction

For the determination of different stress impacts on *MC8* expression levels, wild-type plants were treated with heat, light and UV-A + B using the following methods. For UV A + B stress application, the UV 500 Crosslinker (Hoefer Pharmacia Biotech, San Francisco, CA, USA) was used. It was equipped with three UV-B lamps (type G8T5E, Sankyo Denki, peak wavelength 306 nm) and two UV-A lamps (type TL8WBLB, Philips, Tokyo, Japan, peak wavelength 365 nm). *Arabidopsis thaliana* plants were exposed to a single irradiation dose of 1500 mJ$\cdot$cm^{-2}. Light treatment was performed using a white LED panel with the emission of white light (with 1500 μmol photons m$^{-2}\cdot$s^{-1}) (Photon System Instrument, Brno, Czech Republic) for 2 h. For heat stress treatment, plants were incubated in 40 °C for two hours in the laboratory incubator MOV-212s (Philips, Tokyo, Japan). All analyses described in this study were performed 24 h after stress application. After the stress episode, plants were put back in the growing chamber in the same conditions as they were grown in before. For future experiments, UV A + B were chosen, and wild-type plants and all mutants used in this study were exposed to a single irradiation dose of 1500 mJ$\cdot$cm^{-2}.

4.4. Ion Leakage Measurement

Ion leakage was determined as described before [19,44].

4.5. Determination of H_2O_2 and SA Contents

The concentration of hydrogen peroxide (H_2O_2) was assessed according to the method described before [67], with slight adjustments. A total of 50–100 mg of frozen tissue was homogenized in a TissueLyser LT (Qiagen, Venlo, The Netherlands) for 5 min at 50 Hz and 4 °C, using 300 μL of cold 0.1% trichloroacetic acid (TCA), then centrifuged at 13,000 rpm for 15 min. The resulting supernatant was combined with 10 mM potassium phosphate buffer (pH 7.0) and 1 M potassium iodide (KI) at a 1:1:2 (*v:v:v*) ratio. The absorbance was measured at 390 nm using a microplate reader, Multiscan GO (Thermo Scientific, Waltham, MA, USA), and the H_2O_2 concentration was determined using an appropriate standard curve. Results were quantified and expressed as micromoles of H_2O_2 per 100 mg of fresh weight.

The determination of salicylic acid (SA) followed the protocol described before [68], with the utilization of 2-methoxybenzoic acid (oANI) and 3-hydroxybenzoic acid (pHBA) as internal standards. Salicylic acid was separated using a Luna 5uC18(2)100A150x4.6mm column (Phenomenex, Torrance, CA, USA) at 30 °C for 15 min, employing a Shimadzu HPLC System (Shimadzu, Kyoto, Japan). A low-pressure gradient system was used, utilizing a 20 mM phosphate buffer (pH 2.5; adjusted with 8 M HCl) and acetonitrile

(75:25; v/v) at a flow rate of 1 mL per minute. Results were quantified and expressed as micrograms of SA per gram of fresh weight.

4.6. RNA Isolation, cDNA Synthesis and RT-PCR Analysis

RNA was extracted from frozen tissue previously stored in $-80\ °C$. For RNA isolation, the GeneMaTRIX Universal RNA Purification Kit (EURX, Gdańsk, Poland) with an additional step of on-column DNase digestion was used. RNA concentration and quality were assessed using a spectrometer (Eppendorf, Hamburg, Germany). RNA quality was controlled by electrophoretic separation in 1% agarose gel. cDNa synthesis was performed for equimolar RNA amounts of each sample using a High Capacity cDNa Reverse Transcription Kit (Thermo Fisher Scientific). qPCRs were performed in three technical repetitions for each of the three biological replicates using the Power SYBR Green PCR Master Mix and the aBI 7500 Fast Real-Time PCR System (Thermo Fisher Scientific, Waltham, MA, USA). Two reference genes were used: 5-FORMYLTETRAHYDROFOLATE CYCLOLIGASE (5-FCL, AT5G13050) and PROTEIN PHOSPHATASE 2A SUBUNIT A2 (PP2AA2, aT3G25800).

4.7. Protein Extraction and Western Blot Analysis

Total plant protein extraction was performed as previously described [69], with modifications. Proteins were extracted from 100 mg of ground leaf tissue. The powder was resuspended in 500 μL of 2× Leammli buffer (4% SDS, 20% glycerol, 0.12 M Tris-HCl pH 7.0, 0.02% bromophenol blue and 0.7 M β-mercaptoethanol) and incubated for 10 min at 95 °C, followed by incubation for 10 min in ice [70]. The resuspended samples were centrifuged at $12,000\times g$ for 5 min at 4 °C and the supernatants were used for further steps. Total protein concentration was determined using the RC-DC protein assay kit II (Bio-Rad, Hercules, CA, USA, 5000122). A total of 50 μg of total protein extract was used for 12% SDS-PAGE. Next, the proteins were electrotransferred to an Immobilon P PVDF membrane (Merck, Darmstadt, Germany) using the Trans-Blot Turbo Transfer System (Bio-Rad). The membrane was blocked in 2% skim milk in TBS-T buffer (1× Tris-buffered Saline, 0.1% Tween-20) for at least 1 h and incubated with primary antibodies (diluted at a ratio of 1:10,000, 2% skim milk in TBS-T buffer)—PR1 (AS10 687, Agrisera, Vännäs, Sweden) for 1 h at room temperature, and PR2 (AS12 2366, Agrisera) and PR5 (AS12 2373, Arisera) overnight at 4 °C. Incubation with the goat anti-rabbit horseradish peroxidase-conjugated secondary antibodies (Thermofisher, QG221919; diluted at a ratio of 1:10,000) was performed for 1 h at room temperature. Protein bands were immunodetected using SuperSignal West Dura Extended Duration Substrate (Thermo Scientific, 34075) according to the manufacturer's recommendations, visualized with the ChemiDoc XRS+ System (Bio-Rad) and analyzed with ImageLab Software 5.2.1 (Bio-Rad). Total protein staining of membranes was conducted as described previously [71].

Supplementary Materials: The supporting information can be downloaded at: https://www.mdpi.com/article/10.3390/ijms25063195/s1.

Author Contributions: M.J.B. formed the hypothesis, planned the experiments, wrote the manuscript and was involved in mutants crossing, elative electrolyte leakage measurement, RNA isolation, cDNA synthesis and real-time PCR analysis. A.R. was involved in SA and H_2O_2 determination. K.G. was involved in proteomic analysis. A.B.M.-F. performed the experiment for determination of MC8 levels in response to abiotic stresses. W.C. was involved in drafting the manuscript, and S.M.K. was involved in formulating the hypothesis, planning the experiments and drafting the manuscript. All authors have read and agreed to the published version of the manuscript.

Funding: This study was funded by the "Miniatura 4" project (2020/04/X/NZ3/00829) granted to Maciej Jerzy Bernacki by the National Science Centre and the "OPUS 15" project (UMO-2018/29/B/NZ3/01198) granted to Stanisław Karpiński by the National Science Centre.

Institutional Review Board Statement: Not applicable.

Informed Consent Statement: Not applicable.

Data Availability Statement: All of the data generated or analyzed during this study are included in the published article and its Supplementary Files.

Acknowledgments: We would like to thank Patrick Gallois for providing the *mc8* mutant seeds and for his help and advice during genotyping. We would like to express our gratitude to Aleksandra Lechańska for proofreading as well.

Conflicts of Interest: The authors declare that they have no competing interests.

References

1. Mühlenbock, P.; Plaszczyca, M.; Plaszczyca, M.; Mellerowicz, E.; Karpinski, S. Lysigenous Aerenchyma Formation in Arabidopsis Is Controlled by *LESION SIMULATING DISEASE1*. *Plant Cell* **2007**, *19*, 3819–3830. [CrossRef] [PubMed]
2. Mühlenbock, P.; Szechynska-Hebda, M.; Plaszczyca, M.; Baudo, M.; Mateo, A.; Mullineaux, P.M.; Parker, J.E.; Karpinska, B.; Karpinski, S. Chloroplast Signaling and LESION SIMULATING DISEASE1 Regulate Crosstalk between Light Acclimation and Immunity in Arabidopsis. *Plant Cell* **2008**, *20*, 2339–2356. [CrossRef] [PubMed]
3. Karpiński, S.; Szechyńska-Hebda, M.; Wituszyńska, W.; Burdiak, P. Light Acclimation, Retrograde Signalling, Cell Death and Immune Defences in Plants. *Plant Cell Environ.* **2013**, *36*, 736–744. [CrossRef]
4. Szechyńska-Hebda, M.; Kruk, J.; Górecka, M.; Karpińska, B.; Karpiński, S. Evidence for Light Wavelength-Specific Photoelectrophysiological Signaling and Memory of Excess Light Episodes in Arabidopsis. *Plant Cell* **2010**, *22*, 2201–2218. [CrossRef] [PubMed]
5. Spoel, S.H.; Dong, X. How Do Plants Achieve Immunity? Defence without Specialized Immune Cells. *Nat. Rev. Immunol.* **2012**, *12*, 89–100. [CrossRef]
6. Fukuda, H. Programmed Cell Death of Tracheary Elements as a Paradigm in Plants. *Plant Mol. Biol.* **2000**, *44*, 245–253. [CrossRef]
7. Domínguez, F.; Cejudo, F.J. Programmed Cell Death (PCD): An Essential Process of Cereal Seed Development and Germination. *Front Plant Sci* **2014**, *5*, 366. [CrossRef]
8. Jabs, T.; Dietrich, R.A.; Dangl, J.L. Initiation of Runaway Cell Death in an Arabidopsis Mutant by Extracellular Superoxide. *Science* **1996**, *273*, 1853–1856. [CrossRef]
9. Lorrain, S.; Vailleau, F.; Balagué, C.; Roby, D. Lesion Mimic Mutants: Keys for Deciphering Cell Death and Defense Pathways in Plants? *Trends Plant Sci.* **2003**, *8*, 263–271. [CrossRef]
10. Vandenabeele, S.; Vanderauwera, S.; Vuylsteke, M.; Rombauts, S.; Langebartels, C.; Seidlitz, H.K.; Zabeau, M.; Van Montagu, M.; Inzé, D.; Van Breusegem, F. Catalase Deficiency Drastically Affects Gene Expression Induced by High Light in Arabidopsis Thaliana. *Plant J.* **2004**, *39*, 45–58. [CrossRef]
11. Dietrich, R.A.; Delaney, T.P.; Uknes, S.J.; Ward, E.R.; Ryals, J.A.; Dangl, J.L. Arabidopsis Mutants Simulating Disease Resistance Response. *Cell* **1994**, *77*, 565–577. [CrossRef]
12. Wituszyńska, W.; Karpiński, S. Programmed Cell Death as a Response to High Light, UV and Drought Stress in Plants. In *Abiotic Stress—Plant Responses and Applications in Agriculture*; InTech: Rijeka, Croatia; Shanghai, China, 2013. [CrossRef]
13. Mateo, A.; Funck, D.; Mühlenbock, P.; Kular, B.; Mullineaux, P.M.; Karpinski, S. Controlled Levels of Salicylic Acid Are Required for Optimal Photosynthesis and Redox Homeostasis. *J. Exp. Bot.* **2006**, *57*, 1795–1807. [CrossRef]
14. Chai, T.; Zhou, J.; Liu, J.; Xing, D. LSD1 and HY5 Antagonistically Regulate Red Light Induced-Programmed Cell Death in Arabidopsis. *Front. Plant Sci.* **2015**, *6*, 292. [CrossRef] [PubMed]
15. Bernacki, M.J.; Mielecki, J.; Antczak, A.; Drożdżek, M.; Witoń, D.; Dąbrowska-Bronk, J.; Gawroński, P.; Burdiak, P.; Marchwicka, M.; Rusaczonek, A.; et al. Biotechnological Potential of the Stress Response and Plant Cell Death Regulators Proteins in the Biofuel Industry. *Cells* **2023**, *12*, 2018. [CrossRef] [PubMed]
16. Wituszyńska, W.; Ślesak, I.; Vanderauwera, S.; Szechyńska-Hebda, M.; Kornaś, A.; Kelen, K.V.D.; Mühlenbock, P.; Karpińska, B.; Maćkowski, S.; Breusegem, F.V.; et al. LESION SIMULATING DISEASE1, ENHANCED DISEASE SUSCEPTIBILITY1, and PHYTOALEXIN DEFICIENT4 Conditionally Regulate Cellular Signaling Homeostasis, Photosynthesis, Water Use Efficiency, and Seed Yield in Arabidopsis. *Plant Physiol.* **2013**, *161*, 1795–1805. [CrossRef] [PubMed]
17. Szechyńska-Hebda, M.; Czarnocka, W.; Hebda, M.; Karpiński, S. PAD4, LSD1 and EDS1 Regulate Drought Tolerance, Plant Biomass Production, and Cell Wall Properties. *Plant Cell Rep.* **2016**, *35*, 527–539. [CrossRef] [PubMed]
18. Huang, X.; Li, Y.; Zhang, X.; Zuo, J.; Yang, S. The Arabidopsis LSD1 Gene Plays an Important Role in the Regulation of Low Temperature-Dependent Cell Death. *New Phytol.* **2010**, *187*, 301–312. [CrossRef] [PubMed]
19. Bernacki, M.J.; Rusaczonek, A.; Czarnocka, W.; Karpiński, S. Salicylic Acid Accumulation Controlled by LSD1 Is Essential in Triggering Cell Death in Response to Abiotic Stress. *Cells* **2021**, *10*, 962. [CrossRef] [PubMed]
20. Aviv, D.H.; Rustérucci, C.; Iii, B.F.H.; Dietrich, R.A.; Parker, J.E.; Dangl, J.L. Runaway Cell Death, but Not Basal Disease Resistance, in Lsd1 Is SA- and NIM1/NPR1-Dependent. *Plant J.* **2002**, *29*, 381–391. [CrossRef] [PubMed]
21. Rustérucci, C.; Aviv, D.H.; Holt, B.F.; Dangl, J.L.; Parker, J.E. The Disease Resistance Signaling Components EDS1 and PAD4 Are Essential Regulators of the Cell Death Pathway Controlled by LSD1 in Arabidopsis. *Plant Cell* **2001**, *13*, 2211–2224. [CrossRef]
22. Bernacki, M.J.; Czarnocka, W.; Rusaczonek, A.; Witoń, D.; Kęska, S.; Czyż, J.; Szechyńska-Hebda, M.; Karpiński, S. LSD1, EDS1 and PAD4-dependent conditional correlation among salicylic acid, hydrogen peroxide, water use efficiency, and seed yield in Arabidopsis thaliana. *Physiol. Plant.* **2018**, *165*, 369–382. [CrossRef]

23. Wituszyńska, W.; Szechyńska-Hebda, M.; Sobczak, M.; Rusaczonek, A.; Kozłowska-Makulska, A.; Witoń, D.; Karpiński, S. Lesion Simulating Disease 1 and Enhanced Disease Susceptibility 1 Differentially Regulate UV-C-Induced Photooxidative Stress Signalling and Programmed Cell Death in Arabidopsis Thaliana. *Plant Cell Environ.* **2015**, *38*, 315–330. [CrossRef]
24. Li, Y.; Chen, L.; Mu, J.; Zuo, J. LESION SIMULATING DISEASE1 Interacts with Catalases to Regulate Hypersensitive Cell Death in Arabidopsis1[C][W]. *Plant Physiol.* **2013**, *163*, 1059–1070. [CrossRef]
25. Kliebenstein, D.J.; Dietrich, R.A.; Martin, A.C.; Last, R.L.; Dangl, J.L. LSD1 Regulates Salicylic Acid Induction of Copper Zinc Superoxide Dismutase in Arabidopsis Thaliana. *Mol. Plant. Microbe. Interact.* **1999**, *12*, 1022–1026. [CrossRef]
26. Feys, B.J.; Moisan, L.J.; Newman, M.-A.; Parker, J.E. Direct Interaction between the Arabidopsis Disease Resistance Signaling Proteins, EDS1 and PAD4. *EMBO J.* **2001**, *20*, 5400–5411. [CrossRef]
27. Czarnocka, W.; Van Der Kelen, K.; Willems, P.; Szechyńska-Hebda, M.; Shahnejat-Bushehri, S.; Balazadeh, S.; Rusaczonek, A.; Mueller-Roeber, B.; Van Breusegem, F.; Karpiński, S. The Dual Role of LESION SIMULATING DISEASE 1 as a Condition-Dependent Scaffold Protein and Transcription Regulator. *Plant Cell Environ.* **2017**, *40*, 2644–2662. [CrossRef]
28. Parker, J.E.; Holub, E.B.; Frost, L.N.; Falk, A.; Gunn, N.D.; Daniels, M.J. Characterization of Eds1, a Mutation in Arabidopsis Suppressing Resistance to Peronospora Parasitica Specified by Several Different RPP Genes. *Plant Cell* **1996**, *8*, 2033–2046. [CrossRef] [PubMed]
29. Glazebrook, J.; Rogers, E.E.; Ausubel, F.M. Isolation of Arabidopsis Mutants with Enhanced Disease Susceptibility by Direct Screening. *Genetics* **1996**, *143*, 973–982. [CrossRef] [PubMed]
30. Falk, A.; Feys, B.J.; Frost, L.N.; Jones, J.D.G.; Daniels, M.J.; Parker, J.E. EDS1, an Essential Component of R Gene-Mediated Disease Resistance in Arabidopsis Has Homology to Eukaryotic Lipases. *Proc. Natl. Acad. Sci. USA* **1999**, *96*, 3292–3297. [CrossRef] [PubMed]
31. Jirage, D.; Tootle, T.L.; Reuber, T.L.; Frost, L.N.; Feys, B.J.; Parker, J.E.; Ausubel, F.M.; Glazebrook, J. Arabidopsis Thaliana PAD4 Encodes a Lipase-like Gene That Is Important for Salicylic Acid Signaling. *Proc. Natl. Acad. Sci. USA* **1999**, *96*, 13583–13588. [CrossRef] [PubMed]
32. Mateo, A.; Mühlenbock, P.; Rustérucci, C.; Chang, C.C.-C.; Miszalski, Z.; Karpinska, B.; Parker, J.E.; Mullineaux, P.M.; Karpinski, S. LESION SIMULATING DISEASE 1 Is Required for Acclimation to Conditions That Promote Excess Excitation Energy. *Plant Physiol.* **2004**, *136*, 2818–2830. [CrossRef]
33. Dietrich, R.A.; Richberg, M.H.; Schmidt, R.; Dean, C.; Dangl, J.L. A Novel Zinc Finger Protein Is Encoded by the Arabidopsis LSD1 Gene and Functions as a Negative Regulator of Plant Cell Death. *Cell* **1997**, *88*, 685–694. [CrossRef]
34. Takatsuji, H. Zinc-Finger Transcription Factors in Plants. *CMLS Cell. Mol. Life Sci.* **1998**, *54*, 582–596. [CrossRef]
35. Coll, N.S.; Vercammen, D.; Smidler, A.; Clover, C.; Van Breusegem, F.; Dangl, J.L.; Epple, P. Arabidopsis Type I Metacaspases Control Cell Death. *Science* **2010**, *330*, 1393–1397. [CrossRef]
36. Fagundes, D.; Bohn, B.; Cabreira, C.; Leipelt, F.; Dias, N.; Bodanese-Zanettini, M.H.; Cagliari, A. Caspases in Plants: Metacaspase Gene Family in Plant Stress Responses. *Funct. Integr. Genom.* **2015**, *15*, 639–649. [CrossRef]
37. Vercammen, D.; van de Cotte, B.; De Jaeger, G.; Eeckhout, D.; Casteels, P.; Vandepoele, K.; Vandenberghe, I.; Van Beeumen, J.; Inzé, D.; Van Breusegem, F. Type II Metacaspases Atmc4 and Atmc9 of Arabidopsis Thaliana Cleave Substrates after Arginine and Lysine. *J. Biol. Chem.* **2004**, *279*, 45329–45336. [CrossRef] [PubMed]
38. He, R.; Drury, G.E.; Rotari, V.I.; Gordon, A.; Willer, M.; Farzaneh, T.; Woltering, E.J.; Gallois, P. Metacaspase-8 Modulates Programmed Cell Death Induced by Ultraviolet Light and H_2O_2 in Arabidopsis. *J. Biol. Chem.* **2008**, *283*, 774–783. [CrossRef] [PubMed]
39. Kwon, S.I.; Hwang, D.J. Expression Analysis of the Metacaspase Gene Family in Arabidopsis. *J. Plant Biol.* **2013**, *56*, 391–398. [CrossRef]
40. Tsiatsiani, L.; Van Breusegem, F.; Gallois, P.; Zavialov, A.; Lam, E.; Bozhkov, P.V. Metacaspases. *Cell Death Differ.* **2011**, *18*, 1279–1288. [CrossRef]
41. Glazebrook, J. Genes Controlling Expression of Defense Responses in Arabidopsis—2001 Status. *Curr. Opin. Plant Biol.* **2001**, *4*, 301–308. [CrossRef] [PubMed]
42. Thomma, B.P.; Penninckx, I.A.; Cammue, B.P.; Broekaert, W.F. The Complexity of Disease Signaling in Arabidopsis. *Curr. Opin. Immunol.* **2001**, *13*, 63–68. [CrossRef]
43. Burke, R.; Schwarze, J.; Sherwood, O.L.; Jnaid, Y.; McCabe, P.F.; Kacprzyk, J. Stressed to Death: The Role of Transcription Factors in Plant Programmed Cell Death Induced by Abiotic and Biotic Stimuli. *Front. Plant Sci.* **2020**, *11*, 1235. [CrossRef]
44. Bernacki, M.J.; Czarnocka, W.; Zaborowska, M.; Różańska, E.; Labudda, M.; Rusaczonek, A.; Witoń, D.; Karpiński, S. EDS1-Dependent Cell Death and the Antioxidant System in Arabidopsis Leaves Is Deregulated by the Mammalian Bax. *Cells* **2020**, *9*, 2454. [CrossRef]
45. Lacomme, C.; Cruz, S.S. Bax-Induced Cell Death in Tobacco Is Similar to the Hypersensitive Response. *Proc. Natl. Acad. Sci. USA* **1999**, *96*, 7956–7961. [CrossRef]
46. Danon, A.; Delorme, V.; Mailhac, N.; Gallois, P. Plant Programmed Cell Death: A Common Way to Die. *Plant Physiol. Biochem.* **2000**, *38*, 647–655. [CrossRef]
47. Williams, B.; Dickman, M. Plant Programmed Cell Death: Can't Live with It; Can't Live without It. *Mol. Plant Pathol.* **2008**, *9*, 531–544. [CrossRef] [PubMed]

48. Aarts, N.; Metz, M.; Holub, E.; Staskawicz, B.J.; Daniels, M.J.; Parker, J.E. Different Requirements for EDS1 and NDR1 by Disease Resistance Genes Define at Least Two R Gene-Mediated Signaling Pathways in Arabidopsis. *Proc. Natl. Acad. Sci. USA* **1998**, *95*, 10306–10311. [CrossRef] [PubMed]

49. Cui, H.; Gobbato, E.; Kracher, B.; Qiu, J.; Bautor, J.; Parker, J.E. A Core Function of EDS1 with PAD4 Is to Protect the Salicylic Acid Defense Sector in Arabidopsis Immunity. *New Phytol.* **2017**, *213*, 1802–1817. [CrossRef] [PubMed]

50. Tanaka, R.; Koshino, Y.; Sawa, S.; Ishiguro, S.; Okada, K.; Tanaka, A. Overexpression of Chlorophyllide a Oxygenase (CAO) Enlarges the Antenna Size of Photosystem II in Arabidopsis Thaliana. *Plant J.* **2001**, *26*, 365–373. [CrossRef] [PubMed]

51. Lv, R.; Li, Z.; Li, M.; Dogra, V.; Lv, S.; Liu, R.; Lee, K.P.; Kim, C. Uncoupled Expression of Nuclear and Plastid Photosynthesis-Associated Genes Contributes to Cell Death in a Lesion Mimic Mutant. *Plant Cell* **2019**, *31*, 210–230. [CrossRef] [PubMed]

52. Szechyńska-Hebda, M.; Ghalami, R.Z.; Kamran, M.; Van Breusegem, F.; Karpiński, S. To Be or Not to Be? Are Reactive Oxygen Species, Antioxidants, and Stress Signalling Universal Determinants of Life or Death? *Cells* **2022**, *11*, 4105. [CrossRef] [PubMed]

53. Ahn, G.; Jung, I.J.; Cha, J.-Y.; Jeong, S.Y.; Shin, G.-I.; Ji, M.G.; Kim, M.G.; Lee, S.Y.; Kim, W.-Y. Phytochrome B Positively Regulates Red Light-Mediated ER Stress Response in Arabidopsis. *Front. Plant Sci.* **2022**, *13*, 846294. [CrossRef] [PubMed]

54. Fichman, Y.; Myers, R.J.; Grant, D.G.; Mittler, R. Plasmodesmata-Localized Proteins and ROS Orchestrate Light-Induced Rapid Systemic Signaling in Arabidopsis. *Sci. Signal.* **2021**, *14*, eabf0322. [CrossRef] [PubMed]

55. Kawai-Yamada, M.; Jin, L.; Yoshinaga, K.; Hirata, A.; Uchimiya, H. Mammalian Bax-Induced Plant Cell Death Can Be down-Regulated by Overexpression of Arabidopsis Bax Inhibitor-1 (AtBI-1). *Proc. Natl. Acad. Sci. USA* **2001**, *98*, 12295–12300. [CrossRef] [PubMed]

56. Nawrath, C.; Métraux, J.-P. Salicylic Acid Induction–Deficient Mutants of Arabidopsis Express PR-2 and PR-5 and Accumulate High Levels of Camalexin after Pathogen Inoculation. *Plant Cell* **1999**, *11*, 1393–1404. [CrossRef] [PubMed]

57. Kalbina, I.; Strid, Å. Supplementary Ultraviolet-B Irradiation Reveals Differences in Stress Responses between Arabidopsis Thaliana Ecotypes. *Plant Cell Environ.* **2006**, *29*, 754–763. [CrossRef] [PubMed]

58. Sahoo, A.; Satapathy, K.B.; Panigrahi, G.K. Ectopic Expression of Disease Resistance Protein Promotes Resistance against Pathogen Infection and Drought Stress in Arabidopsis. *Physiol. Mol. Plant Pathol.* **2023**, *124*, 101949. [CrossRef]

59. Czégény, G.; Mátai, A.; Hideg, É. UV-B Effects on Leaves—Oxidative Stress and Acclimation in Controlled Environments. *Plant Sci.* **2016**, *248*, 57–63. [CrossRef]

60. Li, H.; Li, Y.; Deng, H.; Sun, X.; Wang, A.; Tang, X.; Gao, Y.; Zhang, N.; Wang, L.; Yang, S.; et al. Tomato UV-B Receptor SlUVR8 Mediates Plant Acclimation to UV-B Radiation and Enhances Fruit Chloroplast Development via Regulating SlGLK2. *Sci. Rep.* **2018**, *8*, 6097. [CrossRef]

61. Nasibova, A.N. UV-B Radiation Effects on Electron-Transport Reactions in Biomaterials. *Adv. Biol. Earth Sci.* **2022**, *7*, 13–18.

62. Piccini, C.; Cai, G.; Dias, M.C.; Romi, M.; Longo, R.; Cantini, C. UV-B Radiation Affects Photosynthesis-Related Processes of Two Italian Olea Europaea (L.) Varieties Differently. *Plants* **2020**, *9*, 1712. [CrossRef]

63. Mittler, R.; Vanderauwera, S.; Suzuki, N.; Miller, G.; Tognetti, V.B.; Vandepoele, K.; Gollery, M.; Shulaev, V.; Van Breusegem, F. ROS Signaling: The New Wave? *Trends Plant Sci.* **2011**, *16*, 300–309. [CrossRef]

64. Shah, J. The Salicylic Acid Loop in Plant Defense. *Curr. Opin. Plant Biol.* **2003**, *6*, 365–371. [CrossRef] [PubMed]

65. Straus, M.R.; Rietz, S.; Ver Loren van Themaat, E.; Bartsch, M.; Parker, J.E. Salicylic Acid Antagonism of EDS1-Driven Cell Death Is Important for Immune and Oxidative Stress Responses in Arabidopsis. *Plant J.* **2010**, *62*, 628–640. [CrossRef]

66. Mur, L.A.J.; Kenton, P.; Lloyd, A.J.; Ougham, H.; Prats, E. The Hypersensitive Response; the Centenary Is upon Us but How Much Do We Know? *J. Exp. Bot.* **2008**, *59*, 501–520. [CrossRef] [PubMed]

67. Velikova, V.; Sharkey, T.D.; Loreto, F. Stabilization of Thylakoid Membranes in Isoprene-Emitting Plants Reduces Formation of Reactive Oxygen Species. *Plant Signal. Behav.* **2012**, *7*, 139–141. [CrossRef]

68. Meuwly, P.; Métraux, J.P. Ortho-Anisic Acid as Internal Standard for the Simultaneous Quantitation of Salicylic Acid and Its Putative Biosynthetic Precursors in Cucumber Leaves. *Anal. Biochem.* **1993**, *214*, 500–505. [CrossRef]

69. Górecka, M.; Lewandowska, M.; Dąbrowska-Bronk, J.; Białasek, M.; Barczak-Brzyżek, A.; Kulasek, M.; Mielecki, J.; Kozłowska-Makulska, A.; Gawroński, P.; Karpiński, S. Photosystem II 22kDa Protein Level—A Prerequisite for Excess Light-Inducible Memory, Cross-Tolerance to UV-C and Regulation of Electrical Signalling. *Plant Cell Environ.* **2020**, *43*, 649–661. [CrossRef]

70. Laemmli, U.K. Cleavage of Structural Proteins during the Assembly of the Head of Bacteriophage T4. *Nature* **1970**, *227*, 680–685. [CrossRef] [PubMed]

71. Goldman, A.; Harper, S.; Speicher, D.W. Detection of Proteins on Blot Membranes. *Curr. Protoc. Protein Sci.* **2016**, *86*, 10.8.1–10.8.11. [CrossRef]

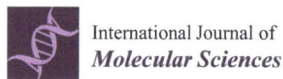

International Journal of
Molecular Sciences

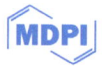

Article

RNAi-Mediated Suppression of *OsBBTI5* Promotes Salt Stress Tolerance in Rice

Zhimin Lin [1,*,†], Xiaoyan Yi [2,†], Muhammad Moaaz Ali [2], Lijuan Zhang [2], Shaojuan Wang [2], Shengnan Tian [2] and Faxing Chen [2,*]

1   Fujian Academy of Agricultural Sciences Biotechnology Institute, Fuzhou 350003, China
2   College of Horticulture, Fujian Agriculture and Forestry University, Fuzhou 350002, China; 1210305019@fafu.edu.cn (X.Y.); moaaz@fafu.edu.cn (M.M.A.); 1210305020@fafu.edu.cn (L.Z.); 3210330057@fafu.edu.cn (S.W.); 3210330052@fafu.edu.cn (S.T.)
*   Correspondence: linzhimin@faas.cn (Z.L.); fxchen@fafu.edu.cn (F.C.)
†   These authors contributed equally to this work.

Abstract: This study explores the impact of RNAi in terms of selectively inhibiting the expression of the *OsBBTI5* gene, with the primary objective of uncovering its involvement in the molecular mechanisms associated with salt tolerance in rice. *OsBBTI5*, belonging to the Bowman–Birk inhibitor (BBI) family gene, is known for its involvement in plant stress responses. The gene was successfully cloned from rice, exhibiting transcriptional self-activation in yeast. A yeast two-hybrid assay confirmed its specific binding to *OsAPX2* (an ascorbate peroxidase gene). Transgenic *OsBBTI5*-RNAi plants displayed insensitivity to varying concentrations of 24-epibrassinolide in the brassinosteroid sensitivity assay. However, they showed reduced root and plant height at high concentrations (10 and 100 μM) of GA_3 immersion. Enzyme activity assays revealed increased peroxidase (POD) and superoxide dismutase (SOD) activities and decreased malondialdehyde (MDA) content under 40–60 mM NaCl. Transcriptomic analysis indicated a significant upregulation of photosynthesis-related genes in transgenic plants under salt stress compared to the wild type. Notably, this study provides novel insights, suggesting that the BBI gene is part of the BR signaling pathway, and that *OsBBTI5* potentially enhances stress tolerance in transgenic plants through interaction with the salt stress-related gene *OsAPX2*.

Keywords: *OsBBTI5*; rice; 24-epibrassinolide; salt tolerance; RNAi; transcriptome

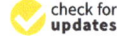

Citation: Lin, Z.; Yi, X.; Ali, M.M.; Zhang, L.; Wang, S.; Tian, S.; Chen, F. RNAi-Mediated Suppression of *OsBBTI5* Promotes Salt Stress Tolerance in Rice. *Int. J. Mol. Sci.* **2024**, *25*, 1284. https://doi.org/10.3390/ijms25021284

Academic Editors: Philippe Jeandet and Mateusz Labudda

Received: 19 October 2023
Revised: 14 January 2024
Accepted: 16 January 2024
Published: 20 January 2024

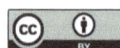
1. Introduction

Abiotic stresses typically exert a direct influence on various facets of plant growth, developmental processes, and ultimate crop yield outcomes [1,2]. Salinity stress is one of the major abiotic stresses [3]. Elevated salinity primarily triggers ionic and osmotic stress in plants, adversely affecting plant cells by disrupting crucial cellular processes such as photosynthesis and promoting the generation of reactive oxygen species (ROS) [4,5]. In the natural environment, dicotyledons exhibit a more extensive range of variation in salinity tolerance compared to monocotyledons. Within the plant kingdom, barley stands out as the most salinity-tolerant species, while wheat typically displays a moderate level of tolerance. Among cereals, rice is notably the most susceptible to salinity stress [6]. Moreover, it is noteworthy that the yield of rice is considerably more affected by salt stress than by the overall growth of the plant [7]. Consequently, there has been a considerable focus on researching salt tolerance in rice, as evidenced by numerous studies [8–10]. Currently, advances in whole genome sequencing, marker-assisted breeding strategies and targeted mutagenesis have greatly improved the tools available for rice breeding [11–15]. Using the whole-genome sequencing analysis of two salt-tolerant (Pokkali and Nona-Bokra) and three salt-sensitive rice varieties (Bengal, Cocodrie and IR64), and employing a combination of quantitative trait locus (QTL) localization and expression profiling data, a total of 396 differentially expressed genes were identified within the coding region [16].

The B-type response regulator *hst1* (hitomebore salt-tolerant 1) controls salinity tolerance in rice by regulating transcription factors and antioxidant mechanisms [17]. The introduction of the *hst1* gene into rice, coupled with the application of single-nucleotide polymorphism (SNP) marker-assisted selection, led to the development of the BC3FC population YNU31-24, which exhibited a genomic similarity of 93.5% to the parental varieties. YNU31-24 seedlings demonstrated enhanced survival and increased plant biomass when exposed to 125 mM NaCl [12]. A deletion mutant exclusively targeting the salt tolerance (*DST* genes) was generated in the indica rice variety MTU1010 through CRISPR-Cas9 gene editing. This modification led to observable phenotypic changes, including broader leaves, diminished stomatal density, heightened leaf water retention, and a discernible tolerance to osmotic stress and high salt stress during the seedling stage of the mutant [18]. In addition, T-DNA insertion mutagenesis and RNAi silencing of target genes are also methods used to improve salt tolerance in rice [19,20].

One of the many important physiological changes during the early evolution of plant cells was the ability to adapt to low levels of Na^+ and K^+ intermediates [21]. Cellular Na^+ toxicity is the ionic toxicity that primarily causes salt stress and usually results in a variety of physiological processes in rice, including K^+ attraction [22]. In rice, intracellular Na+ is mainly transported out of the cell via the SOS1 transporter protein or to the root xylem via the high-affinity potassium transporter proteins (HKT1;4, HKT1;5) to mitigate Na^+ toxicity in the stem [23]. In rice, the role of HKT2;1 may be to provide an entry pathway for Na^+ uptake under K^+ limitations, mainly to support cell expansion and plant growth [24]. In plants, superior K^+ retention in salt-stressed roots is positively correlated with salt tolerance [25]. In rice, the K^+ transporter proteins OsHAK1 and OsHAK5, when induced by salt stress, mediate K^+ uptake and transport, maintaining a high K^+/Na^+ ratio under salt stress [26,27]. Studies have shown that most transcription factors (TFs) are involved in the response to salt stress, such as *AP2/ERF, bHLH, NAC, MYB* and *bZIP* [28–32]. For example, overexpression of rice *AP2/ERF-type* TFs in *Arabidopsis thaliana* showed improved tolerance to drought, salt and cold [33]. In addition, many hormone-like genes in rice are involved in the salt stress response. Overexpression of the rice Aux/IAA TF *OsIAA17* significantly increases salt and drought tolerance in rice [34]. Knockdown of *OsABI5*, a gene downstream of the abscisic acid signaling pathway in rice, resulted in delayed seed germination and reduced seedling salt tolerance [35]. Overexpression of *OsGA2ox5* increased the resistance of rice to high-salinity stress [36].

Brassinolide (BR) is an asterol compound that, when soaked, inhibits the accumulation of ROS, reduces the level of MDA, increases the SPAD of rice seedlings under NaCl stress, and protects the plant's photosynthetic system [37,38].

The Bowman–Birk Inhibitor (BBI) encodes a serine protease inhibitor and has a repetitive cysteine-rich structural domain with a reactive site from the trypsin or chymotrypsin family [39]. BBIs are generally well known in soybeans and their main function is reflected in their role in inhibiting the proliferation of cancer cells [40]. Moreover, BBIs in wheat and maize mainly show strong inhibitory effects on the growth of plant pathogenic fungi [41]. In rice, there are currently 12 *BBI* genes [42], and there is limited understanding of their functions. For instance, the overexpression of the BBI protein APIP4 in rice has been shown to enhance resistance against the fungal pathogen *Magnaporthe oryzae* [43]. The hypothesis of this study is that the newly identified salt-inducible BBI, *OsBBTI5*, plays a crucial role in regulating salt tolerance in rice seedlings. In the current study, *OsBBTI5* gene, when suppressed through RNAi in transgenic plants, produced a positive enhancement of salt tolerance. Our investigation also aimed to understand the molecular mechanisms underlying *OsBBTI5*'s involvement in salt tolerance, particularly its association with the brassinosteroid (BR) pathway. Despite exhibiting insensitivity to BR, *OsBBTI5* showed remarkable sensitivity to the downstream gibberellic acid (GA$_3$), leading to the inhibition of root system growth at high concentrations of GA$_3$. Furthermore, physical interaction of *OsBBTI5* with *OsAPX2* was crucial in mediating its effects on salt tolerance. *OsBBTI5* regulated ROS accumulation and GA_3 synthesis under salt stress conditions, implying a dual role in oxidative stress management and hormonal signaling. Thus, lowering the expression of *OsBBTI5* enhanced salt tolerance in rice seedlings by modulating H_2O_2 and GA_3 signaling pathways. The selection of *OsBBTI5* among other genes was based on its novel identification as a salt-inducible BBI and our preliminary findings suggesting its significant impact on salt tolerance through intricate interactions with hormonal pathways and ROS regulation.

2. Results

2.1. In Silico Analysis of Rice BBI Genes

The full-length coding sequence (CDS) of *OsBBTI5* (Os01g0124401) was cloned based on Rice Genome Annotation Project (http://rice.uga.edu/index.shtml, accessed on 11 January 2023). Using the 12 BBI amino acid sequences of rice (*Oryza sativa* L.) as a query and searching for their homologues in phragmites (*Brachypodium distachyon* L.), maize (*Zea mays* L.) and soybean (*Glycine max* L.), we obtained 5, 5 and 10 homologues, respectively. These proteins, together with *OsBBTI5*, were used to construct the phylogenetic tree (Figure 1A). Phylogenetic analyses showed that *OsBBTI5* had the highest homology with the *OsBBTI4* gene in rice. It is closely related to *BdBBTI3* in *Brachypodium distachyon* L. and to *ZmBBTI5* and *ZmBBTI11* in maize. The *BBI* genes in rice are distributed between 2 and 9 motifs, with *OsBBTI5* having 9 motifs, according to structural domain analysis (Figure 1B). Analysis of the promoter regions of rice *BBI* genes showed that they have a total of 27 transcription factor binding sites, including the common C2H2, Dof, MYB, WRKY, NAC, BES1, bHLH, bZIP, and others (Figure 1C). Structural analysis of the rice *BBI* family genes showed that most of the *BBI* genes had only one exon, including *OsBBTI5*, with the exception of *OsBBTI11*, *OsBBTI12* and *OsBBTI13*, which had two exons, and *OsBBTI10*, which had three exons (Figure 1D).

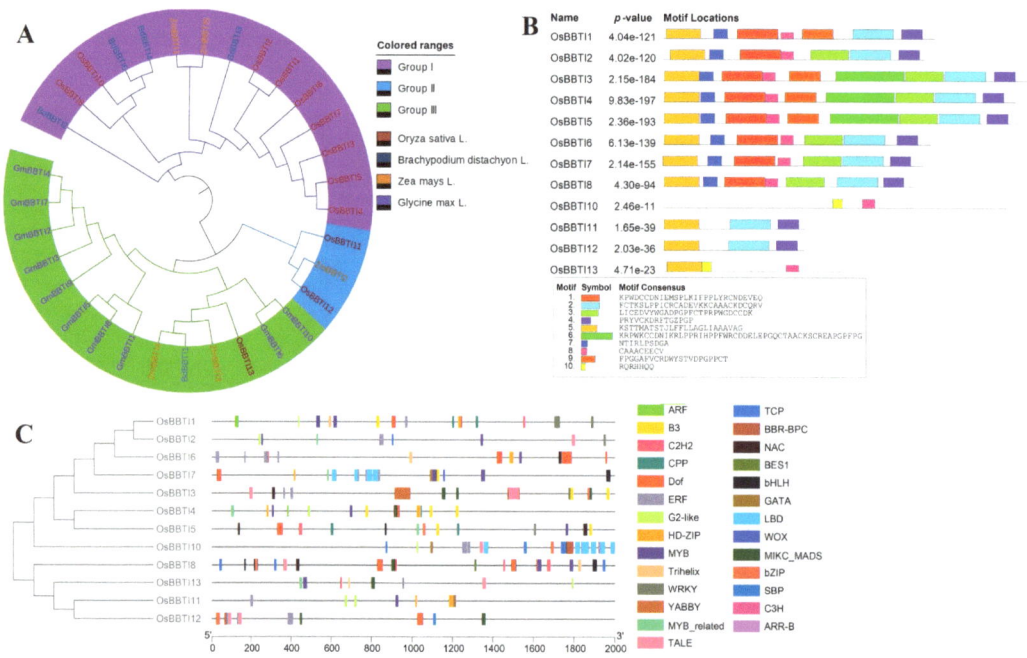

Figure 1. *Cont.*

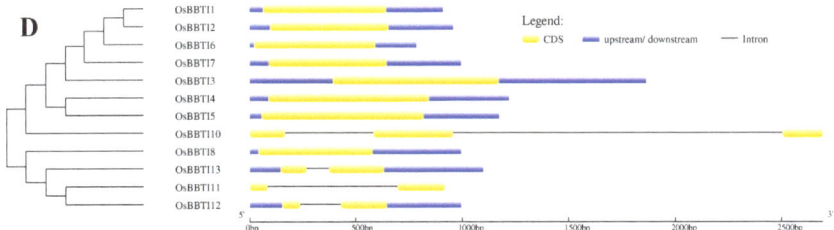

Figure 1. (A) Cluster analysis of the rice *BBI* family with homologs from *Brachypodium distachyon*, *Zea mays* and *Glycine max*. The four species are represented in red, blue, orange, and purple, respectively. **(B)** Structural domain analysis of BBI amino acids in rice. **(C)** Analysis of transcription factor binding sites of *BBI* family genes in rice. **(D)** Exon analysis of rice BBI family genes.

2.2. Sub-Cellular Localization of OsBBTI5

To determine the subcellular localization of *OsBBTI5* protein, the *OsBBTI5*-GFP recombinant plasmid of pCXSN was generated by fusing the *OsBBTI5* cDNA, lacking the termination codon, to the 5′ end of the GFP reporter gene under the control of the CaMV-35S promoter. The results showed that *OsBBTI5* expression in cells was distributed across organelles (Figure 2B), similar to the 35S:GFP (control) (Figure 2A).

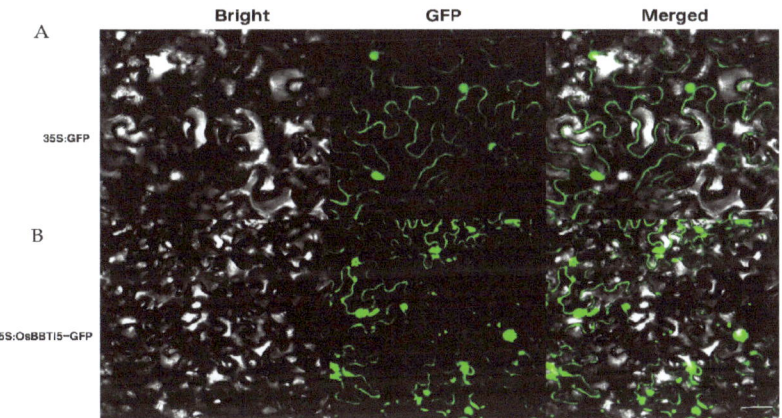

Figure 2. (A) Subcellular localization of the GFP protein in tobacco leaf epidermal cells, scale bar: 20 μm. **(B)** Subcellular localization of the OsBBTI5 protein in tobacco leaf epidermal cells, scale bar: 20 μm.

2.3. Characterization of OsBBTI5-RNAi Lines

To further validate the role of *OsBBTI5* in regulating BR signaling, we generated *OsBBTI5*-RNAi lines through RNAi knockdown technology. A BR sensitivity assay revealed that *OsBBTI5*-RNAi plants exhibited insensitivity to BR compared to the wild type (WT) (Figure 3A,B). Subsequently, seeds from both WT and transgenic plants were germinated and placed on a 0.5 × MS agar medium containing 0, 0.001 μM, 0.01 μM, 0.1 μM, or 1 μM 24-epibrassinolide.

The expression of BR biosynthesis-related genes, including *D11*, *D61*, *DLT*, *OsBBTI5*, *OsBR6ox*, *OsBZR1* and *OsSPY* genes, was analyzed via fluorescence quantitative PCR. The results showed different cumulative transcriptions of BR biosynthesis-related genes in the *OsBBTI5*-RNAi line (Figure 3C).

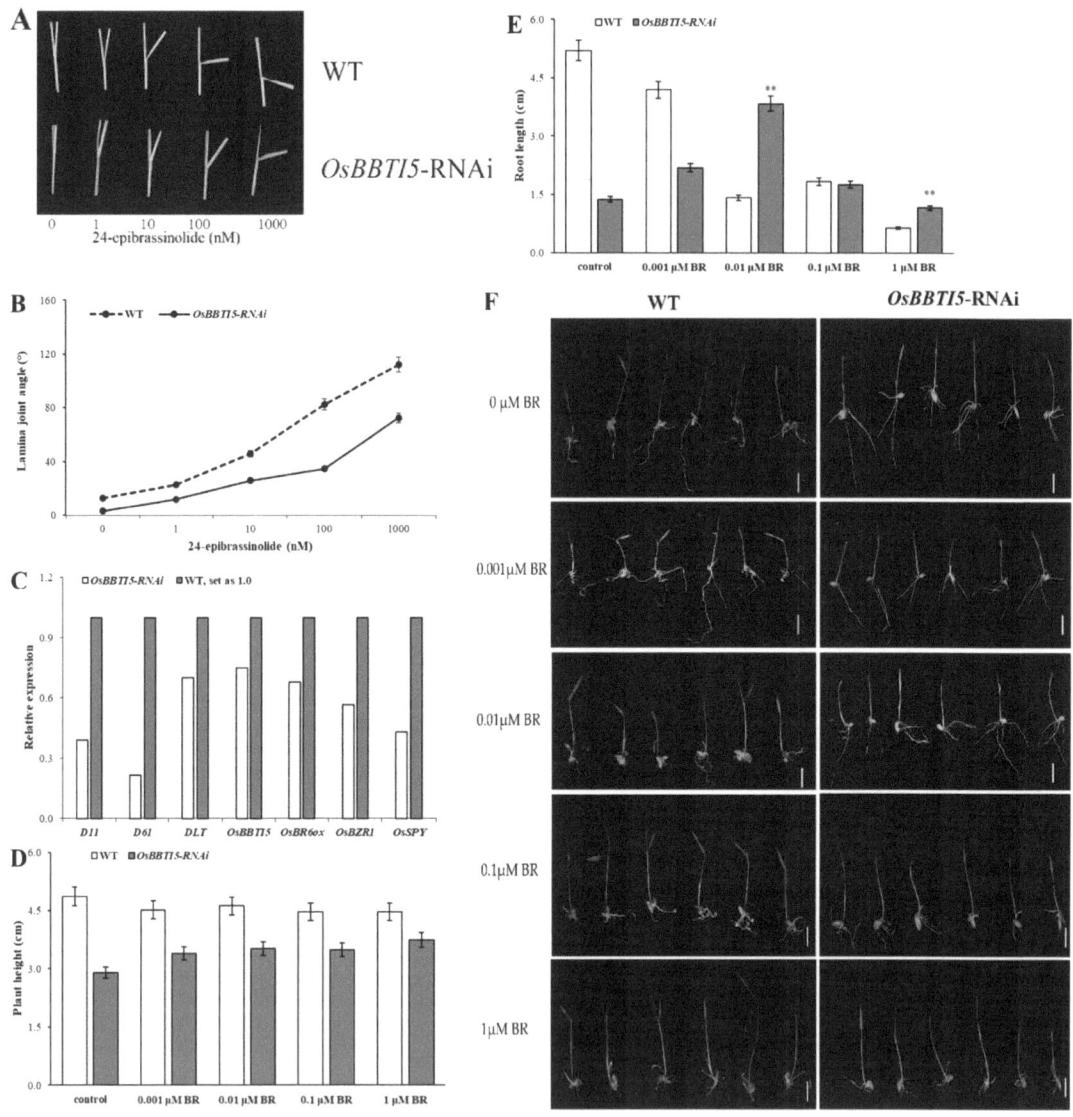

Figure 3. (**A**) The leaf inclination of *OsBBTI5*-RNAi and WT in the presence of indicated concentrations of 24-epibrassinolide. (**B**) Statistical analysis of leaf inclination, data are means ±SE (*n* = 20). (**C**) Comparison of BR-related gene expression between WT and *OsBBTI5*-RNAi. (**D,E**) Measurements of the plant heights and root lengths of WT and *OsBBTI5*-RNAi transgenic seedlings after 7 days of growing on an MS medium containing different 24-epibrassinolide concentrations. Data are means ± SDs (*n* = 30). (**F**) The growth of WT and *OsBBTI5*-RNAi plants grown on an MS medium containing different 24-epibrassinolide concentration after 7 days. ** *p* < 0.01. Scale = 1 cm.

When cultivated on a medium containing 0 and 1 μM 24-epibrassinolide, no discernible differences in plant height or root length were observed between wild-type and transgenic *OsBBTI5*-RNAi plants (Figure 3D,F). However, in terms of root length, the transgenic *OsBBTI5*-RNAi showed significant differences compared to the wild type at 0.01 μM and 1 μM, indicating reduced sensitivity to 24-epibrassinolide (Figure 3E,F).

OsBBTI5-RNAi transgenic plants exhibited slower growth compared to the wild type at 0.1 μM, 1 μM, 10 μM, and 100 μM. Notably, transgenic plants were significantly shorter than the wild type in both plant height and root length when the medium contained 10 μM and 100 μM GA$_3$ (Figure S1A,B). Overall, *OsBBTI5*-RNAi transgenic plants exhibited involvement in the BR pathway, displaying insensitivity to BR and sensitivity to high concentrations of GA$_3$, with a predominant phenotype characterized by the absence of root growth (Figure S1C).

2.4. Effect of NaCl Stress on Seed Germination

To determine salt stress in *OsBBTI5*-RNAi plants, seeds of WT and transgenic plants were germinated and then placed on a half-strength Murashige and Skoog (MS) medium containing 0 mM, 40 mM, 50 mM, or 60 mM NaCl. Under normal conditions, the transgenic seeds germinated faster and had greater plant height and root length than the wild type. The transgenic plants showed greater plant height and root length than WT when grown in different concentrations of salt solution (Figure 4A,B,C).

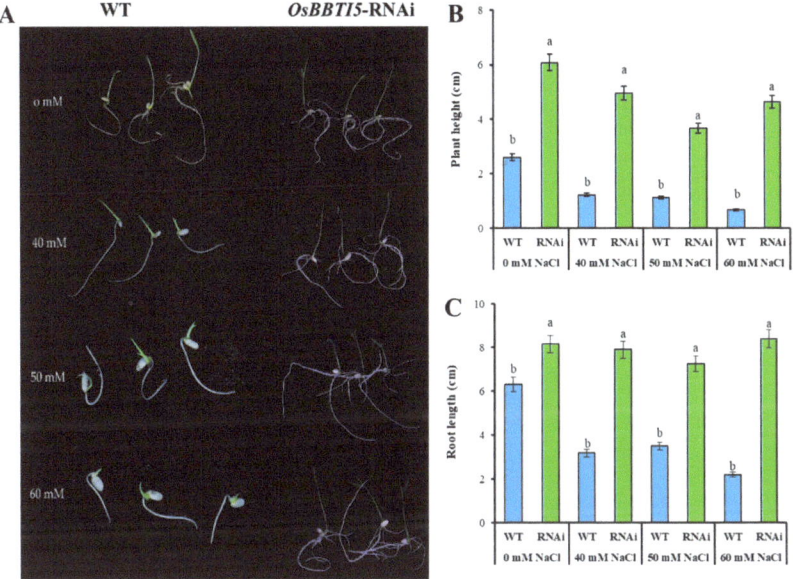

Figure 4. (**A**) Photographs of WT and *OsBBTI5*-RNAi transgenic seedlings supplemented with 0 mM, 40 mM, 50 mM, or 60 mM NaCl after 7 days of initiation. (**B**) Differences in plant height were compared between WT and *OsBBTI5*-RNAi transgenic plants. (**C**) Differences in root length were compared between wild-type and RNAi transgenic plants. Data represent means ± SD (*n* = 3). Different letters indicate significant differences (Tukey's HSD test, *p* ≤ 0.05).

2.5. OsBBTI5-RNAi Enhances Salt Tolerance in Transgenic Rice

OsBBTI5-RNAi plants were exposed to salt stress with different concentrations of NaCl for 7 days. As shown in Figure 5A, transgenic plants showed strong tolerance compared to WT after exposure to salt stress at a concentration of 40 mM. Under normal conditions without salt treatment, peroxidase (POD) and superoxide dismutase (SOD) activities were almost the same in *OsBBTI5*-RNAi and WT plants. Following salt stress treatment, *OsBBTI5*-RNAi plants exposed to 60 mM NaCl exhibited significantly higher activities of peroxidase (POD) and superoxide dismutase (SOD) compared to wild-type plants. However, at 40 mM NaCl, only the activity of POD was higher in *OsBBTI5*-RNAi plants than in the wild-type plants (Figure 5B,D). The activity of another antioxidant enzyme, CAT, was significantly increased in all seedlings at 40 mM NaCl after 7 days of salt treatment compared to control conditions, while the difference was not significant at 60 mM NaCl (Figure 5C). H_2O_2 was significantly higher in both 40 mM NaCl and 60 mM NaCl, whereas it was essentially indistinguishable in the no-salt condition (Figure 5E). Moreover, under normal conditions, the malondialdehyde (MDA) level, serving as an indicator of lipid peroxidation, was higher in *OsBBTI5*-RNAi compared to WT. Furthermore, the MDA content in *OsBBTI5*-RNAi plants was significantly elevated compared to wild-type plants, signifying an increased level of lipid peroxidation in transgenic plants under both 40 mM NaCl and 60 mM NaCl salt stress conditions (Figure 5F).

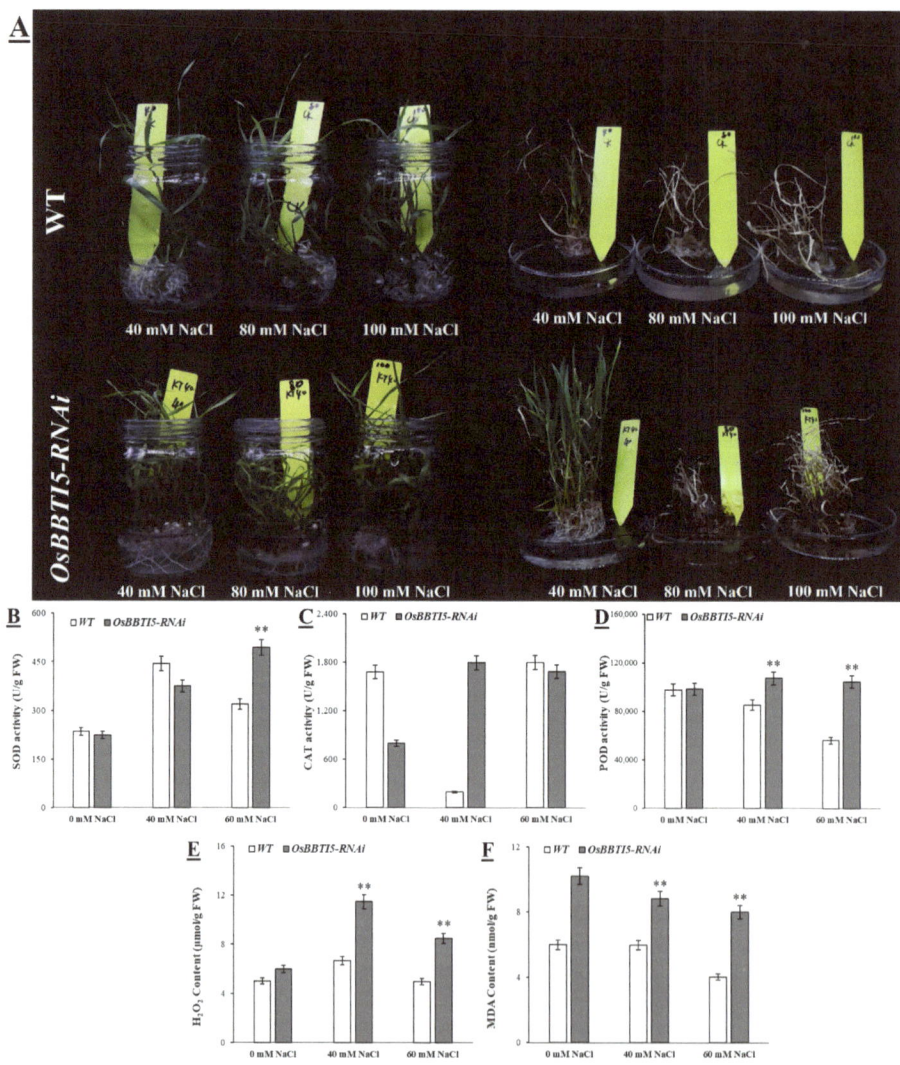

Figure 5. (**A**) Phenotypes of WT and transgenic plants in response to salt stress. (**B**) SOD activity. (**C**) CAT content. (**D**) POD content. (**E**) H_2O_2 content. (**F**) MDA content. Three independent experiments were carried out with similar results. Data represent means ± SD (*n* = 30). ** $p \leq 0.01$.

2.6. Differentially Expressed Genes Regulated by OsBBTI5 in Response to Salt Stress

RNA sequencing primarily involved three treatment groups: the wild-type (WT) group, the wild-type post-40 mM NaCl treatment (CK4), and *OsBBTI5*-RNAi after-40 mM NaCl treatment (KT39). Each sample yielded sequences ranging from 6.02 to 8.66 Gb, which underwent quality control using FASTQC. The results indicated that 92.12% to 95.12% of the sequences exhibited quality scores above Q30, and 62.69% to 95.05% of the reads were uniquely aligned with the genome (Supplementary Table S1). The alignment ratios were found to be similar across the three lines. Consequently, the analysis of differentially expressed genes (DEGs) was carried out using this consistent alignment ratio for further investigation.

DEGs were assessed by comparing the number of reads between the control and salt-treated samples in each line. Heat map analysis revealed significant differences in gene expression between the three lines (Figure 6A). Under 40 mM NaCl treatment, the expression level of *OsBBTI5*-RNAi was twofold higher compared to the salt-stressed WT, as observed in the analysis of DEGs in the WT (Figure 6B). Between salt-stressed WT and non-stressed WT, 2105 genes were upregulated and 2039 genes were downregulated. In contrast, between salt-stressed *OsBBTI5*-RNAi and WT, 5603 genes were upregulated and 6272 genes were downregulated. KEGG pathway enrichment analysis revealed that the phenylpropanoid biosynthesis pathway was best to be regulated under salt stress in rice (Figure 6C,D). Certainly, the most differential pathways between salt-stressed *OsBBTI5*-RNAi and salt-stressed WT were mainly focused on light-related pathways, including photosynthesis and photosynthesis-antenna proteins (Supplementary Tables S2 and S3). In addition, photosynthesis-related genes in particular showed significant upregulated expression (Supplementary Figures S2 and S3). GO enrichment analysis also revealed drastic changes in light-related pathways (Supplementary Figure S4), including photosynthesis, photosystem, and photosystem II. These findings support the hypothesis that distinct pathways are either activated or repressed in response to salt stress in *OsBBTI5*-RNAi compared to the wild type of rice.

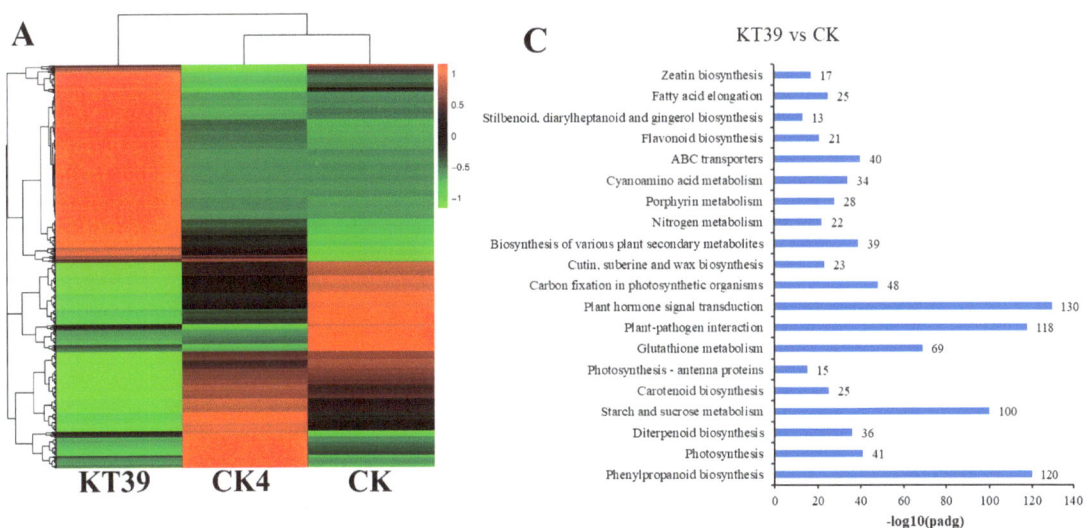

Figure 6. *Cont.*

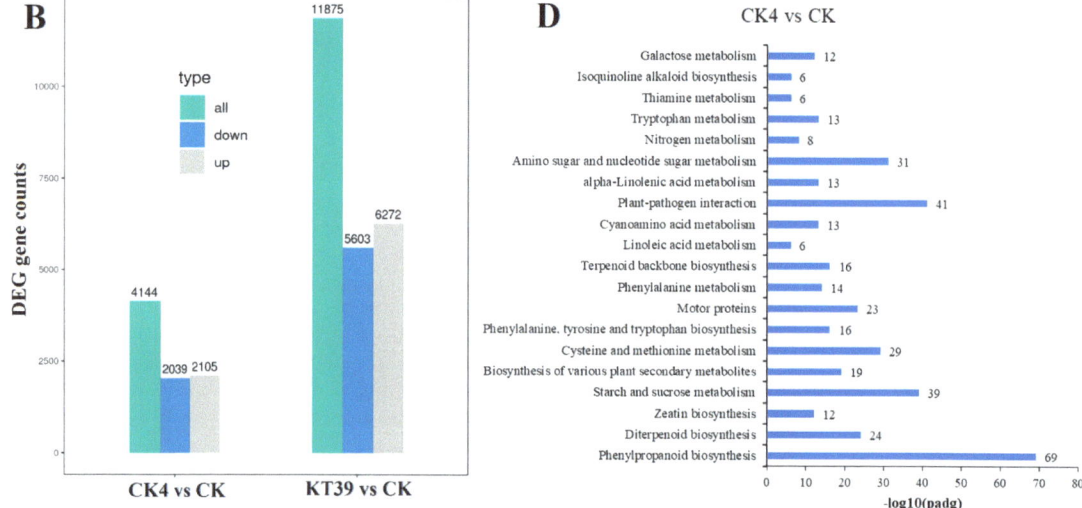

Figure 6. (**A**) Heat map of DEGs' expressions in response to salt stress in two salt-stressed and WT samples. (**B**) Upregulated and downregulated DEGs comparison between two groups. (**C**) KEGG enrichment analysis between KT39 and CK group. (**D**) KEGG enrichment analysis between CK4 and CK group. KT39 is a synonym with the *OsBBTI5*-RNAi lines under 40 mM NaCl treatment; CK4 is a synonym with the wild-type lines under 40 mM NaCl treatment; and CK is a synonym with the wild-type lines under treatment with a normal nutrient solution.

2.7. In Vitro Interaction of OsBBTI5 with OsAPX2

In order to understand whether the *OsBBTI5* gene was self-activating, we carried out its self-activation experiments. On SD/-Trp, SD/-Trp/-His, SD/-Trp/-His/-Ade, and SD/-Trp/-His/-Ade+X-α-gal plates, pGBKT7-B5 was able to grow, whereas pGBKT7-negative was not able to grow, suggesting that there is self-activation of pGBKT7-B5 (Figure 7A). Inhibition experiments of 3-AT showed that the self-activation of pGBKT7-*OsBBTI5* could be effectively inhibited in 3-AT-deficient plates at concentrations higher than 10 mM (Figure 7B). We previously performed an interaction screening of *OsBBTI5* proteins against the rice yeast library and obtained 96 candidate proteins, including *OsAPX2*. To elucidate the molecular mechanism underlying salt tolerance in rice seedlings mediated by *OsBBTI5*, we conducted yeast two-hybrid library screening, using *OsBBTI5* as bait. *OsAPX2*, an ascorbate peroxidase gene in rice, was identified as an *OsBBTI5*-interacting protein by an *OsBBTI5* bait protein screen (Figure 7C,D).

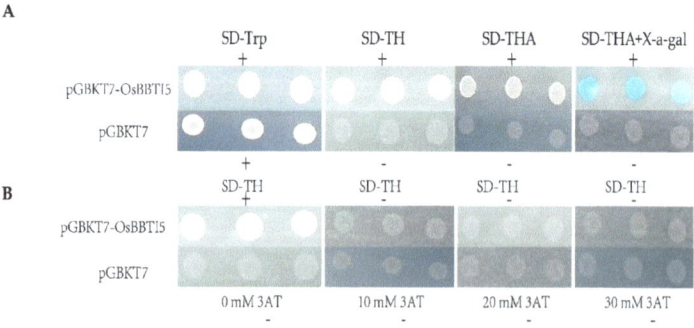

Figure 7. *Cont.*

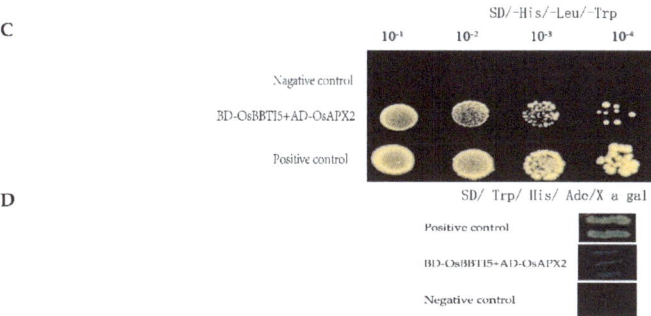

Figure 7. (**A**) Self-activating of *OsBBTI5*. +:pGBKT7-*OsBBTI5* (positive control), −:pGBKT7 (negative control). (**B**) Inhibitory effect of 3-AT. (**C**) Yeast two-hybrid assays for the interaction between *OsBBTI5* and *OsAPX2*. These strains were grown on SD-His-Leu-Trp. (**D**) Yeast two-hybrid assays for the interaction between *OsBBTI5* and *OsAPX2*. These strains were grown on SD-His-Leu-Trp + X-α-Gal.

3. Discussion

The majority of structures within the rice *BBI* genes exhibit conserved coding sequences (CDS) without introns (Figure 1). These inhibitor families operate through specific mechanisms of enzyme hydrolysis and are categorized based on the active amino acid in their reaction center, such as serine, cysteine, aspartic, and metalloproteases [44].

Until now, the sole reported cloning of a Bowman–Birk-type protease inhibitor gene, *WRSI5*, in wheat was achieved using the 5′-race technique, and its overexpression in *Arabidopsis thaliana* demonstrated tolerance to 150 mM NaCl [45]. Recent research on BBI has primarily focused on crops like soybean and wheat, with limited relevance to stress responses in rice. However, our study provides novel insights by demonstrating that the *OsBBTI5* gene, belonging to the BBI family, is associated with the BR signaling pathway. Notably, RNA interference (RNAi) knockdown of this gene enhances salt tolerance in rice. We present, for the first time, a working model illustrating how salt-sensitive OsBBTI5-RNAi promotes salt tolerance (Figure 8).

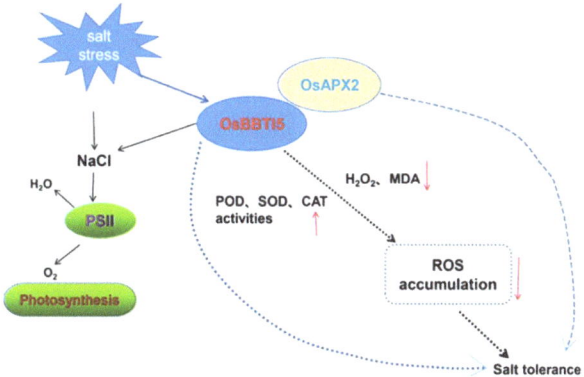

Figure 8. A proposed model illustrating how the *OsBBTI5*-RNAi, responsive to salt stress, enhances salt tolerance in rice.

In the salt tolerance pathway, *OsBBTI5*-RNAi transgenic plants increased the expression of photosystem II (PSII) genes. Additionally, the *OsBBTI5* gene may interact with *OsAPX2* gene, leading to a reduction in the accumulation of ROS and thereby enhancing salt tolerance.

BR biosynthetic enzymes in rice have been studied mainly by phenotyping dwarf mutants, and the results indicate that BR is involved in many physiological processes in rice, including leaf elongation, tiller development, photogenesis, root differentiation, and reproductive growth [46]. BR signaling in *Arabidopsis* and rice (dicot and monocot models, respectively) is mediated by the receptor kinases *BRI1* and *OsBRI1* [47]. BR stimulates the activities of SOD, CAT, POD and APX, thereby reducing cold-induced damage [48]. Brassinolide (BL) improves plant tolerance to abiotic stress. In apples, exogenous BL increases the activities of SOD and CAT, thereby eliminating the salt stress-induced production of ROS [49]. BR immersion significantly increases SPAD, Pn and Tr, as well as Fm, Fv/Fm, and Fv/Fo in rice seedlings under NaCl stress, which protects the photosynthetic system of the plant and increases plant biomass [37]. In our study, the results from the BR assay revealed that rice with *OsBBTI5*-RNAi was less sensitive to exogenous brassinolide. Reducing the expression of *OsBBTI5* showed that a significant increase in POD, SOD, and CAT occurred after salt soaking, while a significant decrease in H_2O_2 and MDA occurred, which reduced the accumulation of ROS and improved the salt tolerance of transgenic plants in rice. In addition, the transcriptomic results indicated that the transgenic plants showed a significant increase in gene expression, mainly in photosynthesis-related and photosynthetic systems after salt immersion, which was an important factor contributing to the increase in salt stress.

Under normal conditions, exposure to NaCl leads to an increase in the activities of ascorbate peroxidase (APX) and glutathione reductase (GR) in rice roots. Simultaneously, the expression of *OsAPX* and *OsGR* is upregulated [50]. Rice has 8 *APX* genes that encode enzymes that function in the cytoplasm (*APX1* and *APX2*), peroxisomes (*APX3* and *APX4*), mitochondria (*APX5* and *APX6*), and chloroplasts (*APX7* and *APX8*) [51,52]. Overexpression of *OsAPX2* increases APX activity and improves stress tolerance. It is also shown that NaCl-induced expression of *OsAPx8* in rice roots requires Na(+) but not Cl(-) [53]. The yeast two-hybrid results in our study suggest that it is possible for *OsBBTI5* to act on stress tolerance through *OsAPX2* interactions.

Brassinosteroid (BR) and gibberellin (GA) are the two main hormones that regulate cell elongation in plants. Rice mutants that are insensitive to BR signaling typically exhibit stem and leaf elongation defects [54]. A member of the *GRAS* family, the *DLT* gene, is insensitive to BR expression, causing leaf bending, and affecting radicle elongation [55]. Coleoptile elongation and root inhibition assays show that rice overexpressing *OsPRA2* is less sensitive to exogenous brassinosteroid. BR regulates cell elongation by modulating GA metabolism in rice. For example, under physiological conditions, BR stimulates cell elongation by regulating the expression of GA metabolism genes, thereby promoting GA accumulation [56]. In addition, mutations in *LEA33* may affect grain size and seed germination in rice by reducing BR accumulation and promoting GA biosynthesis [57]. The overexpression of *OsOFP22* promotes SLR1 protein expression in response to GA-induced accumulation and represses the BR expression of signaling genes that ultimately regulate rice plant and grain size [58]. Similarly, in this study, the growth and development of transgenic plants after the downregulation of *OsBBTI5* expression were affected by high concentrations of GA_3 more than BR.

4. Materials and Methods

4.1. Plant Materials and Growth Conditions

Rice (*Oryza sativa* L. spp. Japonica) seedlings were grown in a greenhouse under standard rice growing conditions. Tobacco was grown in an artificial climate chamber at 26 °C under long-day conditions (16 h light/8 h darkness).

4.2. Vector Construction and Genetic Transformation in Rice

Two sets of specific primers, Os5F1/Os5R1 and Os5F2/Os5R2, were employed to amplify a 765 bp fragment corresponding to the full-length *OsBBTI5* cDNA. Subsequently, the PCR products were cloned into the pTCK303 vector using BamHI/KpnI and SpeI/SacI restriction sites through a two-step cloning process facilitated by a cloning kit (Vazyme, China, code: C113). The resulting plasmid, pTCK303-BBI5, was then introduced into *Agrobacterium tumefaciens* strain LBA4404. The transformation of transgenic rice plants was conducted following established procedures [59]. Briefly, mature seeds were sterilized and placed in an induction medium (NB, 2,4-D 2.5 mg/L, pH 5.8) for dark culturing at 28 °C. Following a two-week healing induction period, Agrobacterium and healing pellets were allowed to incubate in a dark culture at 28 °C for half an hour. Subsequently, the pellets were transferred to a co-culture medium (induction basal medium, AS 100 μM/L, pH 5.8) and underwent 2–3 washes with sterile water over a 3-day period. After the 3-day co-culture, the calli were washed 2–3 times with sterile water and then rinsed once with cephalexin 100 mg/L. These calli were then cultured on a screening medium containing induction medium, hygromycin 30 mg/L, and pH 5.8. Following 15 days of dark culture at 28 °C, the newly formed calli were subjected to an additional 3 days of dark culture at 28 °C. After a total of 15 days, the newborn calli were transferred to a differentiation medium (NB, 1.5 mg/L KT, 0.5 mg/L NAA, pH 5.8) and ultimately cultivated on a rooting medium (1/2 MS, sucrose 5%, Phytagel 2.5 g/L, pH 5.8) for a period ranging from 15 to 30 days. *OsBBTI5*-RNAi lines, exhibiting varying levels of expression, were generated and utilized for subsequent analyses.

4.3. Subcellular Localization

The full-length *OsBBTI5* cDNA without the termination codon and GFP cDNA were amplified using PCR primers Os5F3/Os5R3 and GFF/GFR (Table S4), and the resulting products were inserted into the *Bam*HI/*Hind*III-digested pCXSN (pCXSN-35SBBI5) using cloning kit (Vazyme, Nanjing, China, code: C113). Then, the plasmids of pCXSN35GFP (as positive control) and pCXSN35SBBI5 were, respectively, transformed into *Agrobacterium tumefaciens* strain GV3101.

The single clone was picked and grown in an LB medium (containing rifampicin) on a shaker at 28 °C for 48 h and collected by centrifugation at 4000 rpm for 10 min. It was resuspended with MES resuspension (1 mL 500 mM MES + 1 mL 100 mM MgCl$_2$.6H$_2$O + 10 μL 500 mM AS, add ddH$_2$O to 50 mL, pH 5.8) solution to OD$_{600}$ = 1.0, left at room temperature for 2 h, and injected into tobacco leaves. Then the samples were observed after 2–3 days. The GFP fluorescence was monitored at 488 nm excitation using a laser confocal microscope (Leica SP8 STED, Germany).

4.4. Lamina Joint Assay

Leaf co-determination experiments were conducted by utilizing excised leaf segments, following previously established protocols [60]. Seeds were subjected to dark culture for 7 days in an incubator set at 30 °C, allowing the formation of two leaves. Subsequently, the entire segment, encompassing 1 cm of the second leaf, the leaf node, and 1 cm of the leaf sheath, was immersed in varying concentrations of 24-epibrassinolide for 48 h in the absence of light. The angles of lamina joint bending were measured using ImageJ software version 1.54a (http://rsbweb.nih. gov/ij/, accessed on 12 February 2023).

4.5. Salt Stress Treatment and Phenotypic Analysis of Transgenic Rice

Seeds were cultivated on a Murashige and Skoog (MS) solid medium containing 0, 40 mM, 50 mM, and 60 mM NaCl for a duration of 7 days. Two-week-old seedlings of both wild-type (WT) and *OsBBTI5*-RNAi varieties were cultured in hydroponic solution containing 40 mM, 80 mM, and 100 mM NaCl for 7 days. Additionally, rice seeds were placed on a 0.5× agar medium with varying concentrations of NaCl, 24-epibrassinolide (0.001 μM, 0.01 μM, 0.01 μM, 0.1 μM, 1 μM), or GA3 (0.1 μM, 1 μM, 10 μM, 100 μM) for 7 days, and seedling phenotypes were subsequently assessed. Each treatment was replicated three times, with 30 seedlings per replication.

4.6. RNA Extraction and Transcriptome Data Analysis

Rice seedlings treated with 40 mM NaCl for 3 days were stored into liquid nitrogen. RNA extraction was performed by using RNA-extraction kit (TransGen, Beijing, China, code:DP432). Three distinct samples, namely wild-type (WT), 40 mM NaCl-soaked, and *OsBBTI5*-RNAi samples, were subjected to differential expression analysis to elucidate specific responses.

The determination of differential gene expression involved the utilization of the Cuffdiff utility within the Cufflinks package. Transcripts exhibiting log2-fold changes of ≥ 1 (indicative of upregulated genes) and $\leq (-1)$ (indicative of downregulated genes), with a *p*-value cut-off of ≤ 0.05, were considered significantly differentially expressed [61]. Subsequently, the identified DEGs underwent gene ontology (GO) enrichment analysis. Following the generation of DEGs for each region, as depicted in the Venn diagram analysis [62], the GO enrichment analysis was conducted to unravel the functional significance of the differentially expressed genes.

4.7. Quantitative Real-Time PCR Analysis

qRT-PCR was performed using a Q1 real-time PCR system (Thermo Fisher Scineitific, Waltham, MA, USA). The system is a 10 μL volume: each reaction contains 5 μL of $2 \times$ Taq Pro Universal SYBR qPCR Master Mix (Vazyme, China), 0.4 μL of primers (10 μM), 1 μL of cDNA template, and added 10 μL of ddH2O. The procedure was performed according to the Q1 Semi-quantitative PCR Operation Manual. The rice actin gene was used as an internal reference. Quantitative PCR expression levels were calculated according to the $2^{-\Delta\Delta CT}$ method. All experiments were performed with three biological replicates and three technical replicates.

4.8. Yeast Two-Hybrid Assay

The coding sequences of *OsBBTI5* and *OsAPX2* were, respectively, cloned into the pGBKT7 and pGADT7 vectors (Clontech, Mountain View, CA, USA), which were named pGBKT7-BBI5 and pGADT7-APX2. The resulting constructs and the corresponding empty vectors were then co-transformed into the yeast strain Golden Yeast in various combinations. The screening of the rice yeast library was conducted, resulting in the identification of 96 clones subjected to PCR validation. Upon reversing the validation outcomes, we proceeded to sequence a total of 210 candidate genes to explore potential interactions. Notably, this set included the *OsAPX2* gene. Interactions were detected on SD/-His-Leu-Trp and SD/-His-Leu-Trp+X-gal media. Transformation was performed according to the Yeast Two-Hybrid System User Manual (Clontech, Beijing China). All primers used in this assay are listed in Table S4.

5. Conclusions

This study employed a comprehensive approach to investigate the role of the *OsBBTI5* gene in rice under various conditions, shedding light on its potential functions and molecular interactions. The sequence analysis of *OsBBTI5* provided insights into its evolutionary relationships within the *BBI* gene family, its motif distribution, and the regulatory elements in its promoter region. Subcellular localization studies revealed the widespread distribution of *OsBBTI5* across organelles, suggesting its involvement in cellular processes. The generation of *OsBBTI5*-RNAi lines demonstrated the gene's role in brassinosteroid (BR) signaling, with transgenic plants displaying insensitivity to BR and altered responses to 24-epibrassinolide and gibberellic acid (GA_3). Furthermore, this study explored the impact of *OsBBTI5* on salt stress, revealing enhanced salt tolerance in *OsBBTI5*-RNAi transgenic rice plants. Physiological analyses, including measurements of peroxidase (POD) and superoxide dismutase (SOD) activities, hydrogen peroxide (H_2O_2) levels, and malondialdehyde (MDA) content, provided valuable insights into the mechanisms underlying salt stress responses. RNA sequencing and differential gene expression analysis unveiled distinct regulatory pathways, particularly in light-related processes, indicating the intricate role of *OsBBTI5* in the rice salt stress response. The identification of *OsAPX2* as an interacting partner of *OsBBTI5* through yeast two-hybrid assays suggests a potential molecular mechanism underlying salt tolerance in rice. These findings contribute to our understanding of the multifaceted functions of *OsBBTI5* and its implications in plant growth, development, and stress responses. Overall, this study provides a foundation for further research into the intricate molecular networks governing plant responses to environmental stimuli.

Supplementary Materials: The following supporting information can be downloaded at: https://www.mdpi.com/article/10.3390/ijms25021284/s1.

Author Contributions: Conceptualization, Z.L.; methodology, X.Y., L.Z. and S.W.; software, L.Z., S.T. and X.Y.; validation, Z.L. and X.Y.; formal analysis, X.Y., L.Z. and S.W.; investigation, Z.L. and X.Y.; resources, Z.L.; data curation, Z.L., X.Y., S.T. and F.C.; writing—original draft preparation, Z.L.; writing—review and editing, M.M.A., X.Y., L.Z., S.W., Z.L. and F.C.; visualization, M.M.A.; X.Y., S.W., S.T. and L.Z.; supervision, Z.L., and F.C.; project administration, Z.L.; funding acquisition, Z.L. All authors have read and agreed to the published version of the manuscript.

Funding: This study is supported by the Innovation Platform for Horticultural Biotechnology Genetic Transfusion, Fujian Academy of Agricultural Sciences (CXPT202204), and Enterprise Technology Development (2020-3501-04-001995).

Institutional Review Board Statement: Not applicable.

Informed Consent Statement: Not applicable.

Data Availability Statement: Data are contained within the article and supplementary materials.

Conflicts of Interest: The authors declare no conflicts of interest.

References

1. Nadarajah, K.; Abdul Hamid, N.W.; Abdul Rahman, N.S.N. SA-mediated regulation and control of abiotic stress tolerance in rice. *Int. J. Mol. Sci.* **2021**, 22, 5591. [CrossRef] [PubMed]
2. Mizoi, J.; Yamaguchi-Shinozaki, K. Molecular approaches to improve rice abiotic stress tolerance. *Rice Protoc.* **2013**, 956, 269–283.
3. Ganie, S.A.; Molla, K.A.; Henry, R.J.; Bhat, K.; Mondal, T.K. Advances in understanding salt tolerance in rice. *Theor. Appl. Genet.* **2019**, 132, 851–870. [CrossRef] [PubMed]
4. Jacoby, R.P.; Taylor, N.L.; Millar, A.H. The role of mitochondrial respiration in salinity tolerance. *Trends Plant Sci.* **2011**, 16, 614–623. [CrossRef]
5. Sako, K.; Sunaoshi, Y.; Tanaka, M.; Matsui, A.; Seki, M. The duration of ethanol-induced high-salinity stress tolerance in Arabidopsis thaliana. *Plant Signal. Behav.* **2018**, 13, e1500065. [CrossRef]
6. Munns, R.; Tester, M. Mechanisms of salinity tolerance. *Annu. Rev. Plant Biol.* **2008**, 59, 651–681. [CrossRef]
7. Flowers, T. Improving crop salt tolerance. *J. Exp. Bot.* **2004**, 55, 307–319. [CrossRef]
8. Negrao, S.; Cecília Almadanim, M.; Pires, I.S.S.; Abreu, I.A.; Maroco, J.; Courtois, B.; Gregorio, G.B.; McNally, K.L.; Margarida Oliveira, M. New allelic variants found in key rice salt-tolerance genes: An association study. *Plant Biotechnol. J.* **2013**, 11, 87–100. [CrossRef]
9. Hairmansis, A.; Berger, B.; Tester, M.; Roy, S.J. Image-based phenotyping for non-destructive screening of different salinity tolerance traits in rice. *Rice* **2014**, 7, 16. [CrossRef]
10. Pires, I.S.; Negrão, S.; Oliveira, M.M.; Purugganan, M.D. Comprehensive phenotypic analysis of rice (Oryza sativa) response to salinity stress. *Physiol. Plant.* **2015**, 155, 43–54. [CrossRef]
11. Chen, R.; Cheng, Y.; Han, S.; Van Handel, B.; Dong, L.; Li, X.; Xie, X. Whole genome sequencing and comparative transcriptome analysis of a novel seawater adapted, salt-resistant rice cultivar–sea rice 86. *BMC Genom.* **2017**, 18, 655. [CrossRef] [PubMed]
12. Rana, M.M.; Takamatsu, T.; Baslam, M.; Kaneko, K.; Itoh, K.; Harada, N.; Sugiyama, T.; Ohnishi, T.; Kinoshita, T.; Takagi, H. Salt tolerance improvement in rice through efficient SNP marker-assisted selection coupled with speed-breeding. *Int. J. Mol. Sci.* **2019**, 20, 2585. [CrossRef]
13. Khan, I.; Khan, S.; Zhang, Y.; Zhou, J.; Akhoundian, M.; Jan, S.A. CRISPR-Cas technology based genome editing for modification of salinity stress tolerance responses in rice (Oryza sativa L.). *Mol. Biol. Rep.* **2021**, 48, 3605–3615. [CrossRef] [PubMed]
14. Ganie, S.A.; Wani, S.H.; Henry, R.; Hensel, G. Improving rice salt tolerance by precision breeding in a new era. *Curr. Opin. Plant Biol.* **2021**, 60, 101996. [CrossRef] [PubMed]
15. Farhat, S.; Jain, N.; Singh, N.; Sreevathsa, R.; Dash, P.K.; Rai, R.; Yadav, S.; Kumar, P.; Sarkar, A.K.; Jain, A. CRISPR-Cas9 directed genome engineering for enhancing salt stress tolerance in rice. In *Seminars in Cell & Developmental Biology*; Academic Press: Cambridge, MA, USA, 2019; pp. 91–99.

16. Subudhi, P.K.; Shankar, R.; Jain, M. Whole genome sequence analysis of rice genotypes with contrasting response to salinity stress. *Sci. Rep.* **2020**, *10*, 21259. [CrossRef] [PubMed]
17. Aycan, M.; Nahar, L.; Baslam, M.; Mitsui, T. B-type response regulator hst1 controls salinity tolerance in rice by regulating transcription factors and antioxidant mechanisms. *Plant Physiol. Biochem.* **2023**, *196*, 542–555. [CrossRef] [PubMed]
18. Santosh Kumar, V.; Verma, R.K.; Yadav, S.K.; Yadav, P.; Watts, A.; Rao, M.; Chinnusamy, V. CRISPR-Cas9 mediated genome editing of drought and salt tolerance (OsDST) gene in indica mega rice cultivar MTU1010. *Physiol. Mol. Biol. Plants* **2020**, *26*, 1099–1110. [CrossRef]
19. Paul, P.; Awasthi, A.; Rai, A.K.; Gupta, S.K.; Prasad, R.; Sharma, T.; Dhaliwal, H. Reduced tillering in Basmati rice T-DNA insertional mutant OsTEF1 associates with differential expression of stress related genes and transcription factors. *Funct. Integr. Genom.* **2012**, *12*, 291–304. [CrossRef]
20. Qin, H.; Wang, Y.; Wang, J.; Liu, H.; Zhao, H.; Deng, Z.; Zhang, Z.; Huang, R.; Zhang, Z. Knocking down the expression of GMPase gene OsVTC1-1 decreases salt tolerance of rice at seedling and reproductive stages. *PLoS ONE* **2016**, *11*, e0168650. [CrossRef]
21. Zhang, Y.; Fang, J.; Wu, X.; Dong, L. Na+/K+ balance and transport regulatory mechanisms in weedy and cultivated rice (*Oryza sativa* L.) under salt stress. *BMC Plant Biol.* **2018**, *18*, 375. [CrossRef]
22. Hauser, F.; Horie, T. A conserved primary salt tolerance mechanism mediated by HKT transporters: A mechanism for sodium exclusion and maintenance of high K+/Na+ ratio in leaves during salinity stress. *Plant Cell Environ.* **2010**, *33*, 552–565. [CrossRef] [PubMed]
23. Shi, H.; Quintero, F.J.; Pardo, J.M.; Zhu, J.-K. The putative plasma membrane Na+/H+ antiporter SOS1 controls long-distance Na+ transport in plants. *Plant Cell* **2002**, *14*, 465–477. [CrossRef] [PubMed]
24. Horie, T.; Costa, A.; Kim, T.H.; Han, M.J.; Horie, R.; Leung, H.Y.; Miyao, A.; Hirochika, H.; An, G.; Schroeder, J.I. Rice OsHKT2;1 transporter mediates large Na+ influx component into K+-starved roots for growth. *EMBO J.* **2007**, *26*, 3003–3014. [CrossRef] [PubMed]
25. Liu, J.; Shabala, S.; Shabala, L.; Zhou, M.; Meinke, H.; Venkataraman, G.; Chen, Z.; Zeng, F.; Zhao, Q. Tissue-specific regulation of Na+ and K+ transporters explains genotypic differences in salinity stress tolerance in rice. *Front. Plant Sci.* **2019**, *10*, 1361. [CrossRef]
26. Yang, T.; Zhang, S.; Hu, Y.; Wu, F.; Hu, Q.; Chen, G.; Cai, J.; Wu, T.; Moran, N.; Yu, L. The role of a potassium transporter OsHAK5 in potassium acquisition and transport from roots to shoots in rice at low potassium supply levels. *Plant Physiol.* **2014**, *166*, 945–959. [CrossRef]
27. Chen, G.; Hu, Q.; Luo, L.; Yang, T.; Zhang, S.; Hu, Y.; Yu, L.; Xu, G. Rice potassium transporter O s HAK 1 is essential for maintaining potassium-mediated growth and functions in salt tolerance over low and high potassium concentration ranges. *Plant Cell Environ.* **2015**, *38*, 2747–2765. [CrossRef]
28. Singh, K.B.; Foley, R.C.; Oñate-Sánchez, L. Transcription factors in plant defense and stress responses. *Curr. Opin. Plant Biol.* **2002**, *5*, 430–436. [CrossRef]
29. Verma, D.; Jalmi, S.K.; Bhagat, P.K.; Verma, N.; Sinha, A.K. A bHLH transcription factor, MYC2, imparts salt intolerance by regulating proline biosynthesis in Arabidopsis. *FEBS J.* **2020**, *287*, 2560–2576. [CrossRef]
30. Sun, Y.; Song, K.; Guo, M.; Wu, H.; Ji, X.; Hou, L.; Liu, X.; Lu, S. A NAC transcription factor from 'sea rice 86' enhances salt tolerance by promoting hydrogen sulfide production in rice seedlings. *Int. J. Mol. Sci.* **2022**, *23*, 6435. [CrossRef]
31. Yang, A.; Dai, X.; Zhang, W.-H. A R2R3-type MYB gene, OsMYB2, is involved in salt, cold, and dehydration tolerance in rice. *J. Exp. Bot.* **2012**, *63*, 2541–2556. [CrossRef]
32. Liu, C.; Mao, B.; Ou, S.; Wang, W.; Liu, L.; Wu, Y.; Chu, C.; Wang, X. OsbZIP71, a bZIP transcription factor, confers salinity and drought tolerance in rice. *Plant Mol. Biol.* **2014**, *84*, 19–36. [CrossRef] [PubMed]
33. Sun, S.; Yu, J.-P.; Chen, F.; Zhao, T.-J.; Fang, X.-H.; Li, Y.-Q.; Sui, S.-F. TINY, a dehydration-responsive element (DRE)-binding protein-like transcription factor connecting the DRE-and ethylene-responsive element-mediated signaling pathways in Arabidopsis. *J. Biol. Chem.* **2008**, *283*, 6261–6271. [CrossRef]
34. Wang, F.; Niu, H.; Xin, D.; Long, Y.; Wang, G.; Liu, Z.; Li, G.; Zhang, F.; Qi, M.; Ye, Y. OsIAA18, an Aux/IAA transcription factor gene, is involved in salt and drought tolerance in rice. *Front. Plant Sci.* **2021**, *12*, 738660. [CrossRef]
35. Li, Y.; Zhou, J.; Li, Z.; Qiao, J.; Quan, R.; Wang, J.; Huang, R.; Qin, H. SALT AND ABA RESPONSE ERF1 improves seed germination and salt tolerance by repressing ABA signaling in rice. *Plant Physiol.* **2022**, *189*, 1110–1127. [CrossRef] [PubMed]
36. Shan, C.; Mei, Z.; Duan, J.; Chen, H.; Feng, H.; Cai, W. OsGA2ox5, a gibberellin metabolism enzyme, is involved in plant growth, the root gravity response and salt stress. *PLoS ONE* **2014**, *9*, e87110. [CrossRef] [PubMed]
37. Mu, D.-w.; Feng, N.-j.; Zheng, D.-f.; Zhou, H.; Liu, L.; Chen, G.-j.; Mu, B. Physiological mechanism of exogenous brassinolide alleviating salt stress injury in rice seedlings. *Sci. Rep.* **2022**, *12*, 20439. [CrossRef]
38. Ali, M.M.; Anwar, R.; Malik, A.U.; Khan, A.S.; Ahmad, S.; Hussain, Z.; Hasan, M.U.; Nasir, M.; Chen, F. Plant growth and fruit quality response of strawberry is improved after exogenous application of 24-epibrassinolide. *J. Plant Growth Regul.* **2022**, *41*, 1786–1799. [CrossRef]
39. Qu, L.-J.; Chen, J.; Liu, M.; Pan, N.; Okamoto, H.; Lin, Z.; Li, C.; Li, D.; Wang, J.; Zhu, G. Molecular cloning and functional analysis of a novel type of Bowman-Birk inhibitor gene family in rice. *Plant Physiol.* **2003**, *133*, 560–570. [CrossRef]

40. Fereidunian, A.; Sadeghalvad, M.; Oscoie, M.O.; Mostafaie, A. Soybean Bowman-Birk protease inhibitor (BBI): Identification of the mechanisms of BBI suppressive effect on growth of two adenocarcinoma cell lines: AGS and HT29. *Arch. Med. Res.* **2014**, *45*, 455–461. [CrossRef]

41. Chen, Z.-Y.; Brown, R.L.; Lax, A.R.; Cleveland, T.E.; Russin, J.S. Inhibition of plant-pathogenic fungi by a corn trypsin inhibitor overexpressed in Escherichia coli. *Appl. Environ. Microbiol.* **1999**, *65*, 1320–1324. [CrossRef]

42. Kawahara, Y.; de la Bastide, M.; Hamilton, J.P.; Kanamori, H.; McCombie, W.R.; Ouyang, S.; Schwartz, D.C.; Tanaka, T.; Wu, J.; Zhou, S.; et al. Improvement of the Oryza sativa Nipponbare reference genome using next generation sequence and optical map data. *Rice* **2013**, *6*, 4. [CrossRef] [PubMed]

43. Zhang, C.; Fang, H.; Shi, X.; He, F.; Wang, R.; Fan, J.; Bai, P.; Wang, J.; Park, C.H.; Bellizzi, M. A fungal effector and a rice NLR protein have antagonistic effects on a Bowman–Birk trypsin inhibitor. *Plant Biotechnol. J.* **2020**, *18*, 2354–2363. [CrossRef] [PubMed]

44. Mourão, C.B.; Schwartz, E.F. Protease inhibitors from marine venomous animals and their counterparts in terrestrial venomous animals. *Mar. Drugs* **2013**, *11*, 2069–2112. [CrossRef] [PubMed]

45. Shan, L.; Li, C.; Chen, F.; Zhao, S.; Xia, G. A Bowman-Birk type protease inhibitor is involved in the tolerance to salt stress in wheat. *Plant Cell Environ.* **2008**, *31*, 1128–1137. [CrossRef] [PubMed]

46. Duan, K.; Li, L.; Hu, P.; Xu, S.P.; Xu, Z.H.; Xue, H.W. A brassinolide-suppressed rice MADS-box transcription factor, OsMDP1, has a negative regulatory role in BR signaling. *Plant J.* **2006**, *47*, 519–531. [CrossRef] [PubMed]

47. Müssig, C.; Altmann, T. Brassinosteroid signaling in plants. *Trends Endocrinol. Metab.* **2001**, *12*, 398–402. [CrossRef] [PubMed]

48. Xu, Q.; Wei, Q.; Kong, Y.; Zhu, L.; Tian, W.; Huang, J.; Pan, L.; Jin, Q.; Zhang, J.; Zhu, C. Unearthing the Alleviatory Mechanisms of Brassinolide in Cold Stress in Rice. *Life* **2022**, *12*, 833. [CrossRef]

49. Su, Q.; Zheng, X.; Tian, Y.; Wang, C. Exogenous brassinolide alleviates salt stress in Malus hupehensis Rehd. by regulating the transcription of NHX-Type Na+ (K+)/H+ antiporters. *Front. Plant Sci.* **2020**, *11*, 38. [CrossRef]

50. Tsai, Y.-C.; Hong, C.-Y.; Liu, L.-F.; Kao, C.H. Expression of ascorbate peroxidase and glutathione reductase in roots of rice seedlings in response to NaCl and H2O2. *J. Plant Physiol.* **2005**, *162*, 291–299. [CrossRef]

51. Zhang, Z.; Zhang, Q.; Wu, J.; Zheng, X.; Zheng, S.; Sun, X.; Qiu, Q.; Lu, T. Gene knockout study reveals that cytosolic ascorbate peroxidase 2 (OsAPX2) plays a critical role in growth and reproduction in rice under drought, salt and cold stresses. *PLoS ONE* **2013**, *8*, e57472. [CrossRef]

52. Maruta, T.; Sawa, Y.; Shigeoka, S.; Ishikawa, T. Diversity and evolution of ascorbate peroxidase functions in chloroplasts: More than just a classical antioxidant enzyme? *Plant Cell Physiol.* **2016**, *57*, 1377–1386. [CrossRef] [PubMed]

53. Hong, C.-Y.; Kao, C.H. NaCl-induced expression of ASCORBATE PEROXIDASE 8 in roots of rice (Oryza sativa L.) seedlings is not associated with osmotic component. *Plant Signal. Behav.* **2008**, *3*, 199–201. [CrossRef] [PubMed]

54. Hong, Z.; Ueguchi-Tanaka, M.; Shimizu-Sato, S.; Inukai, Y.; Fujioka, S.; Shimada, Y.; Takatsuto, S.; Agetsuma, M.; Yoshida, S.; Watanabe, Y. Loss-of-function of a rice brassinosteroid biosynthetic enzyme, C-6 oxidase, prevents the organized arrangement and polar elongation of cells in the leaves and stem. *Plant J.* **2002**, *32*, 495–508. [CrossRef] [PubMed]

55. Tong, H.; Jin, Y.; Liu, W.; Li, F.; Fang, J.; Yin, Y.; Qian, Q.; Zhu, L.; Chu, C. DWARF AND LOW-TILLERING, a new member of the GRAS family, plays positive roles in brassinosteroid signaling in rice. *Plant J.* **2009**, *58*, 803–816. [CrossRef] [PubMed]

56. Tong, H.; Xiao, Y.; Liu, D.; Gao, S.; Liu, L.; Yin, Y.; Jin, Y.; Qian, Q.; Chu, C. Brassinosteroid regulates cell elongation by modulating gibberellin metabolism in rice. *Plant Cell* **2014**, *26*, 4376–4393. [CrossRef] [PubMed]

57. Li, Q.-F.; Zhou, Y.; Xiong, M.; Ren, X.-Y.; Han, L.; Wang, J.-D.; Zhang, C.-Q.; Fan, X.-L.; Liu, Q.-Q. Gibberellin recovers seed germination in rice with impaired brassinosteroid signalling. *Plant Sci.* **2020**, *293*, 110435. [CrossRef]

58. Chen, H.; Yu, H.; Jiang, W.; Li, H.; Wu, T.; Chu, J.; Xin, P.; Li, Z.; Wang, R.; Zhou, T. Overexpression of ovate family protein 22 confers multiple morphological changes and represses gibberellin and brassinosteroid signalings in transgenic rice. *Plant Sci.* **2021**, *304*, 110734. [CrossRef]

59. Slamet-Loedin, I.H.; Chadha-Mohanty, P.; Torrizo, L. Agrobacterium-mediated transformation: Rice transformation. *Cereal Genom. Methods Protoc.* **2014**, *1099*, 261–271.

60. Tian, X.; He, M.; Mei, E.; Zhang, B.; Tang, J.; Xu, M.; Liu, J.; Li, X.; Wang, Z.; Tang, W. WRKY53 integrates classic brassinosteroid signaling and the mitogen-activated protein kinase pathway to regulate rice architecture and seed size. *Plant Cell* **2021**, *33*, 2753–2775. [CrossRef]

61. Shankar, R.; Bhattacharjee, A.; Jain, M. Transcriptome analysis in different rice cultivars provides novel insights into desiccation and salinity stress responses. *Sci. Rep.* **2016**, *6*, 23719. [CrossRef]

62. Hsieh, C.; Chen, Y.-H.; Chang, K.-C.; Yang, S.-Y. Transcriptome analysis reveals the mechanisms for mycorrhiza-enhanced salt tolerance in rice. *Front. Plant Sci.* **2022**, *13*, 1072171. [CrossRef] [PubMed]

MDPI AG
Grosspeteranlage 5
4052 Basel
Switzerland
Tel.: +41 61 683 77 34

International Journal of Molecular Sciences Editorial Office
E-mail: ijms@mdpi.com
www.mdpi.com/journal/ijms

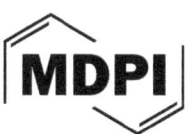

www.ingramcontent.com/pod-product-compliance
Lightning Source LLC
LaVergne TN
LVHW072341090526
838202LV00019B/2452